Botulinum Toxins

Botulinum Toxins

Cosmetic and Clinical Applications

Edited by

Joel L. Cohen, MD (FAAD, FACMS)
Director
AboutSkin Dermatology and DermSurgery
Greenwood Village and Lone Tree
CO, USA

David M. Ozog, MD (FAAD, FACMS)
Chair, Department of Dermatology
C.S. Livingood Chair in Dermatology
Director of Cosmetic Dermatology
Division of Mohs and Dermatological Surgery
Henry Ford Hospital
Detroit, MI, USA

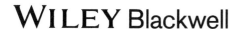

Library of Congress Cataloging-in-Publication Data

Names: Cohen, Joel L. (Dermatologist), editor. | Ozog, David M., editor.
Title: Botulinum toxins : cosmetic and clinical applications / edited by Joel L. Cohen, David M. Ozog.
Description: Chichester, UK ; Hoboken, NJ : John Wiley & Sons Inc., 2017. | Includes

   bibliographical references and index.
Identifiers: LCCN 2017004474 (print) | LCCN 2017005656 (ebook) | ISBN

   9781444338256 (cloth) | ISBN 9781118661864 (Adobe PDF) | ISBN 9781118661857 (ePub)
Subjects: | MESH: Botulinum Toxins, Type A—therapeutic use | Cosmetic Techniques
Classification: LCC RL120.B66 (print) | LCC RL120.B66 (ebook) | NLM QV 140 | DDC 615.7/78—dc23
LC record available at https://lccn.loc.gov/2017004474

Cover image: (Left) © SEBASTIAN KAULITZKI/Gettyimages; (Right) © iconogenic/Gettyimages
Cover design: Wiley

Set in 10/12pt WarnockPro by Aptara Inc., New Delhi, India

Contents

List of Contributors

Alan Ackerman, PhD
Master Medical Scientific Liaison, Retired
Ackerman LLC
Greeley, USA

Ki Young Ahn, MD (PhD)
Director
Dr. Ahn's Aesthetic & Plastic Surgical Clinic
Daegu, South Korea

Murad Alam, MD (MSCI, MBA)
Professor and Vice-Chair
Department of Dermatology
Section of Cutaneous and Aesthetic Surgery
Departments of Dermatology
Otolaryngology, and Surgery
Northwestern University
Chicago, USA

Shawn Allen, MD (FAAD, FACMS)
Director and Founder
Dermatology Specialists
Boulder, USA

Assistant Clinical Professor
University of Colorado
Department of Dermatology
Boulder, USA

Ada Regina Trindade de Almeida, MD
Medical Assistant
Dermatology Clinic
Hospital do Servidor Público Municipal de
São Paulo
São Paulo, Brazil

Cheré Lucas Anthony, MD
Medical Director
Rendon Center for Dermatology and
Aesthetic Medicine
Boca Raton, USA

Voluntary Faculty
Dermatology and Cutaneous Surgery
University of Miami, Miller School of
Medicine
Miami, USA

John P. Arkins, BS
DeNova Research
Chicago, USA

Eileen Axibal, MD
Department of Dermatology
University of Colorado
Aurora, USA

Lakhdar Belhaouari, MD
Director
Centre de Chirurgie Esthétique et Medecine
Esthétique Jules Guesde
Toulouse, France

Anthony V. Benedetto, DO (FACP, FCPP)
Clinical Professor of Dermatology
Perelman School of Medicine
University of Pennsylvania
PA, USA

Medical Director
Dermatologic SurgiCenter
Philadelphia and Drexel Hill
PA, USA

Brian S. Biesman, MD (FACS)
Assistant Clinical Professor Ophthalmology
Dermatology, Otolaryngology
Vanderbilt University Medical Center
Nashville, TN, USA

Donna Bilu Martin, MD (FAAD)
Dermatologist, Premier Dermatology
Aventura, USA

Volunteer Professor of Dermatology and
Cutaneous Surgery
Miller School of Medicine University of
Miami
Miami, USA

Andrew Blitzer, MD (DDS, FACS)
Director
NY Center for Voice and Swallowing
Disorders
Senior Attending Physician
St. Luke's/Roosevelt Hospital
Professor of Clinical Otolaryngology
Columbia University College of Physicians
and Surgeons
New York, USA

Alastair Carruthers, FRCPC
Clinical Professor
Department of Dermatology and Skin
Science
University of British Columbia
Vancouver, Canada

Jean Carruthers, MD (FRCS(C), FRCOphth)
Clinical Professor
Department of Ophthalmology and Visual
Sciences
University of British Columbia
Vancouver, Canada

Lesley F. Childs, MD
Attending Physician
Assistant Professor of Laryngology,
Neurolaryngology, and Professional Voice
UT Southwestern, Dallas, TX

Chinobu Chisaki, MD
Medical Assistant
Dermatology Clinic
Hospital do Servidor Público Municipal de
São Paulo
São Paulo, Brazil

Joel L. Cohen, MD (FAAD, FACMS)
Director
AboutSkin Dermatology and DermSurgery
Greenwood Village and Lone Tree
Colorado, USA

Associate Clinical Professor
University of Colorado Department of
Dermatology
Denver, USA

Assistant Clinical Professor
University of California Irvine Department
of Dermatology
Irvine, USA

Carolee M. Cutler Peck, MD
Ophthalmic and Plastic and Reconstructive
Surgeon
SouthEast Eye Specialists
Knoxville, USA

Steven H. Dayan, MD (FACS)
Clinical Assistant Professor of
Otolaryngology
Chicago Centre for Facial Plastic Surgery
University of Illinois Chicago
Chicago, USA

Koenraad De Boulle, MD
Aalst Dermatology Clinic
Aalst, Belgium

Chérie M. Ditre, MD
Associate Professor
Department of Dermatology
University of Pennsylvania School of
Medicine
Philadelphia, USA

Jason J. Emer, MD
Cosmetic Dermatology and Body
Contouring
Private Practice
Beverly Hills, CA

Ramin Fathi, MD
Resident Physician
Department of Dermatology
University of Colorado
Aurora, USA

Lauren Fine, MD (FAAD)
Associate Dermatologist & Cosmetic Fellow
Advanced Dermatology, LLC
Chicago, USA

Timothy Corcoran Flynn, MD
Clinical Professor of Dermatology
University of North Carolina at Chapel Hill
Chapel Hill, USA

Medical Director
Cary Skin Center
Cary, USA

Conor J. Gallagher, PhD
Executive Director Medical Affairs
Facial Aesthetics
Allergan plc
Irvine, USA

Hayes B. Gladstone, MD
Gladstone Clinic
San Ramon, USA

Dee Anna Glaser, MD
Professor and Interim Chairman
Department of Dermatology
Saint Louis University School of Medicine
Saint Louis, USA

Richard G. Glogau, MD
Clinical Professor of Dermatology
University of California San Francisco
USA

Michael H. Gold, MD
Medical Director
Gold Skin Care Center
Nashville, USA

David J. Goldberg, MD (JD)
Clinical Professor of Dermatology
Department of Dermatology
Icahn School of Medicine at Mount Sinai
New York, USA

Skin Laser and Surgery Specialists of New
York and New Jersey
New York, USA

Timothy M. Greco, MD (FACS)
Clinical Assistant Professor
Department of Otolaryngology-Head and
Neck Surgery
Division of Facial Plastic Surgery
University of Pennsylvania School of
Medicine
Philadelphia, USA

Ryan M. Greene, MD (PhD, FACS)
Director
Plastic Surgery & Laser Center
Fort Lauderdale, USA

James L. Griffith, MD (MSci)
Dermatology Resident
Department of Dermatology
Henry Ford Hospital
Detroit, USA

Camile L. Hexsel, MD (FAAD, FACMS)
Dermatologist and Dermatologic Surgeon
Madison Medical Affiliates
Mohs Surgery
Glendale and Waukesha
USA

Dóris Hexsel, MD
Dermatologist and Dermatologic Surgeon
Brazilian Center for Studies in Dermatology
Porto Alegre, Brazil

Matthias Imhof, MD (DALM)
Board Certified Dermatologist and
Allergologist
Aesthetische Dermatologie im Medico Palais
Bad Soden, Germany

Julia D. Kreger, MD
University of Colorado Dermatology
Colorado, USA

Ulrich Kühne, MD (DALM)
Board Certified Dermatologist and
Allergologist
Aesthetische Dermatologie im Medico
Palais
Bad Soden, Germany

Matteo C. LoPiccolo, MD
Henry Ford Health System
Department of Dermatology
Detroit, USA

Stephen Mandy, MD (FAAD)
Volunteer Professor of Dermatology and
Cutaneous Surgery
Miller School of Medicine University of
Miami
Miami, USA

Premier Dermatology
South Beach Dermatology
Miami Beach, USA

Suveena Manhas-Bhutani, MD
Sadick Dermatology and Research
New York, USA

Ellen S. Marmur, MD (FAAD)
Director, Marmur Medical
Mount Sinai School of Medicine
Department of Dermatology
New York, USA

Adam R. Mattox, DO (MS)
Micrographic Surgery & Dermatologic
Oncology Fellow
Department of Dermatology
Saint Louis University School of Medicine
Saint Louis, USA

Gary D. Monheit, MD
Total Skin and Beauty Dermatology Center
PC Private Practice
Associate Clinical Professor
Department of Dermatology
Department of Ophthalmology
University of Alabama at Birmingham
Birmingham, USA

Girish S. Munavalli, MD (MHS, FACMS)
Medical Director, Dermatology, Laser, and
Vein Specialists of the Carolinas, PLLC
Charlotte, USA

David M. Ozog, MD (FAAD, FACMS)
Chair, Department of Dermatology
C.S. Livingood Chair in Dermatology
Director of Cosmetic Dermatology
Division of Mohs and Dermatological
Surgery
Henry Ford Hospital
Detroit, MI, USA

Mee young Park, MD (PhD)
Department of Neurology
Yeungnam University
College of Medicine
Daegu, South Korea

Dennis A. Porto, MD
Department of Dermatology
Henry Ford Hospital
Detroit, USA

Molly C. Powers, MD
Dermatology Senior Resident
Department of Dermatology
Henry Ford Hospital
Detroit, USA

Marta I. Rendon, MD (FAAD, FACP)
Medical Director, Rendon Center for
Dermatology and Aesthetic Medicine
Boca Raton, USA

Voluntary Associate Clinical Professor
University of Miami
Dermatology Department
Miami, USA

Scott Rickert, MD (FACS)
Attending Physician
Assistant Professor of Otolaryngology,
Pediatrics, and Plastic Surgery
NYU Langone Medical Center
New York, USA

Farhaad R. Riyaz, MD
Henry Ford Health System
Department of Dermatology
Detroit, USA

Neil S. Sadick, MD (FACP, FAAD, FAACS, FACPh)
Clinical Professor
Weill Cornell Medical College
Cornell University
New York, USA

Roberta Sengelmann, MD
President and Owner
Santa Barbara Skin Institute
Associate Clinical Professor
UCI Dermatology
Santa Barbara, USA

Carolina Siega, BSc
Biologist
Brazilian Center for Studies in Dermatology
Porto Alegre, Brazil

Rachel Simmons, MD (FAAD)
Dermatologist
Dermatology Specialists
Boulder, USA

Kevin C. Smith, MD (FRCPC (DERM))
Private Practice Dermatologist
Niagara Falls
Ontario, Canada

Amy Forman Taub, MD
Director
Founder
Advanced Dermatology, LLC
Assistant Professor
Northwestern University Medical School
Chicago, USA

Assistant Clinical Professor
Northwestern University
Lincolnshire, USA

Neal D. Varughese, MD (MBA)
Skin Laser and Surgery Specialists of New
York and New Jersey
New York, USA

Heidi Waldorf, MD
Mount Sinai School of Medicine
Department of Dermatology
New York, USA

About the Companion Website

Don't forget to visit the companion website for this book:

www.wiley.com/go/cohen/botulinum

This site hosts valuable video materials to enhance your learning:

Dr Cohen and Dr Ozog present several patient cases, focusing on patient evaluation, preparation for toxins, and specific injection techniques. Each patient is appraised carefully and optimal injection techniques are discussed, along with methods for avoiding adverse effects, and ways to minimize injection points and related bruising. One week follow up videos will highlight optimization of results.

Video Table of Contents

Foreword: Botulinum Toxins in Dermatology

Alastair Carruthers, FRCPC[1], Jean Carruthers, MD, FRCSC[2]

[1]Clinical Professor, Department of Dermatology and Skin Science, University of British Columbia
[2]Clinical Professor, Department of Ophthalmology and Visual Sciences, University of British Columbia

Clostridium botulinum (C. botulinum), discovered over a century ago as the bacterium responsible for botulism, his risen through medical ranks to become the basis of what is one of the most requested procedures in facial rejuvenation and accepted therapeutic options for use in a variety of clinical scenarios.

Until the 1980s, botulinum toxin (BoNT) was merely a potent toxin with devastating effects and up to a 65% mortality rate. The history of food-borne illness to therapeutic agent is checkered with tainted blood sausages, brilliant clinical scientists, biological warfare and, at the heart of it all, an understanding that this toxin that led to so many deaths and devastated the canning industry in the 1930s, could somehow be of clinical use.

Interestingly, the clinical use of BoNT has proven circular: its initial forays into therapeutics, as a nonsurgical treatment for strabismus and blepharospasm, sparked discoveries in facial rejuvenation; the enormous acceptance of its cosmetic use has in turn fuelled the expansion and tremendous growth in therapeutic fields, leading to an even greater clinical experience and understanding of mechanism of action and potential indications for use.

In the last 5 years, the use of BoNT has grown exponentially and now accounts for about half (along with soft-tissue augmenting agents) of all nonsurgical cosmetic procedures in North America. The reasons for such an enthusiastic response to the toxin may be found in the target populations. As we age, the skin atrophies and sags, bones shift, and lines and wrinkles become more prominent. Ameliorating those wrinkles is one of the primary methods of turning back the clock. The fact that BoNT is able to accomplish this feat with minimal downtime or side effects has contributed greatly to its rise in popularity. Moreover, BoNT may be considered a preventative anti-aging modality, appealing to a younger population in addition to those seeking to eradicate already established rhytides and folds.

Therapeutically, indications for BoNT have progressed beyond movement disorders and spasticity to investigations into potential uses for a multitude of disorders and syndromes, including those involving pain, the endocrine system (sweat, lacrimal, and salivary glands), and the central nervous system, among others. Clinicians from nearly all therapeutic specialists have turned their attention, at least in part, to possible applications of BoNT.

It is becoming more difficult to stay abreast of new developments. This book has been compiled to highlight not only the remarkable history and clinical advance of what was once called "sausage poison, but to include the ever-expanding indications, along with a number of new formulations available and the associated side effects or complications. There is a detailed examination of facial anatomy and BoNT in the upper, mid- and lower face and neck, with additional focus on the more artful role of the toxin's ability to restore symmetry and sculpt the face into more pleasing contours, both alone and in combination with other agents and surgical procedures. Patient considerations are of equal importance, both in choosing the most appropriate candidates, and in predicting outcomes. Evidence shows that BoNT has enormous psychosocial impact in the lives of our patients. This book also includes dermatological BoNT outlying the cosmetic domain, such as benefits of using the neurotoxin to treat hyperhidrosis, skin cancer and traumatic scars, and in conjunction with surgical procedures to aid in wound healing or prolong the aesthetic effect.

A book on the dermatological applications of neurotoxin would not be complete without inclusion of the exciting possibilities. Since its clinical properties were discovered nearly a century ago, it is clear that we have not yet uncovered the full potential of what still is the world's most lethal toxin.

Dr. Joel Cohen has achieved an outstanding international reputation both among his colleagues and his patients. He went to medical school at Mt Sinai School of Medicine, New York and then did his dermatology training at Henry Ford Hospital, Detroit. That was followed by a fellowship in advanced dermatologic surgery in Vancouver, B.C. which is where we first met Joel and his family.

Since he completed his training, Dr. Cohen has appeared in the national media on many occasions and has published extensively in the medical literature. Much of this relates to his interest in botulinum toxin and its use in dermatology. His knowledge in this area as well as his contributions to the field are both extensive and these have contributed to his excellent reputation.

Dr. David Ozog trained in medicine at the University of Rochester, N.Y., did his dermatology residency at Henry Ford Hospital in Detroit and his Mohs and cosmetic surgery fellowship with Dr Ron Moy in Beverly Hills, CA. He remained in academics at Henry Ford as Chairman and Director of Cosmetic Dermatology, where he has been teaching residents both surgery and cosmetics for the past thirteen years. An excellent background! He has proven himself to be an excellent teacher and to have an inquiring mind – both valuable attributes.

It is very appropriate that they edit this book which brings together both their own knowledge as well as that of other experts in the field under their direction. This book is an important contribution to our knowledge about both the basic science and the clinical use of botulinum toxin.

Reference

The American Society for Dermatologic Surgery. (2008.) The American Society for Dermatologic Surgery Releases New Procedure Survey Data. Retrieved July 22, 2010 from http://www.asds.net/ TheAmericanSocietyfor DermatologicSurgeryReleases NewProcedureSurveyData.aspx

History of Botulinum Toxin for Medical and Aesthetic Use

Alastair Carruthers, FRCPC[1] and Jean Carruthers, MD (FRCS(C), FRCOphth)[2]

[1] *Clinical Professor, Department of Dermatology and Skin Science, University of British Columbia, Vancouver, Canada*
[2] *Clinical Professor, Department of Ophthalmology and Visual Sciences, University of British Columbia, Vancouver, Canada*

Sausage Poisoning

In the late 1700s in Europe, outbreaks of a deadly illness from contaminated foods swept across the continent, fueled in part by the poverty from the Napoleonic War (1795–1815) that led to unsanitary food production [1]. The primary source of food-borne illness of the time: smoked blood sausages. One of the biggest outbreaks occurred in 1793 in Wildebrad, Southern Germany; by 1811, the Department of Internal Affairs of the Kingdom of Würtemberg named "prussic acid" as the culprit in sausage poisoning [2]. Intrigued, the district medical officer and poet, Dr. Justinus "Würst" Kerner (1786–1862), began what would become a lifelong quest to uncover the mysteries of the poison. He would later be considered the godfather of botulinum toxin (BoNT) research for his early, intensive work. In 1817 and 1820, Kerner identified and described the first accurate descriptions of botulism (a term coined in 1871 from the Latin *botulus*, meaning "sausage") [2, 3]. In 1822, he compared contaminated sausage ingredients and concluded that the toxin must occur in fat, leading him to call the suspicious substance "sausage poison," "fat poison," or "fatty acid," and published the first complete monograph of the "fatty toxin" from blood sausages [2].

In his monograph, Kerner described the symptoms of botulism – including vomiting, intestinal spasms, mydriasis, ptosis, dysphagia, and respiratory failure – and recommended methods for the treatment and prevention of food poisoning. Through animal and self-experimentation, Kerner observed that the toxin developed under anaerobic conditions and was lethal in small doses. Since the effects of this blood poison were similar to atropine, scopolamine, nicotine, and snake venom, Kerner surmised that sausage poison was likely biological in nature – remarkable in that microscopic pathogens had not yet been discovered at that time – and interrupted signal transmissions within the peripheral and autonomic nervous system. Indeed, some would call Kerner prophetic: he suggested that small amounts of this sausage poison might be used to lower sympathetic nervous system activity associated with movement disorders (i.e., treat St. Vitus' dance or Sydenham's chorea, a disorder characterized by jerky, uncontrollable movements, either of the face or of the arms and legs) and hypersecretion of bodily fluid, as well as to treat ulcers, delusions, rabies, plague, tuberculosis, and yellow fever [4].

Botulinum Toxins: Cosmetic and Clinical Applications, First Edition. Edited by Joel L. Cohen and David M. Ozog.
© 2017 John Wiley & Sons Ltd. Published 2017 by John Wiley & Sons Ltd.
Companion Website: www.wiley.com/go/cohen/botulinum

Identification of *C. botulinum*

Microbiologist Professor Emile Pierre van Ermengem (1851–1922) trained under Robert Koch, who discovered anthrax, tuberculosis, and cholera and was the first researcher to prove that microorganisms could cause disease in animals [5]. In 1897, Van Ermengem identified the bacterium *Clostridium botulinum* (originally called *Bacillus botulinus*) as the causative agent of botulism after examining postmortem tissue of patients in Belgium who had contracted gastroenteritis and died from eating raw, salted pork [6]. Over the next twenty years, different strains of the bacterium that produced serologically distinct types of toxins were recognized; these were eventually classified alphabetically into seven serotypes (A, B, C1, D, E, F and G) [7]. In 1928, Dr. Herman Sommer (University of California, San Francisco) isolated the most potent serotype – BoNT type A (BoNTA) – in purified form as a stable acid precipitate, paving the way for future studies [8].

Biological Weapon of Warfare

During the First World War, Germany unsuccessfully attempted to produce chemical and biological weapons. As World War II approached, the American government learned that multiple countries were engaged in bio-warfare programs. In response, and on orders from President Franklin Roosevelt, the US National Academy of Sciences and Fred Ira Baldwin, chairman of the bacteriology department of the University of Wisconsin, gathered bacteriologists and physicians in a laboratory named Fort Detrick (Maryland). The purpose of Fort Detrick: the investigation of dangerous infectious bacteria and toxins to use as offensive and defensive biological weapons [1].

In 1946, Carl Lamanna and James Duff developed concentration and crystallization techniques for the toxin that were subsequently used by Dr. Edward J. Schantz, a young US army officer stationed at Fort Detrick to produce the first BoNTA lot for human use (the basis of the later clinical product) [9, 10]. The US Office of Strategic Services (OSS) developed a plan using Chinese prostitutes to assassinate high-ranking Japanese officials via gelatin capsules containing the newly purified BoNTA. The government abandoned the plan when test donkeys that received the capsules survived [1]. Ironically, though BoNT today is considered one of the deadliest poisons in the world – 1 g has the potential to kill 1 million people – the toxin is not an ideal biological weapon, since large amounts must be ingested and mortality rates vary).

In 1972, President Richard Nixon signed the Biological and Toxic Weapons Convention, effectively putting an end to all investigations on biological agents for use in war. Schantz took his research to the University of Wisconsin, where he produced a large amount of BoNTA (batch 79–11) that remained in clinical use until December of 1997 [11].

Human Experimentation

Clinical use of the toxin began in the late 1960s and early 1970s, when Dr. Alan Scott (Smith-Kettlewell Eye Research Foundation, San Francisco; Figure 1.1) began experimenting with BoNTA, supplied by Dr. Schantz, and other chemical agents in monkeys, with the hope that one of the compounds could be used for the nonsurgical treatment of strabismus in humans [12, 13]. Scott published his first primate studies proving that BoNTA could weaken extraocular muscles in 1973, and postulated that the toxin could be used for a wide variety of musculoskeletal disorders and spasticity, even before conducting any human studies [13, 14]. In 1978, Scott received Food and Drug Association (FDA) approval to begin testing small amounts of the toxin (then named Oculinum) in human volunteers; his landmark paper, published in 1980 [15], showed that intramuscular injections of BoNTA could correct gaze

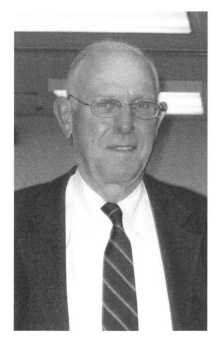

Figure 1.1 Dr Alan Scott, the original user of botulinum toxin A initially in monkeys and then in humans, seen in 2010.

misalignment in humans. In 1989, one year after manufacturer Allergan Inc. (Irvine, CA) acquired the rights to distribute Scott's Oculinum in the United States, BoNTA was approved for the nonsurgical correction of strabismus, blepharospasm, hemifacial spasm, and Meige's syndrome in adults, and clinical use expanded to include the treatment of cervical dystonia and spasmodic torticollis [13, 16, 17]. Shortly thereafter, Allergan bought Scott's company and renamed the toxin. Botox® was born.

The Cosmetic Connection

In the mid-1980s, Dr. Jean Carruthers, an ophthalmologist in Vancouver, Canada, noticed that her patients injected with BoNTA for blepharospasm experienced a reduction in glabellar rhytides, and discussed the findings with both Scott and her dermatologist spouse, Dr. Alastair Carruthers, who was attempting to soften the forehead

wrinkles of his patients using soft-tissue augmenting agents available at that time. Intrigued by the possibilities, the Carruthers used the toxin experimentally in their receptionist's forehead and subsequently published the first report of BoNTA for the treatment of glabellar frown lines in 1992 [18] (Figure 1.2). Other reports soon followed [19, 20], including the first double-blind, placebo-controlled study for the treatment of hyperkinetic facial lines [21].

Properties, Mechanism of Action, and Clinical Effect

Clostridium botulinum is a rod-shaped, gram-positive anaerobic bacterium. Of the seven serotypes, A, B, and E are commonly involved in human botulism [22]. BoNT is a high-molecular-weight protein of 150,000 daltons with nonconvalent proteins protecting it from digestive enzymes, making it a lethal cause of food poisoning [1]. The symptoms of botulism include disturbances in vision, speech, and swallowing, with asphyxia and death sometimes occurring 18–36 hours after ingestion (mortality rate: 10–65%) [22].

Researchers gained an understanding of mechanism of action in the late 1940s, when they discovered that BoNT blocks neurotransmitter release at the neuromuscular junction [23]. The follow-up discovery in the mid-1950s that BoNT blocks the release of acetylcholine from motor nerve endings when injected into hyperactive muscles led to a renewed interest in the neurotoxin as a potential therapeutic agent [3].

Although all seven serotypes block neuromuscular motor transmission by binding to receptor sites on motor nerve terminals and inhibiting the release of acetylcholine, producing temporary chemodenervation of the muscles, each differs with regard to cellular mechanism of action and clinical profile [24, 25]. The commercially available subtypes – type A (BoNTA) and type B (BoNTB) – are both 150 kDa dichain polypeptides

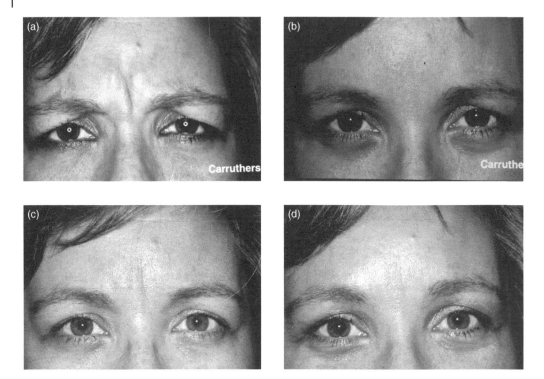

Figure 1.2 The Carruthers' first patient treated in the glabella area for cosmetic reasons alone. Seen (a) before frowning; (b) after frowning; (c) before at rest; (d) after at rest.

comprising heavy and light chains linked by disulfide bonds. The light chain of BoNTA cleaves to a 25 kDa synaptosomal associated protein (SNAP-25), a protein integral to the successful docking and release of acetylcholine from vesicles situated within nerve endings, while the light chain of BoNTB cleaves to vesicle-associated membrane protein (VAMP or synaptobrevin). This difference may be responsible for some of the differences witnessed in the clinical effect of the subtypes [12]. When injected intramuscularly at therapeutic doses, BoNT produces temporary chemical denervation of the muscle, resulting in a localized reduction of muscle activity. The process of cellular recovery after injection of BoNT is only partially understood. Initial recovery of muscle contraction is accompanied by collateral sprouting of active terminal buds near the parent terminal. However, research indicates that these new sprouts are only transitory; neurotransmission is eventually restored at

the original nerve ending, accompanied by the elimination of the dispensable sprouts [26], suggesting that treatment with BoNT does not permanently alter the neuromuscular junction. Recommended doses of injected neurotoxin do not result in systemic clinical effects in patients without other neuromuscular dysfunction. Studies of human and animal tissue show that in the first 2 weeks postinjection with BoNTA, the target muscle begins to atrophy, with changes in individual muscle fibers [27]. The paralytic effect of the toxin is dose-related, with initial effects occurring within 2–3 days and peaking approximately 1–2 weeks after treatment [28]. Atrophy continues for approximately 4 weeks before stabilizing; clinical recovery of function occurs 3–6 months posttreatment [29]. There is an area of denervation associated with each point of injection due to toxin spread of about 1–1.5 cm (diameter, 2–3 cm). Repeated injections can extend the clinical effect for up to 12 months [29]; it is possible that over the course of treatment, individuals alter their habitual use of muscles that cause expression lines. Long-term remodeling of the dermis and epidermis that helps to sustain the cosmetic effects also occurs in most individuals, because the tissue is no longer subjected to the same forces of muscle contraction.

A Multitude of Formulations

Until recently, one product – at least for cosmetic purposes – dominated the market: onabotulinumtoxinA (Botox®/Botox Cosmetic®/Vistabel®/Vistabex®; Allergan, Inc., Irvine, CA). Now, however, a host of other agents have joined the original formulation to fight the signs of aging. Of the formulations of BoNTA available or in development, the original, onabotulinumtoxinA, is the most recognized and discussed in peer-reviewed literature. Botox Cosmetic, which was approved by the US FDA in 2002 for the treatment of glabellar rhytides [30], has gone on to receive approval for 20 indications in more than 75 countries [31]. Now three formulations of botulinumtoxin type A are approved for cosmetic use in North America. The original onabotulinumtoxin A has been joined by abobotulinumtoxinA (Dysport®) and IncobotulinumtoxinA (Xeomin®). Initially approved in over 65 countries for therapeutic indications (Dysport®; Ipsen Ltd., United Kingdom/Medicis, Scottsdale, AZ; and Azzalure® in 15 European countries; Galderma, France), abobotulinumtoxinA received FDA approval for cosmetic applications in North America in 2009 (Dysport®; Ipsen Ltd). Although produced from the same serotype, abobotulinumtoxinA differs from onabotulinumtoxinA in purification procedures, dosing, injection schedules, and clinical effect [32]. Units of abobotulinumtoxinA are less powerful than those of onabotulinumtoxinA; most cosmetic injectors use a multiple of two to three times the number of units. Overall, abobotulinumtoxinA is safe and well tolerated

[33, 34]. A third BoNTA (Xeomin®/NT-201; Merz Pharmaceuticals, Frankfurt, Germany) is approved for therapeutic indications in Germany and other European countries, the United States, Canada, Mexico, and Argentina, and has been approved for the treatment of glabellar rhytides in Argentina and the United States. Clinically, Xeomin and onabotulinumtoxinA appear to behave in a similar fashion, with equal levels of potency, safety, and duration of effect [35–40]. Xeomin is free of complexing proteins, which some believe may result in purer formulations with greater efficacy and a reduced risk of sensitization and antibody formation [37]. One formulation of BoNT type B (BoNTB) is also available in North America. RimabotulinumtoxinB (Myobloc®/NeuroBloc®; Solstice Neurosciences Inc./Eisai Co., Ltd.) was FDA-approved in 2000 for the treatment of cervical dystonia but has been used off-label to treat facial wrinkles with some success [41–44]. BoNTB works faster than but does not last as long as BoNTA [45], although duration has been shown to be dose dependent [46]. BoNTB tends to diffuse more widely than BoNTA and injections can be more painful and may lead to additional side effects [45]; however, a close examination of several doses found all to be safe and effective for cosmetic use [46].

Cosmetic Applications

Hyperkinetic lines result from the repeated contraction of muscles perpendicular to the wrinkles. Weakening or relaxing these muscles with BoNTA can smooth these lines, including horizontal lines on the forehead (from frontalis contraction), vertical lines in the glabellar region between the eyebrows (caused by the corrugator muscles), horizontal creases across the bridge of the nose (from procerus contraction), "crow's feet" and lateral lines along the lower eyelid (caused by contraction of the lateral orbicularis oculi), and perioral lines (from contraction of the orbicularis oris). Deep grooves or folds

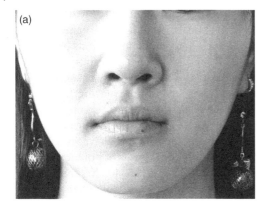 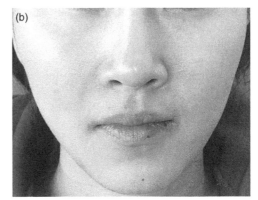

Figure 1.3 Treatment with 25 units to each masseter muscle: (a) before and (b) after.

elsewhere that are exacerbated by muscle activity are also amenable to treatment. Patients 30–50 years of age may be most responsive to BoNTA, because their wrinkles are more likely to be caused by muscle activity than by the loss of skin elasticity that occurs during aging. Clinicians now use the neurotoxin to treat a variety of hyperkinetic facial lines in the upper face, including crow's feet, horizontal forehead lines, and glabellar rhytides, as well as folds and lines in the lower face, neck, and chest with a high level of efficacy and patient satisfaction [12, 47–52].

Facial Sculpting

Facial rejuvenation with BoNT has expanded to involve a more artistic shaping and sculpting of the face. Now, in addition to targeting simple dynamic rhytides, careful injection of

the toxin can be used to lift and shape the brow [53], widen the eyes [12, 54], correct facial asymmetry due to nerve palsies [55], dystonias [17, 20], surgery [56], or trauma [57], and to reduce muscle thickness of the jaw in patients with masseteric hypertrophy (Figure 1.3) [58–61].

Adjunctive Therapy

BoNT is used increasingly in combination with other facial rejuvenation procedures, such as soft-tissue augmentation [28, 62–66] and laser or light-based therapies [12, 28, 67–71], particularly for the treatment of deeper, more static rhytides and folds. BoNT is also used during surgery to prolong or enhance the aesthetic results and as an aid in wound healing and minimizing scars (Figure 1.4) [12, 73–77].

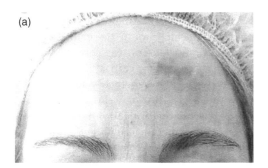 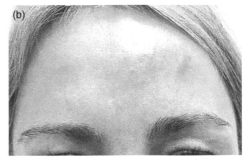

Figure 1.4 Scar forehead (a) shortly after injury and (b) 3 months after BTX. *Source:* Carruthers 1992. Reproduced with permission of Lippincott Williams & Wilkins.

Therapeutic Applications

Intramuscular injections of BoNTA have become the treatment of choice for a number of disorders characterized by muscular hyperactivity, such as strabismus [15], blepharospasm and hemifacial spasm [17], cervical dystonia [78], focal dystonia (writer's cramp) [79], and spasticity due to stroke [80, 81], and cerebral palsy [82]. In addition, the ability of BoNT to block acetylcholine release from autonomic nerve endings innervating glandular tissue or smooth muscle has led to investigation of its use for other indications, including Frey's syndrome [83] and hyperhidrosis [84–89], as well as various gastrointestinal, genitourinary, and sphincter disorders [90], dyshidrotic hand eczema [91, 92], and allergic rhinitis [93, 94]. Flushing of the face and chest can be successfully treated with BoNT due to its ability to regulate blood vessel constriction [95, 96]. Clinicians continue to investigate the use of BoNT for the treatment of chronic pain disorders, including chronic lumbar [97], temporomandibular dysfunction [98], myofascial [99], and neuropathic pain [100], although the toxin's efficacy in the treatment of headache disorders is under debate [101]. More recent research includes applications of BoNT to relieve the pain of arthritis [102, 103].

Future Directions

It is interesting to note that what once began as a potential – rather daring – treatment for a single disorder has translated into a worldwide phenomenon. And one cannot help but wonder what Justinus Kerner would think of his "sausage poison" now that so consumed his time and became his life's research. BoNT has become the treatment of choice for smoothing hyperkinetic lines and shaping the face, alone or in combination with other rejuvenating procedures. Therapeutic applications include a variety of movement, pain, autonomic nervous system, and gastrointestinal and genitourinary disorders, among others. Current recruitment for clinical trials includes everything from arthritis and clubfoot to acne and depression, with new products emerging or on the horizon. Indeed, BoNT seems to have invaded nearly every aspect of clinical medicine, at least in some way, and there is no doubt that the range of indications will only continue to expand.

References

1 Ting PT, Freiman A. The story of *Clostridium botulinum*: From food poisoning to BOTOX. Clin Med 2004;4:258–261.

2 Erbguth FJ, Naumann M. Historical aspects of botulinum toxin: Justinus Kerner (1786–1862) and the "sausage poison." Neurology 1999;53:1850–1853.

3 Hanchanale VS, Rao AR, Martin FL, Matanhelia SS. The unusual history and the urological applications of botulinum neurotoxin. Urol Int 2010:85:125–130.

4 Erbguth FJ. Historical note on the therapeutic use of botulinum toxin in neurological disorders. J Neurol Neurosurg Psychiat 1996;60:151.

5 Koch R. Untersuchungen über Bakterien: V. Die Ätiologie der Milzbrand-Krankheit, begründet auf die Entwicklungsgeschichte des Bacillus anthracis [Investigations into bacteria: V. The etiology of anthrax, based on the ontogenesis of Bacillus anthracis]. Cohns Beitr Biol Pflanzen 1876;2: 277–310.

6 van Ermengem EP. Ueber einen neuen anaëroben Bacillus und seine Beziehungen zum Botulismus. Z Hyg Infektionskr 1897;26:1–56.

7 Burke GS. Notes on *Bacillus botulinus*. J Bacteriol 1919;4:555–565.

8 Snipe PT, Sommer H. Studies on botulinus toxin. 3. Acid precipitation of

botulinus toxin. J Infect Dis 1928;43:152–160.

9 Lamanna C, McElroy OE, Eklund HW. The purification and crystallization of *Clostridium botulinum* type A toxin. Science 1946;103:613–614.

10 Schantz EJ, Johnson EA. Botulinum toxin: The story of its development for the treatment of human disease. Persp Biol Med 1997;40:317–327.

11 Klein AW. Cosmetic therapy with botulinum toxin: Anecdotal memoirs. Dermatol Surg 1996;22:757–759.

12 Carruthers A, Carruthers J. Botulinum toxin type A: History and current cosmetic use in the upper face. Semin Cutan Med Surg 2001;20:71–84.

13 Lipham WJ. A brief history of the clinical applications of botulinum toxin. In: *Cosmetic and Clinical Applications of Botulinum Toxin*. Lipham WJ, ed. Thorofare, NJ: SLACK Incorporated, 2004:1–3.

14 Scott AB, Rosenbaum AL, Collins CC. Pharmacologic weakening of extraocular muscles. Invest Ophthalmol Vis Sci 1973;12:924–927.

15 Scott AB. Botulinum toxin injection into extraocular muscles as an alternative to strabismus surgery. Ophthalmology 1980;87:1044–1049.

16 Tsui JK, Eisen A, Mak E, *et al.* A pilot study on the use of botulinum toxin in spasmodic torticollis. Can J Neurol Sci 1985;12:314–316.

17 Carruthers J, Stubbs HA. Botulinum toxin for benign essential blepharospasm, hemifacial spasm and age-related lower eyelid ectropion. Can J Neurol Sci 1987;14:42–45.

18 Carruthers JDA, Carruthers JA. Treatment of glabellar frown lines with *C. botulinum* A exotoxin. J Dermatol Surg Oncol 1992;18:17–21.

19 Borodic GE, Cheney M, McKenna M. Contralateral injections of botulinum A toxin for the treatment of hemifacial spasm to achieve increased facial symmetry. Plast Reconstr Surg 1992;90:972–7.

20 Blitzer A, Brin MF, Keen MS, Aviv JE. Botulinum toxin for the treatment of hyperfunctional lines of the face. Arch Otolaryngol Head Neck Surg 1993;119:1018–1022.

21 Keen M, Blitzer A, Aviv J, *et al.* Botulinum toxin A for hyperkinetic facial lines: Results of a double-blind, placebo-controlled study. Plast Reconstr Surg 1994;94:94–99.

22 Shapiro RL, Hatheway C, Swerdlow SL. Botulism in the United States: A clinical and epidemiological review. Ann Intern Med 1998;129:221–228.

23 Burgen ASV, Dickens F, Zatman LJ. The action of botulinum toxin on the neuromuscular junction. J Physiol 1949;109:10–24.

24 Aoki KR, Guyer B. Botulinum toxin type A and other botulinum toxin serotypes: a comparative review of biochemical and pharmacological actions. Eur J Neurol 2001;8(suppl 5): 21–29.

25 Dolly JO, Lisk G, Foran PG, *et al.* Insights into the extended duration of neuroparalysis by botulinum neurotoxin A relative to the other shorter-acting serotypes: differences between motor nerve terminals and cultured neurons. In: Brin MF, Jankovic J, Hallett M, eds. *Scientific and Therapeutic Aspects of Botulinum Toxin*. Philadelphia, Pa: Lippincott Williams & Wilkins; 2002:91–102.

26 Meunier FA, Schiavo G, Molgo J. Botulinum neurotxins: From paralysis to recovery of functional neuromuscular transmission. J Physiol Paris 2002;96:105–113.

27 Borodic GE, Ferrante RJ, Pearce LB, *et al.* Pharmacology and histology of the therapeutic application of botulinum toxin. In: Jankovic J, Hallet M. Eds. *Therapy with Botulinum Toxin*. New York: Marcel Dekker, Inc., 1994:119–157.

28 Fagien S, Brandt FS. Primary and adjunctive use of botulinum toxin type A (BOTOX) in facial aesthetic surgery:

Beyond the glabella. Clin Plast Surg 2001;28:127–148.

29 Carruthers A, Carruthers J. Cosmetic uses of botulinum A exotoxin. In: Klein A, ed. *Tissue Augmentation in Clinical Practice: Procedures and Techniques*. New York: Marcel Dekker, Inc., 1998:207–236.

30 Carruthers JA, Lowe NJ, Menter MA, *et al.* A multicenter, double-blind, randomized, placebo-controlled study of the efficacy and safety of botulinum toxin type A in the treatment of glabellar lines. J Am Acad Dermatol 2002;46:840–849.

31 Carruthers J, Carruthers A. The evolution of botulinum neurotoxin type A for cosmetic applications. J Cosmet Laser Ther 2007;9:186–192.

32 Carruthers A, Carruthers J. Botulinum toxin products overview. Skin Therapy Lett 2008;13:1–4.

33 Cohen JL, Schlessinger J, Cox SE, Lin X; Reloxin Investigational Group. An analysis of the long-term safety data of repeat administrations of botulinum neurotoxin type A-ABO for the treatment of glabellar lines. Aesthet Surg J 2009; 29(6 Suppl):S43–S49.

34 Monheit GD, Cohen JL; Reloxin Investigational Group. Long-term safety of repeated administrations of a new formulation of botulinum toxin type A in the treatment of glabellar lines: interim analysis from an open-label extension study. J Am Acad Dermatol 2009;61: 421–425.

35 Dressler D. [Pharmacological aspects of therapeutic botulinum toxin preparations]. [In German]. Nervenarzt 2006;77:912–921.

36 Roggenkamper P, Jost WH, Bihari K, *et al.* Efficacy and safety of a new botulinum toxin type A free of complexing proteins in the treatment of blepharospasm. J Neural Transm 2006;113:303–312.

37 Jost WH, Blumel J, Grafe S. Botulinum neurotoxin type A free of complexing proteins (XEOMIN) in focal dystonia. Drugs 2007;67:669–683.

38 Dressler D. Routine use of Xeomin in patients previously treated with Botox: long term results. Eur J Neurol 2009;16 Suppl 2:2–5.

39 Jankovic J. Clinical efficacy and tolerability of Xeomin in the treatment of blepharospasm. Eur J Neurol 2009;16 Suppl 2:14–18.

40 Dressler D. Comparing Botox and Xeomin for axillary hyperhidrosis. J Neural Transm 2010;117:317–319.

41 Ramirez AL, Reeck J, Maas CS. Botulinum toxin type B (Myobloc) in the management of hyperkinetic facial lines. Otolaryngol Head Neck Surg 2002;126: 459–467.

42 Alster TS, Lupton JR. Botulinum toxin type B for dynamic glabellar rhytides refractory to botulinum toxin type A. Dermatol Surg 2003;29:516–518.

43 Kim EJ, Ramirez AL, Reeck JB, Maas CS. The role of botulinum toxin type B (Myobloc) in the treatment of hyperkinetic facial lines. Plast Reconstr Surg 2003;112(5 Suppl):88S–93S.

44 Sadick NS. Prospective open-label study of botulinum toxin type B (Myobloc) at doses of 2,400 and 3,000 U for the treatment of glabellar wrinkles. Dermatol Surg 2003;29:501–507.

45 Matarasso SL. Comparison of botulinum toxin types A and B: a bilateral and double-blind randomized evaluation in the treatment of canthal rhytides. Dermatol Surg 2003;29:7–13.

46 Carruthers A, Carruthers J, Flynn TC, Leong MS. Dose-finding, safety, and tolerability study of botulinum toxin type B for the treatment of hyperfunctional glabellar lines. Dermatol Surg 2007; 33(1 Spec No.):S60–S68.

47 Becker-Wegerich PM, Rauch L, Ruzicka T. Botulinum toxin A: Successful décolleté rejuvenation. Dermatol Surg 2002;28:168–171.

48 Carruthers J, Carruthers A. Botulinum toxin A in the mid and lower face and neck. Dermatol Clin 2004;22:151–158.

49 Lowe NJ, Yamauchi P. Cosmetic uses of botulinum toxins for lower aspects of the face and neck. Clin Dermatol 2004;22:18–22.

50 Dayan SH, Maas CS. Botulinum toxins for facial wrinkles: beyond glabellar lines. Facial Plast Surg Clin North Am 2007;15:41–49.

51 Fagien S, Carruthers JD. A comprehensive review of patient-reported satisfaction with botulinum toxin type a for aesthetic procedures. Plast Reconstr Surg 2008;122:1915–1925.

52 Carruthers A, Carruthers J, Lei X, *et al.* OnabotulinumtoxinA treatment of mild glabellar lines in repose. Dermatol Surg 2010 Dec:36(Suppl 4):2168–2171.

53 Carruthers A, Carruthers J. Eyebrow height after botulinum toxin type A to the glabella. Dermatol Surg. 2007;33(1 Spec No.):S26–S31.

54 Flynn TC, Carruthers JA, Carruthers JA. Botulinum-A toxin treatment of the lower eyelid improves infraorbital rhytides and widens the eye. Dermatol Surg. 2001;27:703–708.

55 Armstrong MWJ, Mountain RE, Murray JAM. Treatment of facial synkinesis and facial asymmetry with botulinum toxin type A following facial nerve palsy. Clin Otolaryngol Allied Sci 1996;21:15–20.

56 Borodic GE. Botulinum A toxin for (expressionistic) ptosis overcorrection after frontalis sling. Ophthal Plast Reconstr Surg 1992;8:137–142.

57 Carruthers A, Carruthers J. Clinical indications and injection technique for the cosmetic use of botulinum A exotoxin. Dermatol Surg 1998;24:1189–1194.

58 To EW, Ahuja AT, Ho WS, *et al.* A prospective study of the effect of botulinum toxin A on masseteric muscle hypertrophy with ultrasonographic and electromyographic measurement. Br J Plast Surg 2001;54:197–200.

59 von Lindern JJ, Niederhagen B, Appel T, Berge S, Reich RH. Type A botulinum toxin for the treatment of hypertrophy of the masseter and temporal muscle: an alternative treatment. Plast Reconstr Surg 2001;107:327–332.

60 Park MY, Ahn KY, Jung DS. Application of botulinum toxin A for treatment of facial contouring in the lower face. Dermatol Surg 2003;29:477–483.

61 Liew S, Dart A. Nonsurgical reshaping of the lower face. Aesthet Surg J 2008;28:251–257.

62 Coleman KR, Carruthers J. Combination therapy with BOTOX and fillers: The new rejuvenation paradigm. Dermatol Ther 2006;19:177–188.

63 Carruthers J, Carruthers A, Maberley, D. Deep resting glabellar rhytides respond to BTX-A and Hylan B. Dermatol Surg 2003;29:539–544.

64 Carruthers J, Carruthers A. A prospective, randomized, parallel group study analyzing the effect of BTX-A(Botox) and nonanimal sourced hyaluronic acid (NASHA, Restylane) in combination compared with NASHA (Restylane) alone in severe glabellar rhytides in adult female subjects: treatment of severe glabellar rhytides with a hyaluronic acid derivative compared with the derivative and BTX-A. Dermatol Surg 2003;29:802–809.

65 Patel MP, Talmor M, Nolan WB. Botox and collagen for glabellar furrows: Advantages of combination therapy. Ann Plast Surg 2004;52:442–447.

66 Carruthers A, Carruthers J, Monheit GD, *et al.* Multicenter, randomized, parallel-group study of the safety and effectiveness of onabotulinumtoxinA and hyaluronic acid dermal fillers (24-mg/mL smooth, cohesive gel) alone and in combination for lower facial rejuvenation. Dermatol Surg 2010 Dec;36(Suppl 4):2121–2134.

67 Carruthers J, Carruthers A. Combining botulinum toxin injection and laser for facial rhytides. In: Coleman WP, Lawrence N, eds. *Skin Resurfacing.* Baltimore, MD: Williams and Wilkins, 1998:235–243.

68 West TB, Alster TS. Effect of botulinum toxin type A on movement-associated rhytides following CO_2 laser resurfacing. Dermatol Surg 1999;25:259–261.

69 Carruthers J, Carruthers A, Zelichowska A. The power of combined therapies:

Botox and ablative facial laser resurfacing. Am J Cos Surg 2000;17:129–131.

70 Zimbler MS, Holds JB, Kokoska MS, *et al.* Effect of botulinum toxin pretreatment on laser resurfacing results: A prospective, randomized, blinded trial. Arch Facial Plast Surg 2001;3:165–169.

71 Carruthers J, Carruthers A. The effect of full-face broadband light treatments alone and in combination with bilateral crow's feet botulinum toxin type A chemodenervation. Dermatol Surg 2004;30:355–366.

72 Carruthers JDA, Carruthers A. Treatment of glabellar frown lines with *C. botulinum* exotoxin. J Dermatol Surg Oncol 1992;18: 17–21.

73 Sherris DA, Gassner HG. Botulinum toxin to minimize facial scarring. Facial Plast Surg 2002;18:35–39.

74 Gassner HG, Sherris DA. Chemoimmobilization: improving predictability in the treatment of facial scars. Plast Reconstr Surg 2003;112: 1464–1466.

75 Gassner HG, Brissett AE, Otley CC, *et al.* Botulinum toxin to improve facial wound healing: A prospective, blinded, placebo-controlled study. Mayo Clin Proc 2006;81:1023–1028.

76 Wilson AM. Use of botulinum toxin type A to prevent widening of facial scars. Plast Reconstr Surg 2006;117:1758–1766.

77 Flynn TC. Use of intraoperative botulinum toxin in facial reconstruction. Dermatol Surg 2009;35:182–188.

78 Jankovic J, Schwartz K. Botulinum toxin injections for cervical dystonia. Neurology. 1990;40:277–280.

79 Tsui JK, Bhatt M, Calne S, Calne DB. Botulinum toxin in the treatment of writer's cramp: A double-blind study. Neurology 1993;43:183–185.

80 Kaji R, Osako Y, Suvama K, *et al.* Botulinum toxin type A in post-stroke upper limb spasticity. Curr Med Res Opin 2010;26:1983–1992.

81 Kaji R, Osako Y, Suyama K, *et al.* Botulinum toxin type A in post-stroke lower limb spasticity: a multicenter, double-blind, placebo-controlled trial. J Neurol 2010;257:1330–1337.

82 Unlu E, Cevikol A, Bal B, *et al.* Multilevel botulinum toxin type a as a treatment for spasticity in children with cerebral palsy: A retrospective study. Clinics (Sao Paulo) 2010;65:613–619.

83 de Bree R, Duyndam JE, Kuik DJ, Leemans CR. Repeated botulinum toxin type A injections to treat patients with Frey syndrome. Arch Otolaryngol Head Neck Surg 2009;135:287–290.

84 Lowe NJ, Yamauchi PS, Lask GP, *et al.* Efficacy and safety of botulinum toxin type A in the treatment of palmar hyperhidrosis: a double-blind, randomized, placebo-controlled study. Dermatol Surg 2002;28:822–827.

85 Lowe PL, Cerdan-Sanz S, Lowe NJ. Botulinum toxin type A in the treatment of bilateral primary axillary hyperhidrosis: efficacy and duration with repeated treatments. Dermatol Surg 2003;29:545–548.

86 Naumann M, Lowe NJ, Kumar CR, Hamm H. Botulinum toxin type A is a safe and effective treatment for axillary hyperhidrosis over 16 months: a prospective study. Arch Dermatol 2003;139:731–736.

87 Vlahovic TC, Dunn SP, Blau JC, Gauthier C. Injectable botulinum toxin as a treatment for plantar hyperhidrosis: a case study. J Am Podiatr Med Assoc 2008;98:156–159.

88 Lowe NJ, Glaser DA, Eadie N, *et al.* Botulinum toxin type A in the treatment of primary axillary hyperhidrosis: A 52-week multicenter double-blind, randomized, placebo-controlled study of efficacy and safety. J Am Acad Dermatol. 2007;56:604–611.

89 Pérez-Bernal AM, Avalos-Peralta P, Moreno-Ramírez D, Camacho F. Treatment of palmar hyperhidrosis with botulinum toxin type A: 44 months of experience. Cosmet Dermatol 2005;4:163–166.

90 Jankovic J. Botulinum toxin in clinical practice. J Neurol Neurosurg Psychiat 2004;75:951–957.

91 Swartling C, Naver H, Lindberg M, *et al.* Treatment of dyshidrotic hand dermatitis with intradermal botulinum toxin. J Am Acad Dermatol 2002;47:667–671.

92 Wollina U, Karamfilov T. Adjuvant botulinum toxin A in dyshidrotic hand eczema: A controlled prospective pilot study with left–right comparison. J Eur Acad Dermatol Venereol 2002;16:40–42.

93 Yang TY, Jung YG, Kim YH, Jang TY. A comparison of the effects of botulinum toxin A and steroid injection on nasal allergy. Otolaryngol Head Neck Surg 2008;139:367–371.

94 Rohrbach S, Junghans K, Köhler S, Laskawi R. Minimally invasive application of botulinum toxin A in patients with idiopathic rhinitis. Head Face Med 2009 Oct 16;5:18.

95 Yuratisi M, Jacob CI. Botulinum toxin for the treatment of facial flushing. Dermatol Surg 2004;30:102–104.

96 Alexandroff AB, Sinclair SA, Langtry JA. Successful use of botulinum toxin A for the treatment of neck and anterior chest wall flushing. Dermatol Surg 2006;32: 1536.

97 Jabbari B, Ney J, Sichani A, *et al.* Treatment of refractory, chronic low back pain with botulinum neurotoxin A: An open-label, pilot study. Pain Med 2006;7:260–264.

98 von Lindern JJ, Niederhagen B, Bergé S, *et al.* Type A botulinum toxin in the treatment of chronic facial pain associated with masticatory hyperactivity. J Oral Maxillofac Surg 2003;61:774–778.

99 Porta M, Perreti A, Gamba M, *et al.* The rationale and results of treating muscle spasm and myofascial syndromes with botulinum toxin type A. Pain Digest 1998;8:346–352.

100 Rawicki B, Sheean G, Fung VS, *et al.* Botulinum toxin assessment, intervention and aftercare for paediatric and adult niche indications including pain: international consensus statement. Eur J Neurol 2010;17(Suppl 2): 122–134.

101 Naumann M, So Y, Argoff CE, *et al.* Assessment: Botulinum neurotoxin in the treatment of autonomic disorders and pain (an evidence-based review): Report of the Therapeutics and Technology Assessment Subcommittee of the American Academy of Neurology. Neurology 2008;70:1707–1714.

102 Boon AJ, Smith J, Dahm DL, *et al.* Efficacy of intra-articular botulinum toxin type A in painful knee osteoarthritis: A pilot study. PM R 2010;2:268–276.

103 Marchini C, Acler M, Bolognari MA. Efficacy of botulinum toxin type A treatment of functional impairment of degenerative hip joint: Preliminary results. J Rehabil Med 2010;42: 691–693.

2

Anatomy and Aesthetic Principles

Timothy M. Greco, MD (FACS),[1] Chérie M. Ditre, MD,[2] and David M. Ozog, MD (FAAD, FACMS)[3]

[1]*Clinical Assistant Professor, Department of Otolaryngology-Head and Neck Surgery, Division of Facial Plastic Surgery, University of Pennsylvania School of Medicine, Philadelphia, USA*

[2]*Associate Professor, Department of Dermatology, University of Pennsylvania School of Medicine, Philadelphia, USA*

[3]*Chair, Department of Dermatology; C.S. Livingood Chair in Dermatology; Director of Cosmetic Dermatology, Henry Ford Hospital, Detroit, MI, USA*

Anatomy of Youthful versus Aging Skin

Apparent age is readily judged by several factors including the presence and numbers of facial wrinkles, dyschromia, and skin laxity among other anatomic aging skin changes. To understand treatment with neuromodulators, it is important for the reader to familiarize themselves with basic facial skin anatomy as well the anatomy of aging skin and its underlying structures. The neurotoxin injector can then precisely target the intended underlying muscles being treated with an understanding of the expected improvement from the toxin as well as the potential need for adjuvant therapies.

Youthful skin is characteristically smooth in texture, having a dewy luster, even tone, high elasticity, and pleasant balanced contours due to appropriate tissue volume. Rhytides are absent or minimal at rest. Youthful skin is by definition, normal or unaltered in anatomical configuration and histology.

Aging skin, in contrast, exhibits surface irregularities such as textural roughness, sallowness, pigment alterations, and inelasticity as well as the appearance of wrinkles/rhytids. In addition, subsurface changes, namely loss of volume due to dermal atrophy, fat atrophy and redistribution, and biometric volume loss

due to deeper compartmental changes such as bony and cartilaginous resorption, ensue. Aging skin is viewed as an alteration of the skin's normal anatomy.

Wrinkles themselves are one modification of the aging process, but nevertheless are typically the most characteristic hallmark. Despite this, there are few studies dedicated to defining wrinkles both clinically and histologically. These factors have muddied the anatomic and histologic definition of wrinkles.

Kligman attempted to define wrinkles by histologic examination of 58 patients with a variety of wrinkle types from the cheeks, crow's feet, temporal frown lines, upper vertical lip lines and other body areas of crinkling skin such as the abdomen and the back of the neck. He concluded that wrinkles are not a histological entity, as the microanatomic features did not distinguish them from their surrounding skin, but rather a configurational change due to mechanical stresses on the skin. He noted that these changes occurred more prominently in actinically damaged regions due to deterioration of the elastic fibers. Kligman proposed that the facial frown lines occurred primarily through muscular contraction and that the facial muscles are inserted into the overlying skin. Their muscular contraction throws the skin into

Botulinum Toxins: Cosmetic and Clinical Applications, First Edition. Edited by Joel L. Cohen and David M. Ozog.
© 2017 John Wiley & Sons Ltd. Published 2017 by John Wiley & Sons Ltd.
Companion Website: www.wiley.com/go/cohen/botulinum

folds because while the muscles can contract, the skin does not. He stated that in youth, dynamic expression lines disappear immediately when the muscles relax since elastic fibers are not yet altered; however, muscular contractions on a degraded dermal matrix result in permanent wrinkles [1].

Bosset *et al.* analyzed the histological features of the pre-auricular wrinkle compared to retroauricular skin in 16 subjects undergoing face lifts (ages 36–94 years). In doing so, they defined four types of facial skin depressions and classified them based on their depths: (i) invaginations of the skin structures from 250 to 400 μm deep were folds such as nasolabial and melolabial, (ii) permanent wrinkles are invaginations of the skin structures of 100 μm deep, (iii) reducible wrinkles (frown lines, crow lines and preauricular wrinkles) are seen *in vivo* but not after histologic processing, and (iv) microrelief (nonspecific frown lines due to aging) are shallow depressions (10–30 μm deep) involving the horny and granular layers of the epidermis [2]. Histological analysis of the epidermis and dermis of the skin specifically under and surrounding permanent and reducible wrinkles actually demonstrated normal skin morphology; however, deep permanent wrinkles showed a heavier accumulation of basophilic fibers representing actinic elastosis – which involves the entire depth of the superficial dermis in contrast to reducible wrinkles. This suggests that the development of wrinkles could be furthered by actinic elastosis and the disappearance of microfibrils and collagen fibers at the dermal–epidermal junction (DEJ). The authors concluded that a diminished skin resistance at the DEJ and upper superficial dermis due to sun damage is a prerequisite for wrinkle formation.

However, Pierard and Lapiere [3] concluded that the histological changes necessary to produce a wrinkle began with the changes in the hypodermal connective tissue septae below the wrinkles and not actually in the epidermis or dermis. Underneath each wrinkle there were hypodermal septae that were shorter and thicker than those outside the grooves. They postulated that wrinkling was the result of skin remodeling of the hypodermal connective tissue by repetitive mechanical stimuli induced by striated muscle [3].

Facial Fat Compartments

Neuromodulators are frequently injected with filling agents as part of a comprehensive facial rejuvenation plan. Knowledge of facial fat compartments is paramount for expert injectors to properly restore volume with filling agents. Knowledge of cutaneous anatomy in general is necessary to visualize areas in patients that need to be relaxed (neuromodulators), volume restored (fillers), and resurfaced (lasers/chemical peels). This should be the goal of every injector to create a natural, youthful, and rested appearance. Understanding the following key principles regarding fat compartments will help to further that goal (Figure 2.1).

Forehead and Temporal Fat Compartments

Subcutaneous forehead fat is composed of three anatomical units – central, middle and lateral temporal/cheek fat.

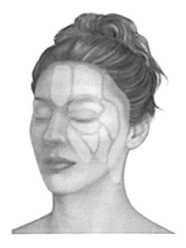

Figure 2.1 Facial fat compartments. *Source:* Rohrich 2007 [14]. Reproduced with permission of Wolters Kluwer Health, Inc.

The central fat is in the midline region of the forehead and is bounded inferiorly at the nasal dorsum and is bounded laterally by a dense fascial plane that appears to be the central temporal septum. This dense fibrous band septum underlies the fascia of the frontalis muscle and inserts into the dermis.

The middle forehead fat sits on either side of the midline central fat, and is medial to the superior temporal septum. The middle forehead fat compartment is bound inferiorly by the orbicularis oculi retaining ligament of the superior orbit.

The lateral temporal/cheek compartment connects the lateral forehead fat to the lateral cheek and cervical fat. The lateral temporal cheek septum spans the forehead with the neck [14].

The Orbital Fat Compartment

There are also three periorbital fat compartments-superior orbital fat, inferior orbital fat, and lateral orbital fat. Loss of periorbital fat contributes to the appearance of rhytids and lax skin, which are treated with combinations of toxins, fillers, and resurfacing.

The superior orbital fat is bounded by the orbicularis oculi retaining ligament of the superior orbit. The orbicularis retaining ligament is circumferential and spans the superior and inferior orbits blending into the medial and lateral canthi; however, the superior and inferior compartments are distinct from each other.

The inferior orbital fat is a thin layer that lies directly below the inferior lid tarsus. It is bounded inferiorly by the orbicularis oculi retaining ligament or malar septum, and medially and laterally by the respective canthi.

The lateral orbital fat is bounded superiorly by the inferior temporal septum and inferiorly by the superior cheek septum. The zygomaticus major muscle adheres to this compartment. To elevate medial cheek fat or jowl fat, one has to traverse the zygomaticus muscle. There is the potential, while chasing inferior crow's feet wrinkles with botulinum toxin, of inadvertently injecting the superior aspect of the zygomaticus muscle, which would then result in depression of the cheek and oral commisure.

The Nasolabial Fat Compartment

Prominence of the nasolabial fold is seen in patients with more severe facial volume loss. The nasolabial fold is one discrete unit with distinct anatomical boundaries. The nasolabial fat compartment lies immediately anterior to the medial compartment of malar cheek fat and overlaps jowl fat. It is bounded superiorly by the orbicularis oculi retaining ligament of the inferior orbit and by the sub-orbicularis fat laterally. The inferior border of the zygomaticus major muscle is tethered to the nasolabial fat compartment. The medial cheek septum separates the nasolabial fat from the medial cheek fat.

The Cheek Fat Compartment

The Malar fat compartment is divided into three units – medial, middle, and lateral temporal cheek fat.

The medial cheek fat is lateral to the nasolabial fold. It is bounded superiorly by the orbicularis oculi retaining ligament of the inferior orbit, laterally by the middle cheek septum and inferiorly by jowl fat. The medial cheek septum then separates the nasolabial fat from the medial cheek fat.

The middle cheek fat lies between the medial and lateral temporal-cheek compartments and is anterior and superficial to the parotid gland. The zygomaticus major muscle adheres to its superior portion. The medial and middle cheek fat compartments abut each other but are clearly separated by the middle cheek septum. Their septal boundaries fuse forming a dense fascial network known as the zygomatic ligament.

The most lateral component of the cheek fat is the lateral temporal-cheek compartment. The lateral temporal cheek fat is directly superficial to the parotid gland connecting the temporal fat to the cervical subcutaneous fat. Anterior to this compartment, the lateral cheek septum appears as a vertical septal barrier. It is the first zone encountered surgically during a face lift procedure after a preauricular incision moving medially.

The Jowl Fat Compartment

Jowl fat is the most inferior facial fat. Nasolabial fat and medial cheek fat are located superiorly to jowl fat. Its medial boundary is the depressor anguli oris (DAO) muscle (lip depressor) while the inferior boundary is the membranous fusion of the platysma. The fusion point of the DAO and the platysma is the mandibular retaining ligament. It is not known how this particular compartment behaves during the aging process, but it is probably the most important with regards to midfacial aging.

Superficial Musculoaponeurotic System

The superficial musculoaponeurotic system (SMAS) is a complex fibromuscular network which serves a distinct role in the face. Superiorly, it is comprised of the galea aponeurotica in the region of the forehead. Here it divides and envelops the frontalis muscle. Laterally, the fascia becomes the temporoparietal fascia as it approaches the zygomatic arch. It is here in the temporoparietal fascia where the temporal branch of the facial nerve resides. This branch is in close relationship to the periosteum of the zygomatic arch. In the cheek, there is a distinct SMAS layer which becomes contiguous with the platysma in the neck. Embryologically the SMAS develops from an upper division comprising the frontalis, orbicularis oculi, lip elevators, and the orbicularis oris. There is also a lower division made up of the actual platysma muscle along with the depressor anguli oris and risorius [16].

The SMAS separates the subcutaneous fat into superficial and deep layers. The superficial layer, as mentioned, is divided into fat compartments. In between these compartments are complex fascial condensations forming a network of retaining ligaments. It is this network that helps to transmit the forces of the fascial musculature to the skin surface – allowing for a myriad of complex facial expressions which characterize the human face as well as being responsible for the formation of hyperfunctional rhytids.

The Facial Nerve

Found below the SMAS in the deep fat layer is the facial nerve. It is this nerve that innervates the distribution of the hyoid arch mesenchyme (second branchial arch) – which is the embryologic precursor of the facial musculature. The facial nerve (seventh cranial nerve) arises from the stylomastoid foramen of the base of the skull. As it exits the foramen it immediately gives off a posterior auricularis branch, which supplies the occipitalis, posterior and superior auricular muscles. It also gives off a branch to the posterior belly of the digastric muscle and the stylohyoid muscle. Next, as the nerve passes as a main trunk anteriorly, it then divides into two main divisions in the body of the parotid gland. The upper division is comprised of the temporofacial segment, and the lower division is comprised of the cervicofacial segment. However, as these divisions proceed more anteriorly, extensive variability of branching patterns may develop with variable patterns of innervation ensuing. The temporal branch runs in the temporoparietal fascia after crossing over the zygomatic arch. It becomes the frontal branch as it enters the lateral and deep aspect of the frontalis muscle. The temporal branch supplies the anterior and superior auricular muscles and the superior portion of the orbicularis oculi as well as the corrugators. The corrugator muscles are also supplied by a branch of the zygomatic nerve.

The zygomatic nerve supplies the lower portion of the orbicularis oculi, the corrugators, the muscles of the nasal aperture including the nasalis and the upper lip elevators. The buccal branch innervates the upper lip sphincteric mechanism with contributions also innervating the upper lip elevators. The marginal mandibular nerve innervates the musculature of the lower lip: the orbicularis oris, the lower lip depressors, depressor anguli oris (DAO), depressor labii inferioris (DLI) and mentalis. The cervical branch innervates the platysma. There is extensive and significant anastomosis between the buccal and zygomatic branches. However, the temporal and marginal branches lack such anastomotic connections. As such, injury to the temporal or marginal nerves during surgery may result in longer lasting paresis. Neurotoxin may be injected into the contralateral musculature to maintain symmetry until the paresis resolves which may or may not occur. For example, if a temporal nerve is unilaterally compromised limiting ipsilateral brow elevation, restoration of symmetry can occur if the neurotoxin is injected into the contralateral frontalis muscle until the temporal nerve function returns on the affected side. The same principle applies to injury of the marginal mandibular nerve and treating the contralateral DAO and DLI muscles to create a more symmetric smile until nerve function returns. If the nerve has been injured and not transected, function usually returns within 6 months to 1 year.

Vasculature of the Face

The vasculature of the face is essentially comprised of branches from the internal and external carotid arteries. Examples include the supratrochlear, supraorbital, infraorbital and mental arteries – which accompany their corresponding nerves and exit the corresponding foramina of the central face.

The external carotid artery feeds primarily the maxilla, mandible, occipital and temporal regions of the face. The main branches of the external carotid artery include the facial, internal maxillary, occipital, superficial temporal, posterior auricular and transverse facial arteries. The internal maxillary artery branches into the infraorbital, the inferior alveolar, which eventually becomes the mental artery, and the posterior superior alveolar arteries. The facial artery branches into the superior and inferior labial arteries and eventually becomes the angular artery as it approaches the lateral aspect of the nose.

The internal carotid artery gives off the ophthalmic artery, which then supplies the supratrochlear and supraorbital vessels. Attention should be given to the watershed area that exists between the supratrocholear arteries in the glabellar region. This area of the glabella is prone to necrosis if injecting large volumes of fillers that, in turn, generates external tamponade of the microvasculature in this watershed region. Direct cannulization of vessels has also occurred with fillers in this area, resulting in complete intravascular occlusion [17].

The venous structures of the face tend to follow the arterial pattern, although the venous pattern may have more variability and less predictability. The venous plexus of the lateral orbital and anterior temporal regions drain into the sentinel veins. Care must be taken when injecting neuromodulator agents in the lateral orbital area for crow's feet treatments to avoid bruising in this region. Magnification and enhanced lighting to identify these vessels as best as possible, as well as injecting tangentially and superficially creating dermal wheals, is the optimal way of injecting this region with botulinum toxin to try to avoid bruising.

Muscles of Facial Expression

To have a successful understanding of the injection technique of neurotoxins for facial reshaping and rhytids, it is imperative to have a working understanding of the muscles of facial expression. Thorough knowledge of muscular anatomy also minimizes complications and allows us to precisely tailor injections to the patient's aesthetic desires. Knowing the origin, insertion, caliber or size,

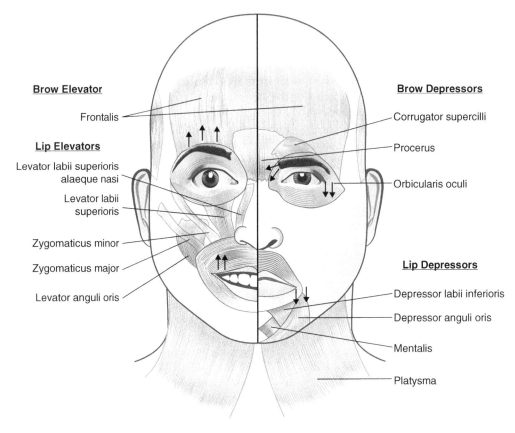

Brow Elevator

Frontalis

Lip Elevators

Levator labii superioris
alaeque nasi

Levator labii
superioris

Zygomaticus minor

Zygomaticus major

Levator anguli oris

Brow Depressors

Corrugator supercilli

Procerus

Orbicularis oculi

Lip Depressors

Depressor labii inferioris

Depressor anguli oris

Mentalis

Platysma

Figure 2.2 Protagonist/antagonist muscles of facial expression. Redrawn based on an original drawing by Margaret Ditré.

course, functional and aesthetic action of each muscle is paramount to successfully treating the facial muscles with neurotoxins. Most facial muscles originate on the facial skeleton and insert on the dermis of the skin with assistance from the superficial musculoaponeurotic system – thus transmitting their forces to the overlying skin and significant facial structures, such as the brows and oral commissures.

The following is an in-depth look at the anatomy of the facial musculature with clinical correlation. The face will be divided into upper, middle, and lower thirds. The neck primarily has the platysma muscle as its major contributor of facial expression and will be discussed last. Although the discussion involves individual analyses, it is important to remember that an intricate interplay

exists between the muscles of facial expression. Each facial expression involves multiple muscles, creating antagonist/protagonist activity to result in a unique expression (Figure 2.2).

The Upper Face

Before discussing the specific muscles of the upper one-third of the face, it is critical to understand the ideal aesthetic position of the overlying skin and soft tissue, particularly the brow. Much media attention has focused on incorrect brow placement after botulinum toxin injection over the past several years. The terms "Nicholson brow," "Spock brow" or "mephisto-look" are now part of the vernacular of those familiar with cosmetic toxin injection, and the astute clinician understands

Figure 2.3 Female and male brow position. Redrawn based on an original drawing by David M. Ozog.

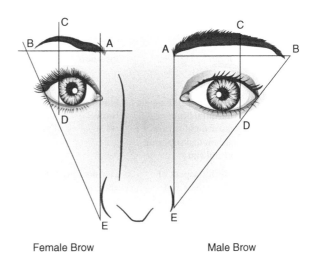

Female Brow   Male Brow

the importance of minimizing this type of appearance.

There are more similarities than differences between the male and female brow (Figure 2.3). The edge of the eyebrow lies in a vertical plane passing through the alar base. The lateral eyebrow ends at an oblique line drawn from the alar base through the lateral canthus. The medial and lateral ends of the eyebrow lie at the same horizontal level in both males and females. The apex of the eyebrow lies vertically above the lateral limbus of the eye at approximately the junction of the medial two thirds and the lateral third of the eyebrow. The main differences are that the eyebrow arches above the supraorbital rim in women and lies at the rim in men and the male eyebrow tends to be heavier and less arched.

The muscles of the upper one-third of the face are critical with respect to the shape and position of the brows and the presence of hyperfunctional rhytids (Table 2.1). These rhytids include the transverse rhytids of the forehead, the vertical and horizontal glabellar frown lines, as well as lateral canthal crow's-feet. The shape and size of the palpebral aperture is intimately associated with function of the orbicularis oculi muscle. The shape and position of the brow exemplifies the antagonist and protagonist relationship

that occurs in the musculature of the upper one-third of the face. The frontalis muscle is a paired muscle that forms the anterior part of the occipitofrontalis (epicranius) muscle. It is connected to the posterior occipitalis muscle via the galea aponeurotica, and therefore does not have a bony origin as most facial muscles do. It inserts into the skin of the lower forehead in the region of the brows and interdigitates with the corrugator, procerus and orbicularis oculi muscles. It is this interdigitation with these muscles that allows it to have a unique role in determining not only the position of the brow but also the shape of the brow. The frontalis muscle is the only elevator of the brow complex, and therefore should be treated conservatively when using neurotoxins. Avoiding injection of neurotoxin to the lower one-third of the frontalis in general is helpful in many patients to preventing brow ptosis and maintaining some brow movement. The frontalis muscle is also responsible for the creation of the transverse rhytids of the forehead. These rhytids may become deeper in time as the frontalis muscle becomes more active to compensate for eyelid ptosis. This hyperfunctional compensatory mechanism is seen in older patients as they try to compensate for ptosis that is occurring from the dis-insertion of the levator aponeurosis from the superior aspect of

Table 2.1 Muscles of the brow complex.

Muscle	Origin	Insertion	Action	Cosmetic consequence
Eyebrow depressors				
Corrugator supercilli	Medial inferior aspect of frontal bone near nasofrontal suture and medial superior orbital rim	Skin above medial brow	Adducts and depresses medial brow	Vertical frown lines of glabella
Procerus	Inferior aspect of nasal bones and upper lateral nasal cartlidges	Dermis of glabella and lower mid forehead	Downward pull on skin of medial forehead	Transverse rhytids between brows
Orbicularis oculi				
– Orbital portion	Medial palpebral ligament, nasal portion of frontal bone and frontal process of maxilla	Cheeks, forehead and temples; interdigitates with surrounding muscles (frontalis and corrugator supercilli)	Depresses medial and lateral aspects of brow; adducts brow	Lateral canthal rhytids (crow's feet)
– Palpebral portion: preseptal and pretarsal	Preseptal: medial palpebral ligament Pretarsal: medial palpebral ligament	Preseptal: lateral palpebral raphe Pretarsal: lateral orbital tubercle	Medial attachments allow for pumping mechanism for tears	Rhytids of lower eyelid
Eyebrow elevators				
Frontalis	Galea aponeurotica	Skin of lower forehead; interdigitates with corrugator, procerus and orbicularis oculi	Elevates brows	Transverse rhytids of forehead

the tarsal plate. Although the frontalis has been classically described as a paired muscle complex, it frequently is contiguous across the forehead, thus explaining the continuous rhytids that are seen in many patients (Figure 2.4). When there is a dehiscence of the muscle, a double arched transverse rhytid pattern may be seen in those patients when raising their eyebrows.

The lateral extent of the frontalis muscle is seen at the temporal fusion line – which is also the medial extent of the temporalis muscle. This is usually the region where the anterior hairline exists. This relationship is important to identify because it explains why

lateral brow ptosis occurs with aging. This will be discussed further in detail later.

The corrugator supercilli muscle originates on the medial inferior aspect of the frontal bone near the nasofrontal suture as well as the medial superior orbital rim. It runs laterally and superiorly to insert onto the skin above the medial brow. Its insertion can be seen as a dimple in the skin above the medial brow as the patient frowns (Figure 2.5). This may be seen medial, at or lateral to the mid-pupillary line – depending on the length of the muscle. There may, in fact, be multiple insertions in this region. This corruguator supercilli muscle runs deep to the procerus, frontalis, and

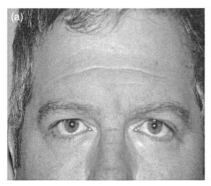 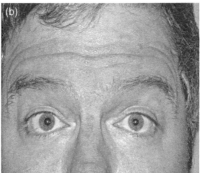

Figure 2.4 Transverse rhytids of the forehead (a) relaxed and (b) in animation showing continuous horizontal rhytids across forehead consistent with contiguous frontalis muscle.

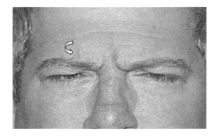

Figure 2.5 Insertion of corrugator supercilli onto dermis of skin of medial brow as depicted by the dimple.

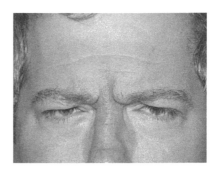

Figure 2.6 Vertical frown lines of glabella created by the action of corrugator supercilli.

orbicularis oculi medially and becomes more superficial as it courses laterally [18]. The supraorbital and supratrochlear neurovascular bundles run through the belly of the corrugator muscle. This explains why migraine headaches may be treated with an injection of the corrugator muscle since the supratrochlear nerve can be considered one of the triggers of migraine headaches [19]. The corrugator muscle functions to adduct and depress the medial brow thus creating vertical frown lines of the glabella (Figure 2.6). The corrugator is innervated by the temporal and zyogomatic branches of the facial nerve.

The procerus muscle is a triangular shaped muscle which originates from the inferior aspect of the nasal bones and upper lateral nasal cartilages and inserts onto the dermis of the skin of the glabella and lower mid forehead. It pulls the skin of the medial forehead downward thus creating transverse

rhytids seen between the brows (Figure 2.7). Although having been described previously, the existence of a distinct depressor supercilli muscle was not identified in the recent anatomic dissections of Macdonald, *et al.* [20].

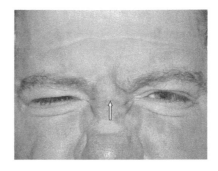

Figure 2.7 Horizontal frown lines of glabella created by the action of the procerus muscle.

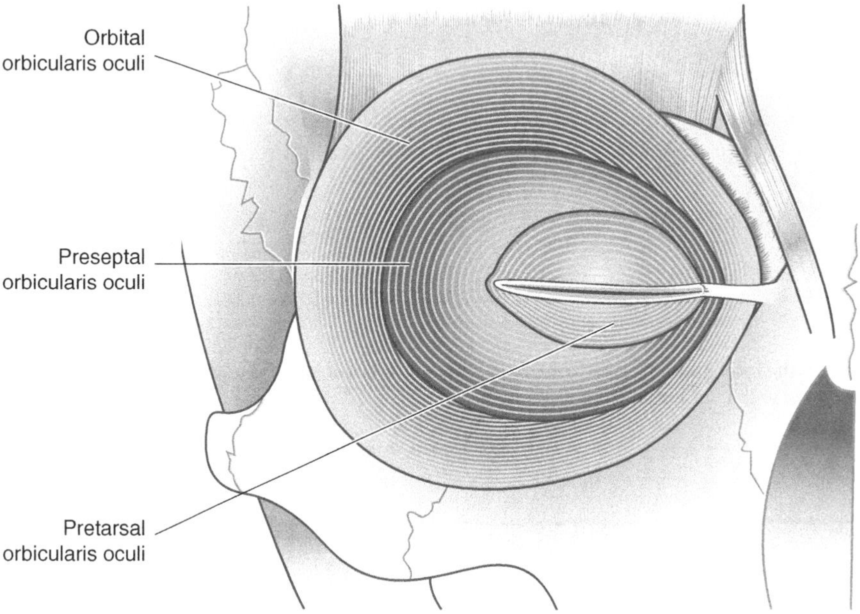

Figure 2.8 Divisions of the orbicularis oculi muscle into orbital and palpebral (preseptal and pretarsal) segments. Redrawn based on an original drawing by Margaret Ditré.

The orbicularis oculi muscle possesses not only critical functional aspects to the eye including eye closure, but also has significant aesthetic influence on the upper one-third of the face. The muscle is divided into orbital and palpebral portions (Figure 2.8). The palpebral portion is then divided into the preseptal and pretarsal segments–named for the muscle fibers that lie over the orbital septum and tarsal plate respectively. This portion is responsible for the gentle closure of the palpebral fissure of the eye. The orbital portion originates from three areas, which include the medial palpebral ligament, nasal portion of the frontal bone and frontal process of the maxilla. The orbital portion extends beyond the orbital rim to the cheeks, forehead and temples and interdigitates with surrounding muscles, including the frontalis and corrugator supercilli muscles. Care should be taken when injecting the lower crow's-feet rhytids so as not to weaken the zygomatic group and cause ptosis to the oral commissure. It is important to recognize that the orbital portion of the orbicularis oculi is considered an accessory muscle to smiling, and is responsible for forceful closure of the palpebral fissure of the eye. The orbital portion of the orbicularis oculi muscle is also responsible for the creation of lateral canthal rhytids (crow's-feet), and depressing the medial and lateral aspects of the brow (Figure 2.9) as well as adducting it. Its influence on depressing the lateral brow owes to the fact that the orbital fibers extend more laterally than the most lateral aspect of the frontalis muscle, thus creating an unopposed downward force vector on the tail of the brow. Chemodenervation of the vertical fibers of the orbital portion of the orbicularis oculi results in a lateral brow lift, as well as improvement in the crow's feet.Persistent adduction of the glabella following neurotoxin injections may occur from recruitment of the orbital portion of the orbicularis oculi.

The palpebral segment of the orbicularis oculi is composed of preseptal and pretarsal components. The preseptal portion overlies the orbital septum and the pretarsal portion overlies the tarsal plate as mentioned earlier.

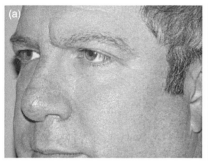 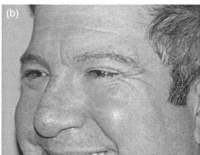

Figure 2.9 (a) Contraction of the orbital portion of the orbicularis oculi resulting in (b) creation of lateral canthal rhytids and depression of tail of brow.

The medial attachments of the preseptal and pretarsal portions onto the anterior and posterior lacrimal crests form a muscle sling surrounding the lacrimal sac – which allows for the pumping mechanism of tears into the canalicular system. Injection of botulinum toxin into the medial eyelid may interfere with this pumping mechanism. Diffusion of neurotoxin onto the medial orbicularis oculi muscle may weaken lid tone and cause punctal eversion and epiphora (tearing). Hypertrophy of the pretarsal orbicularis muscle may be responsible for creating a bulge underneath the ciliary margin of the lower eyelid commonly referred to as the "jellyroll" deformity, as well as a decreased palpebral fissure (Figure 2.10). Unilateral decrease of the palpebral fissure with a hypertonic pretarsal orbicularis oculi muscle is responsible for "Large eye/Small eye syndrome." Application of botulinum toxin to the pretarsal

orbicularis in the mid papillary line 3mm below the ciliary margin can improve this appearance along with improving rhytids of the lower eyelid, as well as providing a subtle widening of the palpebral fissure with smiling. Before injecting the pretarsal orbicularis, a snap test or lid distraction test should be performed to evaluate adequate lid tone. Also, closely examining preinjection photographs to rule out preexisting scleral show is important in patient selection. Patients with impending pseudo-herniation of the lower lid orbital fat should be treated with caution, since relaxation of the preseptal orbicularis oculi may exacerbate this herniation along with interference of the lymphatic drainage system of the lower eyelid. This may also worsen malar festoons which are defined as skin protrusion on the lateral aspect of the malar region caused by aging and inflammation. This injection should also be cautiously considered in patients with dry eye syndrome.

The dynamic antagonists of the orbicularis oculi (lid depressor) in the eyelids are the levator palpebral superioris and Mueller's muscle (lid elevators). The levator palpebral superioris is responsible for the active opening of the eye and has its origin on the lesser wing of the sphenoid. In the region of the superior orbital rim, a ligamentous structure known as Whitnall's ligament acts to convert the anterior posterior vector force to a superior inferior direction, thus providing the appropriate mechanics for opening the eye [21]. The

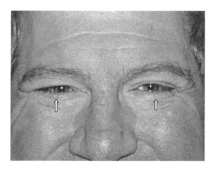

Figure 2.10 Contraction of pretarsal orbicularis oculi creating subtle roll of skin under lower eyelid lashes.

levator palpebral superioris muscle converts into a fibrous aponeurosis before inserting onto the superior border of the upper tarsal plate. Titration of botulinum toxin onto the levator muscle may result in lid ptosis. The orbital septum is a delicate fascial layer that connects the arcus marginalis with the inferior border of the tarsal plate. It acts as a mechanical barrier to the spread of neurotoxin to the levator palpebrae superioris. Patients who have had previous blepharoplasty may have had this septum encroached to remove eyelid fat, and therefore may be theoretically more predisposed to spread of toxin due to comprise of this anatomic barrier. Mueller's muscle runs underneath the levator aponeurosis and has sympathetic innervation. It is also an upper lid elevator that can be stimulated pharmacologically to improve lid ptosis. It provides 2mm of elevation to the upper eyelid and is responsible for the correction of mild ptosis associated with neurotoxin when pharmacologically stimulated with a sympathetic agent (prescription iopidine or even naphazoline hydrochloride).

The anatomic and mechanical relationship of the frontalis, corrugator supercilli, and procerus and orbicularis oculi create a unique antagonistic/protagonistic relationship which determines brow position and shape (Figure 2.11). Thoughtful and careful placement of neurotoxin can result in brow elevation and brow reshaping by selectively altering this relationship.

The Midface

The primary muscle associated with the nose is the nasalis muscle (Table 2.2). This muscle contains both an upper transverse portion (which compresses the cartilage framework of the nose including the upper lateral cartilages and the lower lateral crura), and an alar portion, the dilator naris (which dilates the nares). Both are innervated by the buccal branch of the facial nerve. The transverse portion originates on the maxilla and inserts with the opposite muscle via an aponeurosis in the midline of the dorsum of the nose. The dilator portion originates in the region of the lateral incisor of the maxilla and inserts onto the lower lateral crura. The dilator portion, along with the medial part of the levator labii superioris alaeque nasi muscle, widens or dilates the nostril and can be injected for those with excessive nasal flare (Figure 2.12). The transverse portion is responsible for the oblique expression wrinkles found over the bony dorsum of the nose. It produces the so called "bunny lines," which are exaggerated with scrunching up of the nose (Figure 2.13). Neurotoxins can help soften these lines and may help to improve the recruitment phenomenon of the nasalis – which is sometimes

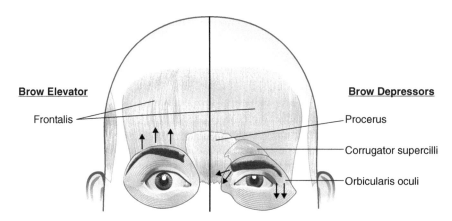

Figure 2.11 Antagonist and protagonist relationship of musculature of upper one-third of face. Redrawn based on an original drawing by Margaret Ditré.

Table 2.2 Additional facial musculature important in neurotoxin injection.

Muscle	Origin	Insertion	Action	Cosmetic consequence
Other				
Nasalis				
– transverse portion	Maxilla	Midline of dorsum of nose	Lifts nares	"Bunny lines"-oblique expression wrinkles over bony dorsum of nose
– dilator portion	Lateral incisor of maxilla	Lower lateral crura	Dilates nares	Flaring of nostrils
Orbicularis oris	Maxilla and mandible	Skin and mucosa of lips	Puckers lips; brings lips together	Vertical lip rhytids
Masseter	Zygomatic arch	Lateral surface of the ramus and angle of the mandible	Mastication	Hypertrophy can result in masculinizing of lower face
Depressor nasi septi	Type 1: orbicularis oris Type II: periosteum of the premaxilla below nasal spine Type III: no discernable muscle	Medial crural footplates of the lower lateral cartilages	Aesthetics of nasal tip and upper lip with smiling	Decreased nasal tip projection, shortening of upper lip, Animation ptosis
Temporalis	Temporal fossa	Coronoid process and ramus of mandible	Primary muscle of mastication	Hypertrophy can result in an unpleasing bulge with mastication in lateral forehead region

seen when the corrugator and procerus muscles are injected for glabellar frown lines.

The depressor nasi septi (DNS) muscle is a delicate paired muscle that can have profound effects on the aesthetics of the nasal tip and upper lip with smiling (Figure 2.14).

Drooping of the nasal tip with smiling (animation ptosis), decreased tip projection and shortening of the upper lip are the primary effects of this muscle on the nasal tip (Table 2.2). Rohrich has described three variations of this muscle [22]. Type I originates

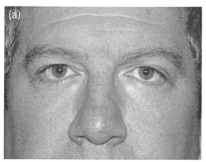
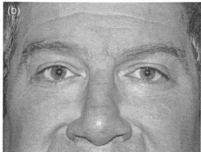

Figure 2.12 Dilation of the nares caused by stimulation of dilator naris and the dilator portion of the levator labii superioris alaeque nasi.

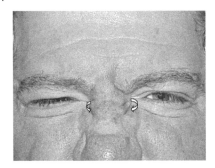

Figure 2.13 Contraction of transverse portion of nasalis muscle creating "bunny lines".

and interdigitates with the orbicularis oris. Type II originates on the periosteum of the premaxilla below the nasal spine and has no discernable relationship with the orbicularis oris. Type III involves little if any discernable muscle. The insertion of the DNS is on the medial crural footplates of the lower lateral cartilages. Injection of the depressor septi muscle can at best result in a subtle upward nasal tip rotation in repose. This is usually performed in the midline of the vertex of the nasolabial angle in the region of the anterior nasal spine. With animation and smiling there is less downward rotation of the nasal tip with loss of tip projection when the DNS is injected. In addition, there is less shortening of the upper lip with smiling.

The primary muscle group in the midface is the elevators of the upper lip (Table 2.3).

Their insertions into the orbicularis oris partially contribute to the formation of the nasolabial fold. These muscles are primarily innervated by the buccal branches of the facial nerve. These muscles all insert into the orbicularis oris, and primarily provide an upward vector force to the upper lip and commissure (Figure 2.15) with the risorius drawing the commissure more posteriorly.

The zygomaticus major muscle arises on the zygoma and courses inferiorly and medially to insert onto the skin and mucosa of the oral commissure in the region of the modiolus (a muscular condensation comprised of multiple muscular insertions) as well as the orbicularis oris muscle sphincter. It is a superficial muscle that can be seen frequently on raising of the skin flap during facelift. It, along with the zygomaticus minor, lifts the oral commissure superiorly and laterally. The zygomaticus minor originates medial to the zygomaticus major on the zygoma, and runs anterior and medial to its larger counterpart and inserts onto the skin, mucosa and orbicularis oris muscle just medial to the zygomaticus major.

The levator labii superiorus originates on the superior aspect of the maxilla just below the margin of the infraorbital rim and above the infraorbital foramen. It courses medially and inferiorly to insert on the lateral aspect of the orbicularis oris, skin and mucosa of the lateral upper lip. As the name

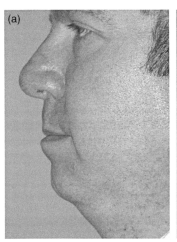
(a)

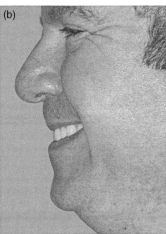
(b)

Figure 2.14 Contraction of depressor septi muscle with resultant derotation (animation ptosis) of nasal tip, decreased tip projection and shortening of the upper lip.

Table 2.3 Elevators and depressors of the lip.

Muscle	Origin	Insertion	Action	Cosmetic Consequence
Lip Elevators				
Levator labii superiorus	Superior aspect of maxilla below infraorbital rim margin and above infraorbital foramen	Lateral aspect of orbicularis oris, skin and mucosa of lateral upper lip	Primary elevator of lip	Contributes to the smile and nasolabial fold formation
Levator anguli oris	Canine fossa	Corner of mouth	Elevates angle of mouth	Contributes to the smile and nasolabial fold formation
Levator labii superioris alaeque nasi	Medial aspect of maxilla	Skin, mucosa and orbicularis oris of medial upper lip	Primary elevator of central upper lip	Contributes to the smile and nasolabial fold formation
Zygomaticus major	Lateral zygoma	Corner of mouth (modiolus)	Elevates oral commisure superiorly and laterally	Contributes to the smile and nasolabial fold formation
Zygomaticus minor	Medial zygoma	Corner of mouth (modiolus) just medial to zygomaticus major	Elevates oral commisure superiorly and laterally	Contributes to the smile and nasolabial fold formation
Lip Depressors				
Depressor anguli oris	Body of mandible between canine and first molar	Skin, mucosa and orbicularis oris at oral commissure (modiolus)	Primary depressor of oral commissure	Marionette folds, parentheses rhytids, prejowl sulcus
Depressor labii inferioris	Anterior aspect of oblique line of mandible	Skin, orbicularis oris and mucosa of lower lip	Depressor of tubercle of lower lip	Lower incisior show
Mentalis	Mandible near lateral incisor	Skin of chin	Protrudes lower lip	Cobblestoning, peau d' orange
Platysma	Deltoid and pectoral fascia	Mandible and depressors of lower lip	Depressor of lip and corners of mouth	Vertical bands, transverse rhytids of neck (necklace lines)

implies, the levator labii superioris is the primary elevator of the upper lip.

The levator anguli oris originates in the region of the canine fossa. It runs deep to the other levators in the area, including the zygomaticus group and levator labii superiorus. It inserts on the corner of the mouth in the region of the modiolus and primarily elevates this structure. The levator labii superioris alaeque nasi muscle is a major elevator of the central upper lip. It originates on the medial aspect of the maxilla just below the infraorbital rim and medial to the origin of levator labii superiorus. It runs

Lip Elevators

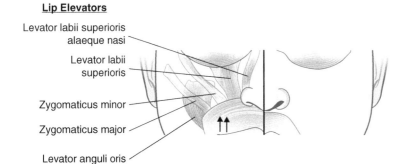

Levator labii superioris alaeque nasi

Levator labii superioris

Zygomaticus minor

Zygomaticus major

Levator anguli oris

Figure 2.15 Elevators of the upper lip. Redrawn based on an original drawing by Margaret Ditré.

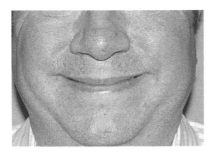

Figure 2.16 Mona Lisa smile secondary to majority of activity of zygomaticus major resulting in elevation of corners of mouth.

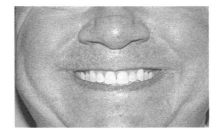

Figure 2.17 Canine smile caused by significant activity of levator labii superioris and levator labii superioris alaeque nasi.

inferiorly along the pyriform aperture. The insertion is into the skin, mucosa and orbicularis oris muscle of the medial upper lip.

In 1974, Rubin characterized the nature of smiles into three types [23]. The first type involves a majority of activity from the zygomaticus major muscle resulting in noticeable elevation of the corners of the mouth and is known as the "Mona Lisa smile" (Figure 2.16). The second smile involves a significant component of the levator labii superioris and levator labii superioris alaeque nasi resulting in elevation of the central upper lip. This is known as the "canine smile" (Figure 2.17). The third type involves the contraction of both the lip elevators and depressors resulting in display of the upper and lower dentition. This smile is referred to as the "full denture smile" (Figure 2.18).

Kane found the canine smile group, especially the gummy smile subset he calls the "extreme canine smile," were the patients who benefited the most from neurotoxin

injection, since relaxation of the levator labii superioris alaeque nasi resulted in significant improvement of the gummy display [24]. It also helped improve the heaviness or sharpness of the medial nasolabial fold. The injection technique involved one injection at the superior aspect of the nasolabial fold in the region of the pyriform aperture. Polo found significant improvement in the gummy smile with injection of the levator labii superioris,

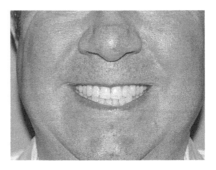

Figure 2.18 Full denture smile resulting from contraction of both lip elevators and depressors.

levator labii superioris alequae nasi, the overlap areas of the levator labii superioris and zygomaticus minor muscles, as well as injection of the depressor septi nasi at the origin of the orbicularis oris muscle [25]. All these injections were performed with low doses (1.25 units of onabotulinum toxin A, Botox).

The risorius plays no significant role in the aesthetic application of neurotoxins. Unlike the bony origin of other muscles in this region, it arises from the layer of tissue above the parotid gland and inserts onto the corner of the mouth and draws the corner of the mouth laterally. The buccinator also plays no significant role in the formation of hyperfunctional rhytids but does play a significant role in mastication. Proper mastication is achieved by the transfer of a bolus of food over the molars, and this is aided by the action of the buccinator muscle. The buccinator muscle is also important in those patients who play wind instruments, since it is responsible for the mouth orientation necessary to generate the force needed to play such instruments. It originates from the posterior aspect of the superior alveolar process and pterygomandibular raphe and passes anteriorly to insert onto the upper and lower portions of the orbicularis oris muscle, skin, and mucosa of the lateral aspects of the mouth.

The masseter muscle is not a muscle of facial expression, but of mastication itself (Table 2). It is derived from the first branchial arch mesoderm as are all the muscles of mastication and is innervated by the trigeminal nerve. However, hypertrophy of this muscle can have a profound effect on the shape of the lower face, particularly masculinizing the lower face in women by making the jawline more "square." The Asian face, particularly Korean, has a greater propensity for this appearance. This condition can also be associated with temporomandibular joint (TMJ) disease and bruxism (grinding of teeth at night). The muscle originates on the zygomatic arch and angles posteriorly to insert onto the lateral surface of the ramus and angle of the mandible. This muscle has two parts – which include a larger superficial belly and

a smaller deeper belly. The muscle is innervated by the third division of the trigeminal nerve and acts primarily to close the jaw and also aids in adducting the jaw to the contralateral side. Both actions are critical to mastication.

The lower lip depressors play an integral role in the function and aesthetics of the lower one-third of the face (Table 3). Despite the fact that fillers and volumization are primarily the means of treatment in this area, neurotoxins play a meaningful role in the rejuvenation of the lower face. The key to successful injection of neurotoxins into the lower face is dependent upon a keen understanding of the facial musculature in this region. There is an intimacy and precision of action of these muscles that is not seen in the upper one-third of the face. This explains why accurate injections of low doses of neurotoxins are of paramount importance in the lower face.

The depressor anguli oris is the primary depressor of the oral commissure and contributes to the dynamic component of the marionette fold (Figure 2.19). This muscle along with the depressor labii inferioris contributes to the antagonistic action on the oral commissure by depressing it (Figure 2.20). The zygomaticus major, zygomatic minor and levator anguli oris are the primary protagonists of the oral commissure. When the antagonistic force vector is negated with neurotoxins, the marionette fold improves in

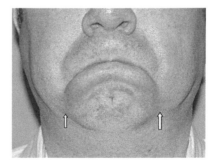

Figure 2.19 Down turning of oral commissures with formation of marionette folds by contraction of depressor anguli oris. Notice also the formation of the prejowl sulcus.

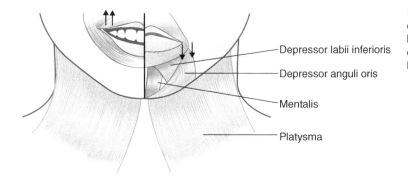

Figure 2.20 Depressors of the lower lip. Redrawn based on an original drawing by Margaret Ditré.

Depressor labii inferioris

Depressor anguli oris

Mentalis

Platysma

appearance and there is a conservative upturn to the corner of the mouth due to a net positive protagonistic effect of the elevators of the commissure. This is enhanced with the addition of fillers into the marionette fold. This is the second example of where antagonist/ protagonist actions are critical to determining the shape and position of aesthetic structures of the face with the first example being the brows.

The depressor anguli oris is a triangular shaped muscle with its base originating from the body of the mandible and between the canine and first molar. It runs superiorly and inserts onto the skin, mucosa and orbicularis oris muscle in the region of the modiolus at the oral commissure. It has intimacy with the platysma muscle laterally and depressor labii inferioris medially. This relationship is important when injecting the depressor anguli oris in that it is important to stay lateral and posterior when injecting this muscle to avoid diffusion of neurotoxin toward the more medial depressor labii inferioris. This diffusion into the region of the depressor labii inferioris can create an upward posture of the lower lip on smiling. This appearance is similar to that seen when there is a marginal paresis – a potential complication of a face-lift procedure. The depressor anguli oris contributes to the formation of the marionette fold, parentheses rhytids found midway between the oral commissure and the margin of the mandible, and the formation of the prejowl sulcus. It is easy to understand why neurotoxin treatments of this

muscle along with fillers in this region can play a significant role in perioral rejuvenation.

The depressor labii inferioris is the second major depressor of the lower lip. Its action is more medial depressing the tubercle of the lower lip resulting in lower incisor show (Figure 2.21). It originates on the anterior aspect in the region of the oblique line of the mandible and runs deep to medial fibers of the depressor anguli oris. It inserts onto the skin, the orbicularis oris, and mucosa of the lower lip in the region of the tubercle. Medial fibers may insert onto the corresponding depressor labii inferioris muscle on the contralateral side. As mentioned, this muscle may be therapeutically injected with neurotoxin if the opposite depressor labii inferioris has been weakened by a malpositioned injection of the depressor anguli oris on the ipsilateral side. This can help to create symmetry with smiling. Also, in patients who

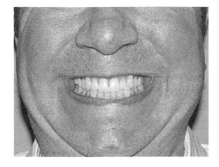

Figure 2.21 Contraction of depressor labii inferioris resulting in depression of lower lip tubercle with mandibular dental show.

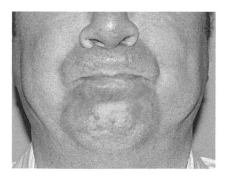

Figure 2.22 Contraction of mentalis muscle with cobblestoning appearance to skin of chin and protrusion of lower lip.

experience marginal paresis after face lifting, a temporary injection of neurotoxin into the contralateral depressor labii inferioris and depressor anguli oris can produce symmetry with smiling until the paresis hopefully resolves.

The mentalis muscle is responsible for protruding the lower lip by elevating the skin of the chin upward. It originates on the mandible in the region of the lateral incisor. It runs inferiorly and medially deep to the depressor labii inferioris and inserts onto the skin of the chin. It is responsible for "cobblestoning" or "peau d'orange" appearance of the chin seen when this muscle contracts (Figure 2.22). Injection of neurotoxin can ameliorate this appearance by relaxing the mentalis.

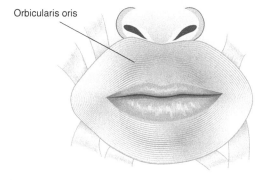

Orbicularis oris

Figure 2.23 Sphincteric fibers of the orbicularis oris. Redrawn based on an original drawing by Margaret Ditré.

These depressors of the lower lip are all innervated by the marginal branch of the facial nerve.

The orbicularis oris muscle, due to the circular nature of its fibers, is a sphincteric muscle which creates a puckering or protruding effect of the lips (Figure 2.23). It also brings the lips together and approximates the corners of the mouth with contraction (Table 2.2). Although the majority of the muscle originates and inserts upon itself because it is circular in nature, deeper fibers originate from the maxilla and mandible to insert onto the deeper aspects of the sphincter. Therefore, the sphincter has both superficial and deep functional units. The levators and depressors of the lips also contribute muscle slips to this sphincter. The buccal and marginal nerves are responsible for its innervation.

The complex and diverse movements of the lips are primarily the result of the complicated interplay between the elevators and depressors of the lips – which insert into the orbicularis oris as well as the skin and mucosa of the lips. These muscles provide a radial vector to the oral sphincter whereas the orbicularis oris provides the circumferential vector. It is the fine interplay of these radial and circumferential forces that create a precision in the perioral area that is really unmatched in the human body. This is what allows for fine movements seen with articulation and mastication. The skin of the lips is closely adherent to the orbicularis oris, and therefore the pursing action of this muscle can readily transmit its force to the skin over the muscle. This leads to the creation of vertical rhytids in the region of the lip (Figure 2.24). Injection of neurotoxin into the superficial aspect of the sphincteric fibers of the orbicularis oris relaxes and softens these rhytids. This effect can be complemented with the use of fillers. The deeper fibers of the orbicularis oris are primarily responsible for maintaining oral competence. It is for this reason that injections for the fine perioral rhytids must be kept superficial to prevent deep diffusion into these muscles, which

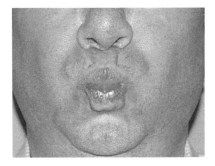

Figure 2.24 Perioral rhytids caused by contraction of the orbicularis oris.

results in incompetence of the oral sphincter, i.e. drooling.

The Platysma

The primary superficial muscle of the neck is the platysma muscle. It originates on the deltoid and pectoral fascia to insert onto the mandible and the depressors of the lower lip. Three separate parts have been described, the pars modiolaris (most lateral and superior inserting into modolaris), the

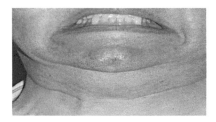

Figure 2.26 Contraction of the platysma with depression of the lower lip and corners of mouth.

pars labialis (inserting into lower lip), and the pars mandibularis (most medial and inferior inserting into chin) (Figure 2.25).

A recent study examining the platysma muscle during deep plane rhytidectomies shows a significant superior extent of the platysma muscle into the midface [26]. It is innervated by the cervical branch of the seventh cranial nerve and is contiguous with the superficial musculoaponeurotic system (SMAS) of the face. It has varying degrees of decussation in relation to the hyoid bone. Its primary action is a depressor of the lower lip and corners of the mouth (Figure 2.26). As this muscle ages, a natural dehiscence may occur centrally. This in combination with the

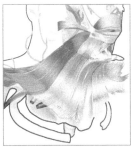

Platysma

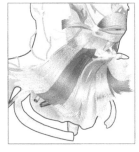

Pars modiolaris
Pars labialis
Pars mandibularis

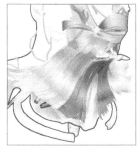

Figure 2.25 Platysma: Pars modiolaris, labialis, and mandibularis.

hypercontraction of the medial borders of the platysma muscle can create vertical cords or bands. Contractile bands may also be present laterally just below the level of the jowl. Injection of neurotoxin into both sets of bands as well as along the margin of the mandible can improve the appearance of the aging neck and jaw line. This effect occurs due to a subtle upward repositioning of the soft tissues of the jaw line secondary to relaxation of the lower extent of the platysma and persistent contraction of the superior extent. This is the premise behind the "Nefertiti lift" [27] to aesthetically improve the appearance of the jawline. Along with the vertical bands, transverse rhytids of the neck (necklace lines) are also caused by a contraction of the platysma muscle. These lines may be conservatively improved with injection of neurotoxin into the muscle in addition to the use of a low-viscosity filler.

The Craniofacial Skeleton

The craniofacial skeleton and the changes that occur as it ages are critical to understanding the art and science of chemodenervation of the muscles of the face since the majority of these muscles take origin here. The primary bones of the facial skeleton include the frontal bone, nasal bones, zygoma, maxilla and mandible. The frontal bone is composed of the vertical aspect of the squama. This is responsible for the shape and extent of the forehead. The caudal portions include the supraorbital rim – with its extensions medially articulating with the paired nasal bones and the extensions laterally articulating with the frontal process of the zygoma. The zygoma forms the major portion of the lateral orbital rim and a portion of the lateral inferior orbital rim where it articulates with the maxilla. The zygoma extends posteriorly as the temple process and articulates with the zygomatic process of the temporal bone. The apex of the zygoma forms the maler eminence (height of the cheek bone). This union of the two processes forms the zygomatic arch – which is where the masseter muscle originates. Running underneath

the arch is the temporalis muscle, a primary muscle of mastication that is innervated by the third division of the trigeminal nerve (Table 2). It originates in the temporal fossa and inserts onto the coronoid process and ramus of the mandible. It, too, can exhibit hypertrophy, particularly in patients with bruxism, and can contribute not only to TMJ symptoms but also create an aesthetically unpleasing bulge with mastication in the lateral forehead region. The maxilla is the primary skeleton of the midface. It is the origin of the majority of the levators of the upper lip. It forms the majority of the inferior and medial orbital rims and articulates with the zygoma and frontal bones respectively. The nasal process of the maxilla articulates with the nasal bones medially and the lacrimal bone laterally. It also forms the lateral and inferior aspects of the pyriform aperture with the superior aspect of the aperture being formed by the inferior borders of the nasal bones. The maxilla houses the superior alveolar ridge, which contains the maxillary dentition. The mandible is the only true mobile bone of the facial skeleton and is critical to the aesthetics of the lower one-third of the face. It is also the origin of the muscles which primarily depress the lip complex. It articulates with the maxilla through the mandibular dentition anteriorly. The relationship of the maxillary dentition to the mandibular dentition defines the concept of occlusion. Angle's classification describes three primary occlusal relationships. Class I is a normal or orthognathic occlusion, with Class II being retrognathic and Class III being prognathic. This occlusal alignment is critical to the aesthetics of the lower one-third of the face. Retrognathic patients have a weak/recessed chin and this relationship not only has a profound effect on the profilimetry of the face but also on the aesthetic relationship of the upper and lower lips, with the upper lip projecting more anteriorly than is seen in the normal occlusion. The prognathic patient has a retrusive maxilla in relation to the mandible and results in over projection of the lower lip on profile. The mandible articulates with the temporal bone posteriorly in the mandibular fossa via the mandibular condyle thus forming the temporomandibular joint.

The changes seen in the aging facial skeleton are profoundly affected by the condition of the mandibular and maxillary dentition. Loss of dentition in either region results in decrease of bony volume as a result of demineralization due to an increase in the osteoclastic activity of the bone, resulting from reduction in transmitted forces to the maxilla and mandible. This is also known as contraction of the facial skeleton. Another significant change in the aging craniofacial skeleton which profoundly affects the appearance of the soft tissues, is the clockwise rotation of the midfacial skeleton in relation to the cranial base as proposed by Lambros and confirmed by Pessa [28]. They showed that there was a continual growth and remodeling of the aging craniofacial skeleton with a resultant clockwise rotation. This was confirmed by measuring the key angles of the face (glabellar, orbital, pyriform, and maxillary) and showing that these angles became more acute with age. These bony changes help define the nature of the ptotic soft tissue changes occurring in the midface and perioral area secondary to loss of structural support of the midface.

Shaw and Kahn confirmed the decrease in maxillary and glabella angles as seen by Pessa [29]. However, they also showed an increase in the surface area of the pyriform aperture with aging, thus signifying that aging has a deteriorating and contracting effect on the maxilla as opposed to a growth and remodeling effect.

Pessa and Chen showed that the nature of the aging orbital aperture is such that curve distortion occurs in the inferior lateral and superior medial regions due to bony remodeling of the orbit with aging [30]. This skeletal change of the orbit is reflected to the eyelids resulting in scleral show and the tear trough deformity seen in the aging eye.

All of the above craniofacial skeleton changes have a profound secondary effect on the overlying soft tissues. Several examples include: soft tissue repositioning which is seen with descent of the cheek fat pad; increased facial muscle tone resulting in greater incidence of hyperfunctional rhytids and aging facial reshaping; and laxity of the key ligaments of the face. This increased facial muscle tone may explain why typically acceptable neurotoxin dosages have less of an effect on older patients in their seventh and eighth decades.

Acknowledgements

The authors would like to thank Joanne Scarpulla and Kristen Whitney D.O., for their tireless effort in the preparation of this chapter. Also, many thanks to Maggie Ditré (Class of 2014, Yale University) for her illustrations for this chapter.

References

1 Kligman AM, Zheng P, Lavker RM. The anatomy and pathogenesis of wrinkles. Br J Dermatol 1985 Jul;113(1):37–42.

2 Bosset S, Barre P, Chalon A, *et al.* Skin ageing: clinical and histopathological study of permanent and reducible wrinkles. Eur J Dermatol 2002 May–Jun;12(3):247–252.

3 Pierard GE, Lapiere CM. The microanatomical basis of facial frown lines. Arch Dermatol 1989 Aug;125(8):1090–1092.

4 Contet-Audonneau JL, Jeanmaire C, Pauly G. A histological study of human wrinkle structures: comparison between sun-exposed areas of the face, with or without wrinkles, and sun-protected areas. Br J Dermatol 1999 Jun;140(6):1038–1047.

5 Fenske NA, Lober CW. Structural and functional changes of normal aging skin. J Am Acad Dermatol 1986 Oct;15(4 Pt 1): 571–585.

6 Cheng CM. Cosmetic use of botulinum toxin type A in the elderly. Clin Interv Aging. 2007;2(1):81–83.

7 Yaar M, Gilchrest BA. Aging of skin In Wolff K, Goldsmith LA, Katz SI, *et al.* eds, *Dermatology in General Medicine*, 7th edn. http://www.accessmedicine.com/content.aspx?aID=2963698.

8 Kurban RS, Bhawan J. Histologic changes in skin associated with aging. J Dermatol Surg Oncol 1990 Oct;16(10):908–914.

9 Bhawan J, Andersen W, Lee J, *et al.* Photoaging versus intrinsic aging: a morphologic assessment of facial skin. J Cutan Pathol. 1995 Apr;22(2):154–159.

10 Carruthers A, Carruthers J. *Botulinum toxin: Procedures in Cosmetic Dermatology*. 2nd edn. Philadelphia, Saunders Elsevier, 2008.

11 Benedetto AV. *Botulinum Toxin in Clinical Dermatology*. London, New York: Taylor and Francis; 2006.

12 Rabe JH, Mamelak AJ, McElqunn PJ. Photoaging: mechanisms and repair. J Am Acad Dermatol 2006 Jul;55(1):1–19.

13 Dessy LA, Mazzocchi M, Rubino C, *et al.* An objective assessment of botulinum toxin A effect of superficial skin texture. Ann Plast Surg 2007 May;58(5):469–473.

14 Rohrich RJ, Pessa JE. The fat compartments of the face: anatomy and clinical implications for cosmetic surgery. Plast Reconstr Surg 2007 Jun;119(7):2219–2227.

15 Rohrich RJ, Pessa JE. The retaining system of the face: histologic evaluation of the septal boundaries of the subcutaneous fat compartments. Plast Reconstr Surg 2008 May;121(5):1804–1809.

16 Larrabee WF, Makielski KH. *Anatomic Systems.Surgical Anatomy of the Face.* New York: Raven Press; 1993:21–102.

17 Glaich AS, Cohen JL, Goldberg LH. Injection necrosis of the glabella: protocol for prevention and treatment after use of dermal fillers. Dermatol Surg 2006 Feb;32(2):276–281.

18 Hollinshead WH. *The Face.Anatomy for Surgeons: The Head and Neck*: Volume 1. 3rd edn. Philadelphia: Harper & Row; 1982:291–323.

19 Guyuron B, Tucker T, Davis J. Surgical treatment of migraine headaches. Plast Reconstr Surg 2002 Jun;109(7):2183–2189.

20 Macdonald MR, Spiegel JH, Raven RB, *et al.* An anatomical approach to glabellar rhytids. Arch Otolaryngol Head Neck Surg 1998 Dec;124(12):1315–1320.

21 McCord CD, Codman M. *Classical Surgical Eyelid Anatomy. Eyelid and Periorbital Surgery*. St. Louis, Missouri: Quality Medical Publishing, Inc.; 2008: 3–46.

22 Rohrich RJ, Adams WP, Huynh BH, Muzafter AR. Importance of the depressor nasi septi muscle: an anatomic study and clinical application. In *Dallas Rhinoplasty Nasal Surgery by the Masters*. St. Louis, Missouri: Quality Medical Publishing, Inc; 2007:1071–1080.

23 Rubin LR. The anatomy of a smile: its importance in the treatment of facial paralysis. Plast Reconstr Surg 1974 Apr; 53(4):384–387.

24 Kane M. The effect of botulinum toxin injections on the nasolabial folds. Plast Reconstr Surg 2003 Oct;112(5 Suppl.):66–74.

25 Polo M. Botulinum toxin type A in the treatment of excessive gingival display. Am J Orthod Dentofacial Orthop 2005 Feb; 127(2):214–218.

26 Shah AR, Rosenberg D. Defining the facial extent of the platysma muscle. A review of 71 consecutive face-lifts. Arch Facial Plast Surg 2009 Nov–Dec;11(6):405–408.

27 Levy PM. The "Nefertiti lift": A new technique for specific re-contouring of the jawline. J Cosmet Laser Ther 2007 Dec; 9(4):249–252.

28 Pessa JE. An algorithm of facial aging: verification of lambros's theory by

three-dimensional stereolithography, with reference to the pathogenesis of midfacial aging, scleral show, and the lateral suborbital trough deformity. Plast Reconstr Surg 2000 Aug;106(2):479–488.

29 Shaw RB, Kahn DM. Aging of the midface bony elements: a three-dimensional computed tomographic study. Plast Reconstr Surg 2007 Feb;119(2):675–681.

30 Pessa JE, Chen Y. Curve analysis of the aging orbital aperture. Plast Reconstr Surg 2002 Feb;109(2):751–755.

3

Botulinum Toxin: From Molecule to Medicine

Conor J. Gallagher, PhD[1] and Alan Ackerman, PhD[2]

[1] Executive Director Medical Affairs, Facial Aesthetics, Allergan plc, Irvine, USA
[2] Master Medical Scientific Liaison, Retired, Ackerman LLC, Greeley, USA

Introduction

Exocytosis of neurotransmitters forms the physiological basis for linking our sensory inputs and cognitive processes to muscle contraction. This mechanism underlies our ability to voluntarily move and interact with our environment, to express facial emotions and in neurally-initiated involuntary muscle or glandular activity The exocytotic processes that accomplish the conversion of sensory/environmental inputs to actions are highly conserved across multiple species and constitute the mechanism by which neurotransmitter-containing vesicles are induced to release their contents into the synaptic cleft, triggering muscle contraction [1]. The bacterium *Clostridium botulinum* produces a neurotoxin that specifically disrupts this vital process, specifically SNAP-25 (synaptosomal associated protein, 25 kDa) mediated exocytosis. In deciphering the mechanism by which botulinum toxin acts, scientists have unlocked a useful tool for the management of clinical disorders of muscle hyperactivity [2]. Many biological processes besides muscle contraction rely on neurotransmitter release and, through scientific experimentation, many additional clinical conditions amenable to botulinum toxin therapy have been reported [3–5].

This chapter will review the state of our knowledge on the mechanism of action of botulinum toxin that underlies its clinical use in therapeutic and aesthetic indications.

Botulinum Toxin

Clostridium botulinum is ubiquitous in soil where it typically lies dormant as a spore. Under optimal conditions, including low oxygen, the bacterial spores germinate and produce neurotoxin [6]. Seven immunologically distinct serotypes of botulinum toxin have been identified, categorized as A–G [7]. Each serotype has distinct pharmacological characteristics [8,9], and only products containing type A or type B botulinum toxin have ever been approved for human use.

In nature, botulinum toxins are produced by the bacteria as protein complexes, consisting of two elements: the core neurotoxin that contains the protease moiety responsible for the intracellular biological activity of the neurotoxin, and a number of nontoxin accessory proteins [10, 11]. The core neurotoxin molecule always has a molecular weight of approximately 150 kDa, and while there is only approximately 30–40% protein homology [12] between serotypes, a high degree of structural similarity has been observed based on crystal structures [13].

The number and identity of the accessory proteins can vary depending on the strain of bacteria, the serotype of neurotoxin, and the

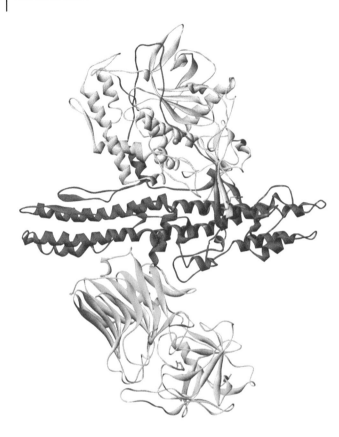

Figure 3.1 Molecular structure of the botulinum toxin type A 150 kDa core neurotoxin. The three functional domains are color coded: Yellow: light chain catalytic domain with a zinc atom shown in blue; Red: heavy chain translocation domain; Green: heavy chain binding domain. *Source:* Image courtesy of Lance E. Steward (Allergan plc.).

growth conditions. In general, three neuro-toxin "complex" (core neurotoxin plus accessory proteins) sizes have been identified with molecular weights of approximately 300, 500 and 900 kDa respectively [14]. Each complex consists of the 150 kDa neurotoxin with the balance of the molecular weight made up of the accessory proteins. In nature, the accessory proteins are known to have a protective role, helping to preserve the activity of the neurotoxin against exposure to proteolytic enzymes and extremes of pH and temperature [11, 15–19]. This is particularly important in the oral route of intoxication, as the neurotoxin is exposed to both changes in pH and proteolytic enzymes. It has been shown that when given orally the type A neurotoxin complex is 350 times more potent than the unprotected 150 kDa neurotoxin alone due to the protective actions of the accessory proteins [20] (Figure 3.1).

Mechanism of Action

In the therapeutic or aesthetic application of botulinum toxin products, minute doses (picograms to nanograms) are administered to induce a focal weakening of the injected muscle leading to a reduction of tone in a hypertonic muscle or to reduce neuronally evoked secretions at exocrine glands. The exquisitely specific action of botulinum toxin at the presynaptic nerve terminal is a function of the 150 kD protein we refer to as the core neurotoxin: a protein in which structure and function are intimately and elegantly linked [2].

The structure and modular organization of the core neurotoxin is generally conserved among the different serotypes; however, small differences in several regions lead to the different receptor and substrate specificities of each of these proteins [21, 22]. The core

Figure 3.2 The botulinum neurotoxin type A complex. Shown here is the deduced crystal structure of the botulinum toxin type A complex, consisting of the core neurotoxin of 150 kDa botulinum toxin type A (labeled BoNT/A, purple) in relation to its nontoxic associated neurotoxin proteins. The close association to the non-toxic non-hemeagglutinin protein (NTNH unit, pink) is evident. The other hemagglutinins assemble in a trefoil arrangement as illustrated. Each arm consists of one HA70 (two are visible in this illustration, colored green and blue), one HA 17 (yellow) and two HA33 subunits (orange). The molecular dimensions of the complex are shown in Angstroms – Å. *Source:* Lee 2013 [107]. Used under CC BY 4.0.

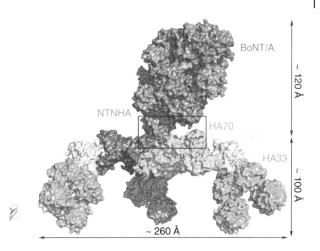

neurotoxin itself can be divided, both structurally and functionally, into three distinct regions: the binding domain, the translocation domain and the catalytic domain. The binding and translocation domains make up the heavy chain, while the light chain contains the catalytic domain (Figure 3.2).

The cellular action of botulinum toxin begins with the specific binding of the neurotoxin to a neuronal cell membrane. The binding domain of the core neurotoxin is located at the C-terminal end of the protein [23]. The presence of specific receptors on neurons that are recognized by this binding domain accounts for the selectivity of the neurotoxin for a neuronal membrane rather than the membrane of any other cell. The complexity of this interaction has only recently begun to be unraveled. The C-terminus of the core neurotoxin first binds to large sugar molecules known as gangliosides [24], which are ubiquitous on the surface of motor nerve terminals. While it was initially thought that gangliosides served as the sole receptor for type A botulinum toxin, it now appears that their primary function may be to retain the neurotoxin molecule close to the cell membrane to increase the probability of the molecule encountering its serotype specific protein receptor.

Identification of SV2 (Synaptic Vesicle 2) 23 as the protein receptor for botulinum toxin type A in 2006 [25] provided a key to unlock some of the earliest experimental findings on the physiology of botulinum toxins, such as the increase in rate and magnitude of muscle weakening with increasing frequency of phrenic nerve stimulation *in vitro* [26]. As its name suggests, SV2 is a protein located on neurotransmitter and neuropeptide containing vesicles within nerve terminals [27, 28]. It therefore follows that the fusion of vesicles and release of neurotransmitter is required to bring SV2 to the cell membrane and allow interaction with the neurotoxin molecule. The more neurotransmitter exocytosis that is actively occurring, the more SV2 will be present on the cell surface – thus, the most active motor neurons should be the most susceptible to the neurotoxin [29]. From an evolutionary perspective, this serves to preferentially target neurotoxin to the most active neurons. The binding region for SV2 is adjacent to the ganglioside binding region on the C-terminus of the heavy chain of the core neurotoxin [30]. In vitro, botulinum toxin type A also binds to fibroblast growth factor receptor-3 (FGFR3), although the *in vivo* significance of this finding is not yet known [31].

Following the binding step, the neurotoxin is internalized into the neuron in a recycling endosome, where the C-terminal portion of the heavy chain embeds in the endosomal

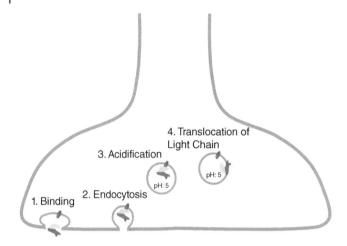

4. Translocation of
Light Chain

3. Acidification

pH: 5

pH: 5

1. Binding

2. Endocytosis

Figure 3.3 Multiple steps in the mechanism of action of botulinum toxin type A. This figure illustrates the steps in the mechanism of action of type A botulinum toxin. (1) Following binding to SV2 (pink), the 150 kDa core neurotoxin is internalized into the neuron via a process of endocytosis. (2) The endosome is acidified (3), which facilitates the translocation of the light chain into the neuronal cytosol (4). Once in the neuronal cytosol the light chain of type A botulinum toxin (yellow) cleaves the membrane-associated SNAP-25, one component of the SNARE complex. Another neurotoxin serotype, type B, botulinum toxin cleaves a different protein known as synaptobrevin or vesicle associated membrane protein (VAMP).

wall. The interior of the endosome is acidified, causing a conformational change in the neurotoxin protein molecule – which then allows the light chain to traverse the endosomal wall and enter the neuronal cytosol [32]. Once in the cytosol, the disulphide bond tethering the light chain and heavy chain together is reduced releasing the light chain [2] (Figure 3.3).

In the neuronal cytosol, the light chain, a zinc dependent endoprotease, is free to interact with its specific substrate [33]. Each serotype of botulinum toxin has a defined target protein and a highly specific molecular location for proteolytic cleavage. Each molecular target is a component of the cellular machinery responsible for the docking of synaptic vesicles and the calcium-dependent release of neurotransmitter. These exocytotic proteins are collectively referred to as the synaptic NSF attachment receptor (SNARE) complex [108]. The SNARE complex consists of two discrete components: those associated with the vesicle and those associated with the cell membrane. Interactions between the vesicle-bound and

membrane-associated SNARE proteins hold the two in apposition. Upon neuronal depolarization, the SNARE proteins sense the increase in intracellular calcium and respond by fusing the neurotransmitter vesicle with the membrane [34]. The membrane-bound SNARE protein SNAP-25 is the target for type A neurotoxin, cleaving it near its C-terminus [35]. SNAP-25 is also the target for types C and E, with type C toxin additionally cleaving Syntaxin. Types B, D and F neurotoxins target the vesicle associated protein Synaptobrevin [36]. The disruption of the specific target protein and subsequent effect on the SNARE complex prevents the fusion of synaptic vesicles with the neuronal membrane, significantly reducing the capability to release neurotransmitter (Figure 3.4).

Although there is general structural similarity between the core neurotoxin in different serotypes of botulinum toxins, significant differences between them occur primarily in the heavy chain C-terminal region, accounting for the differences in receptors for cellular recognition and binding [21, 22].

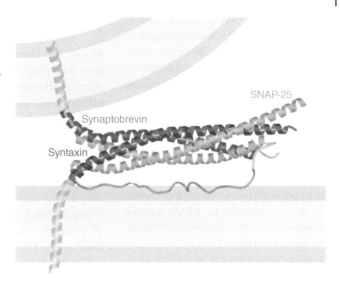

Figure 3.4 SNARE Complex. Crystal structure of a core synaptic fusion complex at 2.4 Å resolution. *Source:* Sutton 1998 [109]. Reproduced with permission of Nature Publishing Group.

The duration of botulinum neurotoxin effect is influenced by several factors, including serotype [37, 38] and somatic vs. autonomic site of action [3, 5, 39]. The long duration of effect following a single focal application of type A botulinum toxin is likely related to two factors. Firstly, the cleaved SNAP-25 likely escapes the normal degradation pathway for damaged proteins. The portion of the SNAP-25 molecule cleaved by the type A light chain is large enough to disrupt normal exocytosis, but small enough that the SNARE complex is preserved and the cell likely does not recognize that the protein has been damaged [40]. Secondly, the light chain of type A toxin appears to evade detection by cellular sentinels by 'hiding' close to the cell membrane [41]. These properties are in sharp contrast to the short-acting type E botulinum toxin. The type E light chain displays a lack of discrete localization in cells and distributed throughout the cytoplasm, making it more vulnerable to degradation [41] Furthermore, type E cleaves SNAP-25 at a more upstream (proximal) location than type A, taking a bigger 'bite' out of the molecule, destabilizing the SNARE complex [2] and allowing the E-cleaved SNAP-25 to be more readily targeted for degradation [38, 41–43].

The effects of botulinum toxin are reversible, and recovery from denervation is gradual. It has been demonstrated, in animal models, that denervation stimulates the muscle to produce growth factors, such as insulin-like growth factor-1 (IGF-1) [44], that trigger the sprouting of new branches from the silent motor neuron. These new branches make contact with the denervated muscle, establish new neuromuscular junctions and become active, contributing to the restoration of muscle function [45] while the originally affected neuron recovers [46]. Full recovery of neuromuscular transmission is not regained until the affected nerve terminals regain their activity. The actual persistence time of catalytically active light chain in motor neurons, *in vivo*, is currently unknown, although, in cell culture, cleaved SNAP-25 has been found 80 days postexposure to type A botulinum toxin [47].

Following clinical administration of botulinum toxin type A into striated muscle, the duration of focal muscle weakening is typically on the order of 12–16 weeks [48, 49], while muscle and glands under autonomic control generally remain inhibited for 26 weeks or longer [3, 5]. The clinical effectiveness of one botulinum toxin product (onabotulinumtoxinA) has been demonstrated to persist for at least 6 months following intra-detrusor application in patients with neurogenic detrusor overactivity [50] or when injected intradermally in individuals with severe primary axillary hyperhidrosis [5]. This may reflect different metabolic characteristics of autonomic cholinergic neurons allowing the active light chain to persist longer than in somatic motor neurons. Alternatively, it may reflect a lack of regenerative nerve sprouting in these tissues. The latter hypothesis has some support from studies of human bladder in which axonal sprouting was only rarely observed following botulinum toxin treatment [51].

Botulinum neurotoxins act to reduce exocytosis from somatic nerves at both of the locations where they innervate striated muscle. Alpha motor neurons directly contact the muscle fibers, triggering muscle contraction when activated, while A-gamma motor neurons innervate the muscle spindles. Muscle spindles are intrafusal muscle fibers responsible for setting the degree of tone and stretch sensitivity of skeletal muscle [52]. As A-gamma neurons also release acetylcholine at their peripheral terminals, botulinum toxin will reduce neurotransmission at this synapse, modulating the output of the spindle afferents and thus the level of muscle tone [53–55], perhaps augmenting the induced relaxation of the injected muscle [56]. At least some muscles of facial expression are reported to lack muscle spindles [57]; therefore, the contribution of this effect in the aesthetic applications of botulinum toxin in the face is unclear.

Beyond the neuromuscular junction, botulinum toxins are effective in treating neuroglandular overactivity. Several conditions such as hyperhidrosis of the axillae [5] and palms [59] and sialorrhea [59] have been demonstrated to be responsive to botulinum toxin following intradermal injection in the case of hyperhidrosis or directly into the salivary glands in the case of sialorrhea. This suggests that the exocytosis of acetylcholine at these post-ganglionic autonomic neurons can also be inhibited by botulinum toxin treatment.

Sensory Mechanism of Action

A role for botulinum toxin in pain reduction was proposed following early trials in cervical dystonia [60–63], and efficacy has subsequently been investigated in a number of other painful conditions such as chronic migraine [64], neuropathic pain [65], myofascial pain [66] and lateral epicondylitis [67]. Although several botulinum toxin products have been reported to reduce the pain associated with cervical dystonia, only onabotulinumtoxinA is approved for the treatment of pain associated with chronic migraine [66].

Recent years have brought a significant increase in the understanding of the mechanisms by which botulinum toxin reduces the perception of pain. Results of a number of clinical and preclinical studies have demonstrated that the highly selective disruption of exocytosis by botulinum toxin also occurs in the sensory system [69–74]. Botulinum toxin type A was shown to block the stimulated release of neuropeptide calcitonin gene-related peptide (CGRP) from cultured trigeminal ganglion neurons (TGNs) and substance P from both rat dorsal root ganglion neurons and TGNs [69, 71]. These proinflammatory neuropeptides are released from the peripheral terminals of nociceptive neurons using the SNARE proteins in response to stimulation, and are known to also trigger the release of other inflammatory mediators such as bradykinin, glutamate, prostaglandins and histamine [75]. Peripherally administered botulinum toxin type A significantly attenuated the release of glutamate in rat hindpaw in a dose-dependent manner following formalin administration [70,76,77].

In addition, several human models have demonstrated that pretreatment with botulinum toxin type A can reduce the flare, wheal, and cutaneous allodynia associated with the topical application of capsaicin or ultraviolet light [78].

More recently, it has been shown that transport of the transient receptor potential vanilloid type 1 (TRPV1) channel, to the cell membrane is significantly reduced by botulinum toxin type A [79, 80].

TRPV1 is an ion channel activated by several classes of painful stimuli and its expression is known to be upregulated in chronic pain and inflammation. Thus, the local effects of botulinum toxin on the peripheral components of the nociceptive system may reduce peripheral sensitization and consequently reduce central sensitization through the reduction in the release of algogenic chemical mediators or by altering the sensitivity of nociceptive neurons [81]. It is important to note that neither the large, myelinated (A-beta) nerve fibers that mediate light touch, vibration and proprioceptive sensation, nor the lightly myelinated nociceptive fibers (A-delta) that mediate acute pain appear to be affected by botulinum toxin type A and therefore botulinum toxin does not alter proprioception or induce cutaneous anesthesia or interfere with the normal perception of acute pain [82].

Retrograde Axonal Transport

The profound and long lasting effects of botulinum toxin on muscle tone in dystonia and spasticity, and the demonstration that treating cervical dystonia with botulinum toxin can result in a reorganization of cortical sensory-motor integration [83, 84], has led some to postulate that there may be a direct central effect of botulinum toxin within the central nervous system (CNS) [85]. Precedent for this phenomenon exists by analogy, as tetanus neurotoxin (also a clostridial neurotoxin that targets SNARE proteins) is retrogradely transported in motor neurons from the periphery to the spinal cord where it transcytoses to central interneurons, blocking the release of the central neurotransmitters GABA and glycine [86]. A single experiment using an extremely high dose of botulinum toxin type A has purported to show a similar phenomenon in a rat whisker model [85]. It is possible that, at non-clinical doses in animal model experiments, botulinum toxin may overwhelm the normal handling

mechanism and be non-specifically trafficked to the neuronal cell body, likely for lysosomal degradation. However, there remains yet no clear evidence for the transfer of the neurotoxin protein from a primary motor neuron to a central neuron.

There is general consensus that at doses used in therapeutic or aesthetic applications of botulinum toxin type A, there is unlikely to be any direct central effect of the neurotoxin [87–89]. Supporting this consensus are the observations that clinical botulism, characterized by exposure to massive amounts of botulinum toxin, is vastly different in presentation than clinical tetanus, with botulism producing a flaccid paralysis characteristic of a lower motor neuron effect, while tetanus presents as a spastic paralysis characteristic of an upper motor neuron effect [90], suggesting that botulinum toxin does not gain access to central neurons through transcytocis.

Immunogenicity

As with all protein biologics, the injection of botulinum toxin may result in activation of the immune system and the formation of antibodies [91, 92]. While any component of the botulinum toxin molecule may elicit antibody formation, only those antibodies that block the biological activity of the neurotoxin (neutralizing antibodies) will lead to treatment failure if present in sufficient amounts [93]. A meta-analysis reported that the incidence of neutralizing antibody formation following treatment with onabotulinumtoxinA in clinical trials was less than 0.3% [94].

The classification of botulinum toxins by serotype is an immunologic categorization, and therefore it stands to reason that neutralizing antibodies produced against a product of one serotype will block responses to other products of the same serotype. Conversely, treatment with another serotype may be employed in cases of true antibody-mediated non-response [95].

As compared to most protein biologics, the amount of protein injected during treatment with any of the currently approved type A botulinum toxins is extremely low. For example, a 20 U dose of onabotulinumtoxinA contains 1 ng of neurotoxin complex and is usually administered every 4 months, whereas the monoclonal antibody adalimumab, used to treat chronic plaque psoriasis, is typically administered at a dose of 40 mg twice a month [96]. On a yearly basis this is 3 ng versus 960 mg load or a difference of 3,200,000-fold in dose by weight. The extremely small amounts of botulinum neurotoxin protein administered may account for the relatively low rate of antibody-induced treatment failure observed with botulinum toxin type A products. It is also important to note that some botulinum toxin products may contain residual bacterial contaminants [97] that might increase the likelihood of developing an immune reaction.

Products and Pharmacology

Following the first approval of onabotulinumtoxinA for clinical use by the US FDA in 1989, several other botulinum toxin type A products have become available. The most widely known other products are abobotulinumtoxinA (Ipsen, Ltd, first approved in the UK in 1990) and incobotulinumtoxinA (Merz, GmbH, first approved in Germany in 2005). Although the biological activity of all of these products resides in a common 150 kD core neurotoxin, they have differing pharmacologic profiles [98]. Each of these products has a unique molecular structure, a different mix of excipients and different definition of a unit, based on proprietary methodologies for conducting the LD50 assay used to define a unit of biological activity. These differences are outlined in the Table 3.1.

Table 3.1   Summary of differences between botulinum neurotoxin type A products.

Non-proprietary name	onabotulinumtoxinA	abobotulinumtoxinA	incobotulinumtoxinA
Manufacturer	Allergan Inc	Ipsen Ltd	Merz GmbH
Molecular weight (kDa)	~900 [68]	<500 [99]	150 [100]
Excipients	HSA[a] 500 µg (100 U vial) NaCl[b] 0.9 mg	HSA 125 µg (500 U vial) Lactose 2.5 mg	HSA 1000 µg (100 U vial) Sucrose 5 mg
Potency assay Diluent	Cell-based potency assay Saline [101]	Mouse LD50 Gelatin phosphate [102]	Mouse LD50 Non-saline stabilizer [103]
150 kDa neurotoxin (ng)	0.73 (100 U vial) [108]	3.24 (500 U vial) [108]	0.44 (100 U vial) [108]
FDA approved clinical indications	Cervical dystonia Blepharospasm Axillary hyperhidrosis Upper limb spasticity Lower limb spasticity Chronic migraine Neurogenic detrusor Overactivity Idiopathic overactive bladder Strabismus Glabellar Lines Crow's feet lines	Cervical dystonia Upper limb spasticity Glabellar lines	Cervical dystonia Blepharospasm in patients previously treated with onabotulinumtoxinA Upper limb spasticity Glabellar lines

[a] HSA, human serum albumin.
[b] NaCl, sodium chloride.

It is important to note that, unlike some other biologics such as insulin, erythropoietin, vaccines, and many other agents, there is no international reference preparation for botulinum toxin products [104] and therefore no "International unit" (i.u.). Therefore, the definition of a unit is not a standardized measure and the units and potency of each product is independent of all others. Potency is determined in relation to an in-house reference standard held by each manufacturer and using their unique and proprietary LD50 assay. Significant differences are reported to exist in, for example, diluents used to perform the potency assay: Allergan uses a saline diluent [101], Ipsen use a gelatin phosphate diluent [102], while Merz utilizes undefined stabilizers [103] in the diluent used to define the potency of incobotulinumtoxinA. Testing of onabotulinumtoxinA and incobotulinumtoxinA using different assay methodologies has demonstrated differences in how each manufacturer defines a unit, as would be expected given the differences reported in assays and reference standards and the differing amounts of core neurotoxin protein in each product. Recognition of these differences is reflected in each product label in the US [68, 100, 105, 106] and in other countries, and forms the basis for the unique non-proprietary names for each FDA approved botulinum toxin product [101].

Allergan has developed a novel cell-based potency assay as an alternative methodology for release testing of onabotulinumtoxinA. This methodology is specific to onabotulinumtoxinA, highly sensitive, and extensively cross-validated against the LD50 assay and was approved by the US FDA in 2011 and subsequently in most markets globally.

Due to the complex interplay of manufacturing, formulation and potency definition, there are no generics or biosimilars in this class of drug. All botulinum toxin products should be considered unique and not interchangeable, and should be dosed and injected according to the manufacturers recommendations.

Summary

In this chapter we provide a brief overview of the known mechanisms of action of botulinum toxin. Botulinum toxin has been shown, in clinical and preclinical studies, to modulate vesicular release of neurotransmitters at both alpha and gamma neurons within the somatic motor system, producing consistent, repeatable benefits in conditions of muscular overactivity. Additionally, effects and clinical utility for botulinum toxins have been demonstrated in the autonomic motor system and the peripheral nociceptive system.

The specificity of the effect of botulinum toxins on vesicular neurotransmitter release forms the basis for the wide variety of documented clinical applications of this agent. With a greater depth of understanding of the structure and pharmacology of botulinum toxins combined with increased insight into the workings of the nervous system, it is likely that the range of clinical indications for botulinum toxin will continue to grow in the future.

References

1 Sudhof TC. The synaptic vesicle cycle. Annu Rev Neurosci 2004;27:509–547.
2 Montal M. Botulinum neurotoxin: a marvel of protein design. Annu Rev Biochem 2010;79:591–617.
3 Dmochowski R, Chapple C, Nitti VW, *et al.* Efficacy and safety of onabotulinumtoxinA for idiopathic overactive bladder: a double-blind, placebo controlled, randomized, dose ranging trial. J Urol 2010;184:2416–2422.
4 Aurora SK, Dodick DW, Turkel CC, *et al.* OnabotulinumtoxinA for treatment of chronic migraine: results from the

double-blind, randomized, placebo-controlled phase of the PREEMPT 1 trial. Cephalalgia 2010;30:793–803.

5 Lowe NJ, Glaser DA, Eadie N, *et al.* Botulinum toxin type A in the treatment of primary axillary hyperhidrosis: a 52-week multicenter double-blind, randomized, placebo-controlled study of efficacy and safety. J Am Acad Dermatol 2007;56:604–611.

6 Sobel J, Tucker N, Sulka A, McLaughlin J, Maslanka S. Foodborne botulism in the United States, 1990–2000. Emerg Infect Dis 2004;10:1606–1611.

7 Hatheway CL. Clostridium-botulinum and other clostridia that produce botulinum neurotoxin. In: A. H. W. Hauschild and K. L. Dodds (eds). Clostridium Botulinum: Ecology and Control in Foods. New York: Marcel Dekker, Inc. 1993.

8 Comella CL, Jankovic J, Shannon KM, *et al.* Comparison of botulinum toxin serotypes A and B for the treatment of cervical dystonia. Neurology 2005;65: 1423–1429.

9 Aoki KR. A comparison of the safety margins of botulinum neurotoxin serotypes A, B, and F in mice. Toxicon 2001;39:1815–1820.

10 Johnson EA, Bradshaw M. Clostridium botulinum and its neurotoxins: a metabolic and cellular perspective. Toxicon 2001;39:1703–1722.

11 Popoff MR, Marvaud JC. Structural and genomic features of clostridial neurotoxins. In: J. E. Alouf and J. H. Freer (eds). The Comprehensive Source Book of Bacterial Protein Toxins. London: Academic Press 1999.

12 Smith TJ, Lou J, Geren IN, *et al.* Sequence variation within botulinum neurotoxin serotypes impacts antibody binding and neutralization. Infect Immun 2005;73: 5450–5457.

13 Swaminathan S. Molecular structures and functional relationships of botulinum neurotoxins. In: H. Jankovic, A. Albanese, M. Z. Atassi, *et al.* (eds). Botulinum Toxin: Therapeutic Clinical Practise and Science. Philadelphia: Saunders Elsevier 2009.

14 Oguma K, Fujinaga Y, Inoue K. Structure and function of Clostridium botulinum toxins. Microbiol Immunol 1995;39: 161–168.

15 Chen F, Kuziemko GM, Stevens RC. Biophysical characterization of the stability of the 150-kilodalton botulinum toxin, the nontoxic component, and the 900-kilodalton botulinum toxin complex species. Infect Immun 1998;66: 2420–2425.

16 Hanson MA, Stevens RC. Structural view of botulinum neurotoxin in numerous functional states. In: M. F. Brin, J. Jankovic and M. Hallett (eds). Scienfitic and Therapeutic Aspects of Botulinum Toxin. Philadelphia: Lippincott Williams & Wilkins 2002.

17 Sharma SK, Singh BR. Enhancement of the endopeptidase activity of purified botulinum neurotoxins A and E by an isolated component of the native neurotoxin associated proteins. Biochemistry 2004;43:4791–4798.

18 Ohishi I, Sugii S, Sakaguchi G. Oral toxicities of Clostridium botulinum toxins in response to molecular size. Infect Immun 1977;16:107–109.

19 Brandau DT, Joshi SB, Smalter AM, *et al.* Stability of the Clostridium botulinum type A neurotoxin complex: an empirical phase diagram based approach. Mol Pharm 2007;4:571–582.

20 Sakaguchi G, Kozaki S, I. O. Structure and function of botulinum toxins. In: J. E. AIouf (eds). Bacterial Protein Toxins. London: Academic Press. 1984.

21 Lacy DB, Stevens RC. Sequence homology and structural analysis of the clostridial neurotoxins. J Mol Biol 1999;291: 1091–1104.

22 Rummel A, Hafner K, Mahrhold S, *et al.* Botulinum neurotoxins C, E and F bind gangliosides via a conserved binding site prior to stimulation-dependent uptake with botulinum neurotoxin F utilising the

three isoforms of SV2 as second receptor. J Neurochem 2009;110:1942–1954.

23 Brunger AT, Rummel A. Receptor and substrate interactions of clostridial neurotoxins. Toxicon 2009;54:550–560.

24 Rossetto O, Montecucco C. Peculiar binding of botulinum neurotoxins. ACS Chem Biol 2007;2:96–98.

25 Dong M, Yeh F, Tepp WH, *et al.* SV2 is the protein receptor for botulinum neurotoxin A. Science 2006;312:592–596.

26 Hughes R, Whaler BC. Influence of nerve-ending activity and of drugs on the rate of paralysis of rat diaphragm preparations by Cl. botulinum type A toxin. J Physiol 1962;160:221–233.

27 Wan QF, Zhou ZY, Thakur P, *et al.* SV2 acts via presynaptic calcium to regulate neurotransmitter release. Neuron 2010;66:884–895.

28 Janz R, Goda Y, Geppert M, Missler M, Sudhof TC. SV2A and SV2B function as redundant Ca2+ regulators in neurotransmitter release. Neuron 1999;24:1003–1016.

29 Jahn R. Neuroscience. A neuronal receptor for botulinum toxin. Science 2006;312:540–541.

30 Brunger AT, Jin R, Breidenbach MA. Highly specific interactions between botulinum neurotoxins and synaptic vesicle proteins. Cell Mol Life Sci 2008;65:2296–2306.

31 Jacky BP, Garay PE, Dupuy J, *et al.* Identification of fibroblast growth factor receptor 3 (FGFR3) as a protein receptor for botulinum neurotoxin serotype A (BoNT/A). PLoS pathogens 2013;9(5): e1003369.

32 Lai B, Agarwal R, Nelson LD, Swaminathan S, London E. Low pH-induced pore formation by the T domain of botulinum toxin type A is dependent upon NaCl concentration. J Membr Biol 2010;236:191–201.

33 Montal M. Translocation of botulinum neurotoxin light chain protease by the heavy chain protein-conducting channel. Toxicon 2009;54:565–569.

34 Jahn R, Sudhof TC. Membrane fusion and exocytosis. Annu Rev Biochem 1999;68: 863–911.

35 Blasi J, Chapman ER, Link E, *et al.* Botulinum neurotoxin A selectively cleaves the synaptic protein SNAP-25. Nature 1993;365:160–163.

36 Simpson LL. Identification of the major steps in botulinum toxin action. Annu Rev Pharmacol Toxicol 2004;44:167–193.

37 Eleopra R, Tugnoli V, Rossetto O, De Grandis D, Montecucco C. Different time courses of recovery after poisoning with botulinum neurotoxin serotypes A and E in humans. Neurosci Lett 1998;256: 135–138.

38 Foran PG, Mohammed N, Lisk GO, *et al.* Evaluation of the therapeutic usefulness of botulinum neurotoxin B, C1, E, and F compared with the long lasting type A. Basis for distinct durations of inhibition of exocytosis in central neurons. J Biol Chem 2003;278:1363–1371.

39 Maia FM, Kanashiro AK, Chien HF, Goncalves LR, Barbosa ER. Clinical changes of cervical dystonia pattern in long-term botulinum toxin treated patients. Parkinsonism Relat Disord 2010;16:8–11.

40 Bajohrs M, Rickman C, Binz T, Davletov B. A molecular basis underlying differences in the toxicity of botulinum serotypes A and E. EMBO Rep 2004;5: 1090–1095.

41 Fernandez-Salas E, Steward LE, Ho H, *et al.* Plasma membrane localization signals in the light chain of botulinum neurotoxin. Proc Natl Acad Sci U S A 2004;101:3208–3213.

42 Dolly JO, Aoki KR. The structure and mode of action of different botulinum toxins. Eur J Neurol 2006;13 Suppl 4:1–9.

43 Rickman C, Meunier FA, Binz T, Davletov B. High affinity interaction of syntaxin and SNAP-25 on the plasma membrane is abolished by botulinum toxin E. J Biol Chem 2004;279:644–651.

44 Shen J, Ma J, Lee C, *et al.* How muscles recover from paresis and atrophy after

intramuscular injection of botulinum toxin A: Study in juvenile rats. J Orthop Res 2006;24:1128–1135.

45 Rogozhin AA, Pang KK, Bukharaeva E, Young C, Slater CR. Recovery of mouse neuromuscular junctions from single and repeated injections of botulinum neurotoxin A. J Physiol 2008;586: 3163–3182.

46 de Paiva A, Meunier FA, Molgo J, Aoki KR, Dolly JO. Functional repair of motor endplates after botulinum neurotoxin type A poisoning: biphasic switch of synaptic activity between nerve sprouts and their parent terminals. Proc Natl Acad Sci USA 1999;96:3200–3205.

47 Keller JE, Neale EA, Oyler G, Adler M. Persistence of botulinum neurotoxin action in cultured spinal cord cells. FEBS Lett 1999;456:137–142.

48 Brashear A, Watts MW, Marchetti A, et al. Duration of effect of botulinum toxin type A in adult patients with cervical dystonia: a retrospective chart review. Clin Ther 2000;22:1516–1524.

49 Naumann M, Yakovleff A, Durif F. A randomized, double-masked, crossover comparison of the efficacy and safety of botulinum toxin type A produced from the original bulk toxin source and current bulk toxin source for the treatment of cervical dystonia. J Neurol 2002;249: 57–63.

50 Herschorn S, Gajewski J, Ethans K, et al. Efficacy of botulinum toxin A injection for neurogenic detrusor overactivity and urinary incontinence: a randomized, double-blind trial. J Urol 2011;

51 Haferkamp A, Schurch B, Reitz A, et al. Lack of ultrastructural detrusor changes following endoscopic injection of botulinum toxin type a in overactive neurogenic bladder. Eur Urol 2004;46: 784–791.

52 Hulliger M. The mammalian muscle spindle and its central control. Rev Physiol Biochem Pharmacol 1984;101:1–110.

53 Trompetto C, Curra A, Buccolieri A, et al. Botulinum toxin changes intrafusal

feedback in dystonia: a study with the tonic vibration reflex. Mov Disord 2006;21:777–782.

54 Trompetto C, Bove M, Avanzino L, et al. Intrafusal effects of botulinum toxin in post-stroke upper limb spasticity. Eur J Neurol 2008;15:367–370.

55 Rosales RL, Arimura K, Takenaga S, Osame M. Extrafusal and intrafusal muscle effects in experimental botulinum toxin-A injection. Muscle Nerve 1996;19: 488–496.

56 Filippi GM, Errico P, Santarelli R, Bagolini B, Manni E. Botulinum A toxin effects on rat jaw muscle spindles. Acta Otolaryngol 1993;113:400–404.

57 Goodmurphy CW, Ovalle WK. Morphological study of two human facial muscles: orbicularis oculi and corrugator supercilii. Clin Anat 1999;12:1–11.

58 Saadia D, Voustianiouk A, Wang AK, Kaufmann H. Botulinum toxin type A in primary palmar hyperhidrosis: randomized, single-blind, two-dose study. Neurology 2001;57:2095–2099.

59 Lagalla G, Millevolte M, Capecci M, Provinciali L, Ceravolo MG. Botulinum toxin type A for drooling in Parkinson's disease: a double-blind, randomized, placebo-controlled study. Mov Disord 2006;21:704–707.

60 Tsui JK, Fross RD, Calne S, Calne DB. Local treatment of spasmodic torticollis with botulinum toxin. Can J Neurol Sci 1987;14:533–535.

61 Poewe W, Schelosky L, Kleedorfer B, et al. Treatment of spasmodic torticollis with local injections of botulinum toxin. One-year follow-up in 37 patients. J Neurol 1992;239:21–25.

62 Odergren T, Tollback A, Borg J. Efficacy of botulinum toxin for cervical dystonia. A comparison of methods for evaluation. Scand J Rehabil Med 1994;26:191–195.

63 Brin et al. Movement Disorders Vol 2(4) p237–254.

64 Dodick DW, Turkel CC, DeGryse RE, et al. OnabotulinumtoxinA for treatment of chronic migraine: pooled results from

the double-blind, randomized, placebo-controlled phases of the PREEMPT clinical program. Headache 2010;50:921–936.

65 Ranoux D, Attal N, Morain F, Bouhassira D. Botulinum toxin type A induces direct analgesic effects in chronic neuropathic pain. Ann Neurol 2008;64:274–283.

66 Foster L, Clapp L, Erickson M, Jabbari B. Botulinum toxin A and chronic low back pain: a randomized, double-blind study. Neurology 2001;56:1290–1293.

67 Placzek R, Drescher W, Deuretzbacher G, Hempfing A, Meiss AL. Treatment of chronic radial epicondylitis with botulinum toxin A. A double-blind, placebo-controlled, randomized multicenter study. J Bone Joint Surg Am 2007;89:255–260.

68 BOTOX® (onabotulinumtoxinA) Prescribing Information. Allergan, Inc. Irvine, CA, October, 2010.

69 Durham PL, Cady R, Cady R. Regulation of calcitonin gene-related peptide secretion from trigeminal nerve cells by botulinum toxin type A: implications for migraine therapy. Headache 2004;44:35–42;discussion 42–33.

70 Cui M, Khanijou S, Rubino J, Aoki KR. Subcutaneous administration of botulinum toxin A reduces formalin-induced pain. Pain 2004;107: 125–133.

71 Purkiss J, Welch M, Doward S, Foster K. Capsaicin-stimulated release of substance P from cultured dorsal root ganglion neurons: involvement of two distinct mechanisms. Biochem Pharmacol 2000;59:1403–1406.

72 Gazerani P, Au S, Dong X, *et al.* Botulinum neurotoxin type A (BoNTA) decreases the mechanical sensitivity of nociceptors and inhibits neurogenic vasodilation in a craniofacial muscle targeted for migraine prophylaxis. Pain 2010;151:606–616.

73 Gazerani P, Staahl C, Drewes AM, Arendt-Nielsen L. The effects of botulinum toxin type A on

capsaicin-evoked pain, flare, and secondary hyperalgesia in an experimental human model of trigeminal sensitization. Pain 2006;122:315–325.

74 Gazerani P, Staahl C, Drewes AM, Arendt-Nielsen L. Botulinum toxin type A reduces capsaicin-evoked sensory and vasomotor responses in human skin. Neurotox Res 2006;9: ABS-P13.

75 McMahon SB, Bennett DLH, Bevan Bennett S. Inflammatory mediators and modulators of pain. In: S. McMahon and M. Koltzenburg (eds). Wall and Melzack's Textbook of Pain. New York: Churchill Livingstone 2005.

76 Gazerani P, Pedersen NS, Staahl C, Drewes AM, Arendt-Nielsen L. Pain 2009 Jan;141(1–2):60–9.

77 Tugnoli V, Capone JG, Eleopra R, Quatrale R, Sensi M, Gastaldo E, Tola MR, Geppetti P. Pain 2007 Jul;130(1–2):76–83.

78 The UVB cutaneous inflammatory pain model: a reproducibility study in healthy volunteers. Carsten Dahl Mørch, Parisa Gazerani, Thomas A Nielsen, Lars Arendt-Nielsen. Int J Physiol Pathophysiol Pharmacol 2013;5(4):203–215. Published online 2013 December 15.

79 TNFα induces co-trafficking of TRPV1/TRPA1 in VAMP1-containing vesicles to the plasmalemma via Munc18–1/syntaxin1/SNAP-25 mediated fusion. Meng J, Wang J, Steinhoff M, Dolly JO. Sci Rep 2016 Feb 18;6:21226. doi: 10.1038/srep21226.

80 Morenilla-Palao C, Planells-Cases R, Garcia-Sanz N, Ferrer-Montiel A. Regulated exocytosis contributes to protein kinase C potentiation of vanilloid receptor activity. J Biol Chem 2004;279: 25665–25672.

81 Aoki KR. Review of a proposed mechanism for the antinociceptive action of botulinum toxin type A. Neurotoxicology 2005;26:785–793.

82 Gazerani P, Pedersen NS, Staahl C, Drewes AM, Arendt-Nielsen L. Subcutaneous Botulinum toxin type A reduces capsaicin-induced trigeminal pain

and vasomotor reactions in human skin. Pain 2009;141:60–69.

83 Walsh R, Hutchinson M. Molding the sensory cortex: spatial acuity improves after botulinum toxin treatment for cervical dystonia. Mov Disord 2007;22: 2443–2446.

84 Thickbroom GW, Byrnes ML, Stell R, Mastaglia FL. Reversible reorganisation of the motor cortical representation of the hand in cervical dystonia. Mov Disord 2003;18:395–402.

85 Antonucci F, Rossi C, Gianfranceschi L, Rossetto O, Caleo M. Long-distance retrograde effects of botulinum neurotoxin A. J Neurosci 2008;28: 3689–3696.

86 Lalli G, Bohnert S, Deinhardt K, Verastegui C, Schiavo G. The journey of tetanus and botulinum neurotoxins in neurons. Trends Microbiol 2003;11: 431–437.

87 Curra A, Berardelli A. Do the unintended actions of botulinum toxin at distant sites have clinical implications? Neurology 2009;72:1095–1099.

88 Caleo M, Schiavo G. Central effects of tetanus and botulinum neurotoxins. Toxicon 2009;54:593–599.

89 Caleo M, Antonucci F, Restani L, Mazzocchio R. A reappraisal of the central effects of botulinum neurotoxin type A: by what mechanism? J Neurochem 2009;109: 15–24.

90 Humeau Y, Doussau F, Grant NJ, Poulain B. How botulinum and tetanus neurotoxins block neurotransmitter release. Biochimie 2000;82:427–446.

91 Schellekens HH. Immunogenicity of therapeutic proteins. Clin Ther 2002;24: 1720–1740.

92 Shankar G, Pendley C, Stein KE. A risk-based bioanalytical strategy for the assessment of antibody immune responses against biological drugs. Nat Biotechnol 2007;25:555–561.

93 Goschel H, Wohlfarth K, Frevert J, Dengler R, Bigalke H. Botulinum A toxin therapy: neutralizing and nonneutralizing

antibodies – therapeutic consequences. Exp Neurol 1997;147:96–102.

94 Naumann M, Carruthers A, Carruthers J, et al. Meta-analysis of neutralizing antibody conversion with onabotulinumtoxinA (BOTOX(R)) across multiple indications. Mov Disord 2010;25:2211–2218.

95 Brin MF, Lew MF, Adler CH, et al. Safety and efficacy of NeuroBloc (botulinum toxin type B) in type A-resistant cervical dystonia. Neurology 1999;53:1431–1438.

96 Humira® (adalimumab) Injection Prescribing Information. Abbott Laboratories. North Chicago, IL. March, 2011.

97 Panjwani N, O'Keeffe R, Pickett A. Biochemical, functional and potency characteristics of type A botulinum toxin in clinical use. Botulinum J 2008;1: 153–166.

98 Foster KA, Bigalke H, Aoki KR. Botulinum neurotoxin – from laboratory to bedside. Neurotox Res 2006;9:133–140.

99 Hambleton P. Clostridium botulinum toxins: a general review of involvement in disease, structure, mode of action and preparation for clinical use. J Neurol 1992;239:16–20.

100 Xeomin® (incobotulinumtoxinA) Prescribing Information. Merz Pharmaceuticals, LLC. August, 2010.

101 Schantz EJ, Johnson EA. Properties and use of botulinum toxin and other microbial neurotoxins in medicine. Microbiol Rev 1992;56:80–99.

102 Hambleton P, Pickett AM. Potency equivalence of botulinum toxin preparations. J R Soc Med 1994;87: 719.

103 Mander G, Fink K, Vey M. Experimental conditions substantially influence botulinum toxin potency testing. Clin Neuropharmacol 2009;32:234;author reply 235.

104 Adler S, Bicker G, Bigalke H, et al. The current scientific and legal status of alternative methods to the LD50 test for botulinum neurotoxin potency testing.

The report and recommendations of a ZEBET Expert Meeting. Altern Lab Anim 2010;38:315–330.

105 Myobloc® (rimabotulinumtoxinB) Prescribing Information. Solstice Neurosciences, Inc. South San Francisco, CA, May, 2010.

106 Dysport® (abobotulinumtoxinA) Prescribing Information. Ipsen Biopharm Ltd., April, 2010.

107 Lee K, Gu S, Jin L, Le TTN, Cheng LW, *et al.* (2013) Structure of a bimodular botulinum neurotoxin complex provides insights into its oral toxicity. PLoS Pathog 9(10): e1003690. doi:10.1371/journal .ppat.1003690

108 Frevert, J., Content of Botulinum Neurotoxin in Botox_/Vistabel, Dysport_/Azzalure and Xeomin_/ Bocouture_ Drugs R D 2010;10 (2):67–73

109 Sutton, B., Fasshauer, D., Jahn. R., Brünger. A.T. (1998) Crystal structure of a core synaptic fusion complex *Nature* 395, 347–353.

4

Myobloc

Neil S. Sadick, MD (FACP, FAAD, FAACS, FACPh)[1,2] *and Suveena Manhas-Bhutani, MD*[2]

[1] *Clinical Professor, Weill Cornell Medical College, Cornell University, New York, USA*
[2] *Sadick Dermatology and Research, New York, USA*

The use of botulinum toxins for the improvement of fine lines and facial wrinkles has become increasingly popular over the past several years. By utilizing toxins to target hyperfunctional facial rhytids, physicians are able to successfully treat aging skin, yielding aesthetically younger, smoother looking skin to patients [1–10]. The occurrence of glabellar lines is due to the constant pulling of the skin by the musculature below. Active muscle movement of the transverse head of the corrugator supercilii results in the vertical glabellar lines, while the oblique head of the corrugator supercilii and the depressor supercilii along with the orbicularis oculi muscles contribute to the formation of the oblique glabellar line [11]. The approach to treatment includes minimizing the appearance of the glabellar lines by considering options of microdermabrasion, chemical peel, injections of collagen, silicone, autologous fat or dermal fillers. There are also surgical venues of endoscopy or limited incision to modify function of the corrugator supercilii and procerus muscle and direct incision of the glabellar line (Figure 4.1 and Figure 4.2).

In 1992, Carruthers and Carruthers evaluated the use of *Clostridium botulinum* type A purified neurotoxin complex (BTX-A; Botox®, Allergan Inc., Irvine, CA) to eradicate glabellar rhytids by chemically denervating the corrugator supercilii [5]. Findings included that botulinum toxin blocked the release of acetylcholine from motor nerve endings, resulting in a decrease in muscle tone and over-activity that was dose-dependent. It was also noted that botulinum toxin provided a safe treatment that targeted the muscle activity that contributed to the formation of wrinkle lines. Since then, myriad of other studies have yielded similar results, and the BTX-A is currently FDA-cleared for cosmetic use in moderate to severe glabellar lines and crow's feet.

Botulinum toxin type B (BTX-B; Myobloc in the USA and Neurobloc in Europe; otherwise identified as Myobloc henceforth, Solstice Neurosciences, South San Francisco, CA) was FDA-cleared in 2000 for the treatment of abnormal head position and pain related to cervical dystonia. Currently its clinical utility is being investigated for a variety of other medical disorders, such as hyperhidrosis and siallorhea, as well as in the setting of cosmetic dermatology. It is readily available in a liquid formulation, which requires no preparation or reconstitution unlike BTX-A [8, 12–15].

Pharmacology of Botulinum Toxin B

The molecular weight of the BTX-A complex is around 900 kDa whereas that of Myobloc is approximately 700 kDa. Both these

Botulinum Toxins: Cosmetic and Clinical Applications, First Edition. Edited by Joel L. Cohen and David M. Ozog.
© 2017 John Wiley & Sons Ltd. Published 2017 by John Wiley & Sons Ltd.
Companion Website: www.wiley.com/go/cohen/botulinum

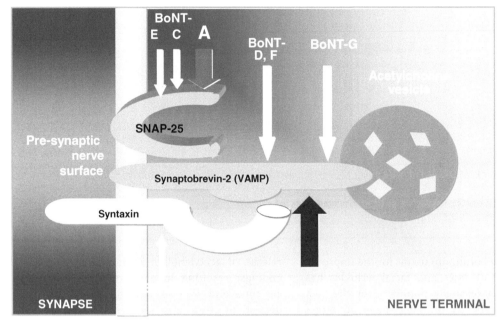

SNARE Proteins

Figure 4.1 Pharmacology of botulinum toxins at the neuromuscular junction. SNAP-25 is the target for the type A toxin (red arrow), synaptobrevin is the target for the type B toxin (black arrow).

complexes are found to be stable in acidic conditions. The large neurotoxin complex is composed of proteins such as a hemagglutinin and a non-toxic, non-hemagglutinin moiety. The active neurotoxin is a 150 Da dimer consisting of heavy chain (100 kDa) and a light chain (50 kDa) moiety linked together by a disulfide bond.

The mechanism of action of botulinum toxin B on the nervous system is similar to that of all other botulinum toxins and involves a series of cellular actions

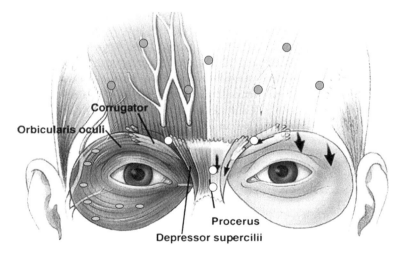

Figure 4.2 Schemata showing the most common sites of botulinum toxin injections in the upper face. Injections in (a) the glabella; (b) the forehead; (c) the crow's feet. The author prefers to use the conversion of 150 U of type B toxin for 1 U of type A toxin.

including binding, internalization, and inhibition of acetylcholine release (Figure 4.1). The heavy chain contributes to the irreversible binding of the toxin to the serotype-specific protein within the soluble N-ethyl maleimide-sensitive factor attachment protein receptor (SNARE) complex, which is involved in release of acetylcholine containing vesicles from the presynaptic neuron. Flaccid paralysis associated with botulism is due to the light chain-mediated proteolysis of SNARE proteins and the subsequent inhibition of synaptic vesicle fusion to the presynaptic membrane of the human motor neurons Tis. A specific residue on one of the N-ethyl maleimide-sensitive factor attachment proteins is cleaved by each serotype. Myobloc cleaves vesicle associated membrane protein (VAMP), also known as synaptobrevin. Serotypes F, G, D also cleave VAMP, but at various locations. It is found that the various sites of action of various serotypes may contribute to the differences in clinical effectiveness. SNARE proteins may be the only intracellular targets of BTX serotypes. The remarkable specificity of the BTX light chain cleavage is due to the light chain recognizing unusually long SNARE sequences (~30–50 residues indicated by the specific serotype) [16–22] (Table 4.1).

Immunogenicity of Myobloc

The injection of any botulinum toxin may elicit an immune response since it is considered a foreign protein injected into the body [16]. Patients that are treated with any toxin can develop neutralizing antibodies that blunt clinical effectiveness [23]. When these antibodies are present, the therapeutic effect may be significantly reduced or completely nullified, based on retrospective studies by Dresseler and Bigalke [13] and Dolimbek *et al.* [6], where 3–5% of patients were treated with dose a of 100–1200 U of BTX-A for cervical dystonia. Formation of antibodies to other parts of the complex is not believed to affect clinical performance of these products. The adverse

Table 4.1 Pharmacology of botulinum toxin serotypes by target/cleavage sizes.

Serotype	Target size	Cleaves at
A	SNAP-25[a]	Gln197-Arg198
B	VAMP[b]	Glu76-Phe77
C	Syntaxin	Lys253-Ala254
		Lys252-Ala252
	SNAP-25[a]	Arg198-Ala199
D	VAMP[b]	Ala67-Asp68
		Lys59-Leu60
E	SNAP-25[a]	Arg180-Ile181
F	VAMP[b]	Gln58-Lys59
G	VAMP[b]	Ala81-Ala82

[a]SNAP-25 is soluble NSF attachment protein of 25,000 kDa.
[b]VAMP is vesicle-associated membrane protein (synaptobrevin).

events are considered significantly lower in patients treated for aesthetic purposes as compared to those patients being treated for cervical dystonia as lower doses are utilized to treat cosmetic issues [24]. When patients become resistant to one particular serotype, another serotype can be used, as botulinum toxin serotypes are not able to undergo cross – neutralization. In various studies conducted on patients with cervical dystonia, those resistant to BTX-A responded to treatment with Myobloc. Furthermore, patients resistant to Myobloc can achieve positive results from BTX-A or any other botulinum toxin serotype. Recent research suggests that resistance to one serotype may potentiate resistance to the other following repeat and multiple injections. Risks associated with cross-antibody resistance include treatment with high doses of toxin, increased frequency of administration, and the high amount of neurotoxin protein per injection [23–25].

Liquid Formulation of Myobloc

Myobloc is prepared in a ready-to-use formulation, which is stabilized at a pH of 5.6. It may be slightly more painful than

BTX-A due to its higher level of acidity [12]. Vials of Myobloc are found in 2,500, 5,000, and 10,000 U, each with concentrations of 5,000 U/ml or 500 U/0.1 ml [26]. Berman *et al.* [24] noted that this preparation can be diluted up to sixfold without losing its viability. Although, one unit equates to the amount of toxin that is detrimental in 50% of female Swiss–Webster mice after intraperitoneal injections (Mouse LD50 bioassay) it is imperative to understand the sensitivity of different species to each toxin serotype. Furthermore, the differences in the potency assays employed and different toxin products cannot be compared on a unit-by-unit basis [27]. Specific dose ranging studies in humans are essential for each toxin serotype and for each indication, and it is important to understand that dose conversion should not be attempted as noted in the package instructions for BTX -A and Myobloc [24].

Storage and refrigeration of Myobloc is beneficial at 2–8°C in a constant environment for up to 3 years. It is stable for at least 9 months at a room temperature of 25°C and remains biologically active when stored in refrigeration for 21 months and then moved back to room temperature for 6 months and then moved to 4°C. Myobloc diluted up to sixfold with either non-preserved or preserved saline can sustain potency for at least 24 h at room temperature [12,17,26,28,29].

Myobloc in the Aesthetics Practice

Although its primary use for the treatment of cervical dystonia, increasing demand for cosmetic improvements such as effective treatment of facial rhytids, have expanded the off-label use of Botulinum Toxin B to a variety of other aesthetic indications. Several peer-reviewed clinical studies and trials have demonstrated the safety and efficacy of BTX-B use in aesthetic medicine, mostly focusing on establishing therapeutic protocols and doses [7].

Alster and Lupton treated 20 female patients with vertical glabellar rhytids who had minimal response to BTX-A (less than 50% reduction in contraction of the muscles treated with BTX-A). Subjects were treated with Myobloc at five standardized intramuscular sites (procerus, inferomedial corrugators and superior medial corrugators) at a total dose of 2,500 U [1]. Improvement of wrinkles occurred in all individuals with peak response at 1 month and complete dissolution of effect at month 4.

Flynn and Clark showed an increased rate of onset and widespread diffusion of Myobloc versus BTX-A in a single centre study of 24 patients with symmetrical, moderate to severe forehead wrinkles [19]. Subjects received type A (BOTOX®) 5 U on one side and type B (Myobloc®) 500 U on the other side of the forehead. Measurements of radius of diffusion and time until full effect took place were taken. Myobloc was found to have a slightly faster rate of onset than type A. A greater radius of diffusion was consistently observed with type B as measured by the greater area of wrinkle reduction at the doses used.

Ramirez *et al.* evaluated Myobloc in 24 subjects with facial wrinkles [31]. Eighty-two percent had been treated with BTX-A previously, but not for 6 months prior to the study. Each subject received 200–400 U of Myobloc per unilateral injection site (total dose, 400–800 U). Three sites were injected, including the frontalis, the corrugators, and the orbicularis oculi. Improvement in facial wrinkles was assessed using two scales: the Wrinkle Improvement Scale (WIS; 0 indicates no improvement and 3 indicates significant improvement) and the Rated Numeric Kinetic Line Scale (RNKLS). The latter scale describes wrinkles both at rest and at maximum frown. It ranges from a score of 1, reflecting no wrinkles at rest that become fine lines with facial animation, to a score of 4, denoting deep lines at rest that become deep furrows with facial animation. Subject response was evaluated before injection and after injection at visits, that is weeks 1, 2, 4, 8, and 12. Photographs were also documented. All subjects exhibited rapid onset of target muscle effect within 72 hours and, in some cases, within 24 hours. Scores on the WIS and RNKLS were moderately to significantly improved by two to three points after Myobloc treatment; however, the duration of effect was suboptimal (mean of 8 weeks). No subjects reported side effects of dysphagia, dyspepsia, or dry mouth, which are commonly seen in treatment of cervical dystonia. Eyelid ptosis, brow ptosis, and dry eye were not measured. This preliminary study showed that Myobloc is effective in treating facial lines of the glabella, forehead, and crow's feet areas, but the authors concluded that doses higher than 400–800 U would be necessary for a longer duration of action.

This study also evaluated the subjects for pain associated with injection, using the McGill Pain Scale. Pain experienced upon injection, usually described as a slight stinging sensation, has been reported to occur with botulinum toxin injections. The McGill Pain Scale is a validated scale ranging from 0, signifying no pain to 5, signifying excruciating pain. At the time of treatment, subjects were asked to rate the pain of Myobloc injection and to rate by memory the pain of BTX-A injection. On average, Myobloc was found to be slightly more painful than the memory of BTX-A injection (2.3 vs. 1.6 respectively), although all subjects indicated that the injection pain would not prevent them from undergoing a repeat injection with Myobloc. A recent study by Lowe and Lowe [32], showed that injection pain of the acidic solution of BTX-B neurotoxin was reduced and efficacy not compromised by changing the pH of BTX-B solution to pH 7.5.

Sadick conducted two open-label studies using higher doses of BTX-B for treatment of glabellar wrinkles [10, 30]. Both studies were similar in design, but the first study evaluated BTX-B 1,800 U ($N = 30$), and the second study evaluated 2,400 U ($N = 16$) and 3,000 U ($N = 18$). Doses were divided equally among six sites; two in the procerus and two in each corrugator supercilii and orbicularis oculi muscle bilaterally. Most of the subjects

had not been previously treated with BTX-A. In the first study, clinical photography and a clinical scoring system was used by both subjects and physicians to evaluate efficacy; 0 denoted marked frowning ability, 1 denoted partial frowning ability, and 2 denoted complete inability to frown because of paralysis. The second study also used the RNKLS. Subjects returned to the office daily postinjection until the effects of BTX-B were observed and weekly thereafter. Both studies found BTX-B to be effective in treating glabellar frown lines, based on photography, patient satisfaction, and improvements in assessment scores. Overall, BTX-B had a very rapid onset of action. Comparing the results of both studies also suggest that the duration of response is dose related. The mean duration of effect was 8.0 weeks with 1,800 U, 9.6 weeks with 2,400 U, and 10.4 weeks with 3,000 U. Lid ptosis was reported in one patient who received 2,400 U and in one patient who received 3,000 U. Headaches and mild pain upon injection were also reported. Overall, BTX-B was very safe, and there was no increase in adverse effects with the higher doses.

In a dosing study, Lowe et al. assessed 13 subjects injected with Myobloc in two different dose schedules versus BTX-A in the corrugator-procerus complex. One subgroup received a conversion of 50 U of Myobloc (total 1,000) to 1 U of BTX-A, while others received a conversion factor of 100 U of Myobloc (total 2,000) to 1 U BTX-A. Patients treated with BTX-A received a total of 20 U. Both types of botulinum toxins were noted to be effective in improving glabellar frown lines. The onset of action was more rapid (2–3 days) with Myobloc than with BTX-A (3–7 days). Duration of effect with BTX-A was at least 16 weeks. While the 1,000 U Myobloc doses, duration was 6–8 weeks and with the 2,000 U Myobloc doses the duration was 10–12 weeks [33].

Kim investigated an escalating dosage formula of 400–800 U to 1,600–2,000 U and 2,500–3,000 U per site treating the bilateral frontalis, corrugator or orbicularis oculi using a WIS and RNKLS, found Myobloc to be clinically effective for up to 8 weeks for treatment of hyperkinetic facial lines and up to week 12 at the higher dosage [34]. The patients exhibited excellent skin smoothing, which was felt to be secondary to an enhanced diffusion effect of Myobloc. Reported side effects included headaches (40%), brow ptosis (7%), dry eyes (5%) and dry mouth (13%).

It is observed from the various clinical assessments on Myobloc that the highest dose to be used for aesthetic means is 3,125 U for glabellar lines and 3,750 U for the frontalis region. In an open-label study, 26 subjects received low (1,875 U), medium (2,500 U), or high (3,125 U) doses of Myobloc for glabellar lines; 18 subjects received a low (2,250 U), medium (3,000 U), or high (3,750 U) dose of Myobloc in the frontalis. Results were similar to other studies of Myobloc for wrinkles in that it has a very rapid onset of effect and a dose-related duration of effect. There were no reports of lid ptosis. Myobloc was reported to yield a very uniform paralysis and a smooth aesthetic effect. This effect has also been observed by the author, as well as by others, and may reflect the diffusion characteristics of Myobloc, which may differ from those of BTX-A. Compared with BTX-A, Myobloc appears to diffuse more within the injected muscle [35].

Studies of Myobloc for the treatment of facial wrinkles demonstrate its effectiveness, rapid onset of action, and dose-dependent duration of effect. In clinical studies of cervical dystonia, the calculated duration of the effect of Myobloc was 12–16 weeks, which is comparable to that seen with BTX-A. These trials demonstrated a dose–response relationship in the duration of effect when treating glabellar lines. It is anticipated that higher doses of Myobloc can be safely and effectively administered to produce an even longer duration of response in the treatment of facial wrinkles. Further studies at higher doses are recommended to determine optimal dosing of Myobloc, without compromising its safety profile [36–38].

Treatment Considerations for Myobloc

Previous studies have been used as a basis to establish initial approximates for effective doses of Myobloc in the treatment of facial rhytids [1, 3–5, 8, 10, 11, 31, 34, 39–52] (Table 4.2).

The procerus complex and corrugators supercilii muscles are treated to eradicate glabellar lines. A dose totaling 20–30 U of BTX-A is divided and equally injected into five sites compared to the Myobloc treatment, which requires 2,000–3,000 U divided among only four injection sites resulting in comparable results (Figure 4.2). The injection of the frontalis utilizes 15–30 U of BTX-A distributed evenly over five to six injection sites and provides satisfactory results while the Myobloc in quantities of 1,000–2,500 U per side yields similar results as well. To achieve effective results in the lifting of the brow, injections of 1,500 U are directed to the corrugator supercilii, the procerus complex and the medial portion of the orbicularis oculi muscle. For the treatment of crow's feet injecting 10–15 U of BTX-A divided into two to three sites per side yields similar results as employing 1,000–1,500 U per side of Myobloc, while diffusion characteristics of Myobloc taken into consideration in this scenario [4, 8, 10, 11, 19, 31, 33, 34, 46–48, 51–53] (Figure 4.3, Figure 4.4, Figure 4.5 and Figure 4.6).

Table 4.2 Provisional dosing guidelines for botulinum toxin B injections for facial rhytids.

Muscle site	BTX-B (Myobloc®) (units)	No. of injections
Glabella	2,000–3,000	3
Frontalis	1,000–2,500	3–6
Brow lift	300–500 per side	1 per side
Periorbital	1,000–1,500 per side	1–2 per side

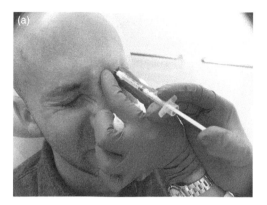 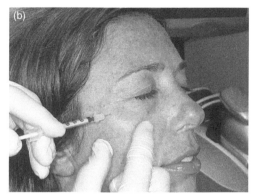

Figure 4.3 Technique of (a) glabella and (b) lateral canthal line injections.

Adverse Events

Complication profiles for BTX-A versus Myobloc are quite similar with temporary mild bruising and headaches. Rarely, potential complications include eyelid and brow ptosis, and asymmetric brow elevation (Figure 4.7). It is imperative to see a fully qualified and skilled physician with a thorough understanding of injection points and dosages for optimal results and minimal complications [43, 54, 55].

Conclusion

In recent years, there has been a strong surge in demand from patients for safe and effective aesthetic solutions to combat signs of

aging manifested by the formation of facial rhytids in the glabellar, forehead and periorbital regions. The overactive nature of

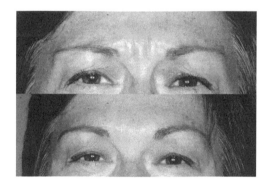

Figure 4.5 Before (a) and after (b) 12 weeks after treatment with 3,000 U of botulinum toxin type B to the glabella.

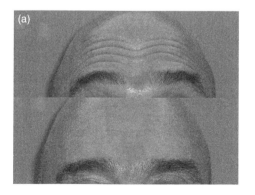 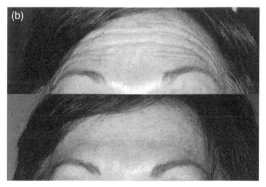

Figure 4.4 Treatment of frontalis muscle in (a) a male patient and (b) a female patient with 3,000 U of botulinum toxin type A.

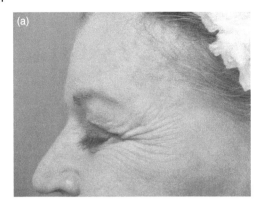
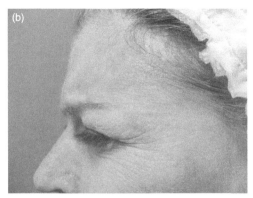

Figure 4.6 Before (a) and after (b) 12 weeks after treatment with 3,000 U of botulinum toxin type B to lateral canthal lines.

the underlying facial muscles has been successfully treated by botulinum toxins, which weaken the muscles and cause paralysis, and are particularly effective for patients with prominent hyperfunctional facial lines. BTX-A and Myobloc are two serotype formulations of botulinum toxin that are available in the United States. Each has its own unique mechanism of action, binds serotype-specific receptors, and targets specific intracellular proteins. Myobloc comes as a ready-to-use liquid formulation compared to the BTX-A, which is found in stable powder form requiring reconstitution before injecting. Although both toxins can elicit an

immune response, further clinical studies are needed to demonstrate which toxin is more prone to provoke an immune response. BTX-A has been used in aesthetic medicine for several years, with numerous clinical studies substantiating its efficacy, whereas Myobloc has only recently been used for aesthetic indications. Nevertheless, initial findings on Myobloc indicate that it can deliver more rapid and greater results in paralysing muscles. The safety profile of Myobloc and BTX-A is favorable and the likelihood of serious adverse effects is low; albeit both toxins are highly potent and extreme care should be taken, especially when increasing doses in patients. When there is excess enthusiasm from the physician's part to deliver formidable aesthetic results by using toxins vigorously (especially in the lower face), the side effects become prevalent and troublesome. Thus, for a practicing clinician in the aesthetic field, patient safety through a deep understanding of best practice and procedure is more paramount to avoid posttreatment complications than securing patient satisfaction. As studies continue to advance our understanding of the the mechanism of action, durability, and safety of Myobloc, the aesthetic indications and treatment protocols are bound to expand, capitalizing on its efficacy while minimizing any potential adverse effects.

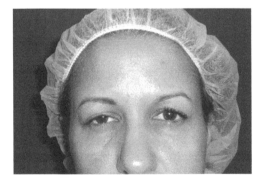

Figure 4.7 Drooping of the left upper eyelid after botulinum toxin type B injection in the glabella. Apraclonidine (0.5%) drops, 3 drops to the affected eye three times a day produces temporary relief of this problem until it completely resolves.

References

1 Alster TS, Lupton JR. Botulinum toxin type B for dynamic glabellar rhytides refractory to botulinum toxin type A. Dermatol Surg 2003. 29(5):516–518.

2 Blitzer A, Brin MF, Keen MS, Aviv JE. Botulinum toxin for the treatment of hyperfunctional lines of the face. Arch Otolaryngol Head Neck Surg 1993;119(9): 1018–1022.

3 Brandt FS, Bellman B. Cosmetic use of botulinum A exotoxin for the aging neck. Dermatol Surg 1998;24(11):1232–1234.

4 Carruthers J, Carruthers A. BOTOX use in the mid and lower face and neck. Semin Cutan Med Surg 2001;20(2):85–92.

5 Carruthers JD, Carruthers JA. Treatment of glabellar frown lines with C. botulinum-A exotoxin. J Dermatol Surg Oncol 1992; 18(1):17–21.

6 Dolimbek BZ, Jankovic J, Atassi MZ. Cross reaction of tetanus and botulinum neurotoxins A and B and the boosting effect of botulinum neurotoxins A and B on a primary anti-tetanus antibody response. Immunol Invest 2002;31(3–4):247–262.

7 Guyuron B, Huddleston SW. Aesthetic indications for botulinum toxin injection. Plast Reconstr Surg 1994;93(5):913–918.

8 Jacob CI. Botulinum neurotoxin type B – a rapid wrinkle reducer. Semin Cutan Med Surg 2003;22(2):131–135.

9 Matarasso A, Matarasso SL, Brandt FS, Bellman B. Botulinum A exotoxin for the management of platysma bands. Plast Reconstr Surg 1999;103(2):645–652; discussion 653–655.

10 Sadick NS, Fellows of the American Academy of Cosmetic Surgeons. Botulinum toxin type B for glabellar wrinkles: a prospective open-label response study. Dermatol Surg 2002;28(9):817–821.

11 Pierard GE, Lapiere CM. The microanatomical basis of facial frown lines. Arch Dermatol 1989;125(8):1090–1092.

12 Callaway JE, Arezzo JC, Grethlein AJ. Botulinum toxin type B: an overview of its biochemistry and preclinical pharmacology. Semin Cutan Med Surg 2001;20(2):127–136.

13 Dressler D, Bigalke H. Botulinum toxin type B de novo therapy of cervical dystonia: frequency of antibody induced therapy failure. J Neurol 2005;252(8):904–907.

14 Han Y, Stevens AL, Dashtipour K, et al. A mixed treatment comparison to compare the efficacy and safety of botulinum toxin treatments for cervical dystonia. J Neurol 2016;263(4):772–780.

15 Hosp C, Naumann MK, Hamm H. Botulinum toxin treatment of autonomic disorders: focal hyperhidrosis and sialorrhea. Semin Neurol 2016;36(1):20–28.

16 Aoki KR. Pharmacology and immunology of botulinum neurotoxins. Int Ophthalmol Clin 2005;45(3):25–37.

17 Callaway JE, Arezzo JC, Grethlein AJ. Botulinum toxin type B: an overview of its biochemistry and preclinical pharmacology. Dis Mon 2002;48(5): 367–383.

18 Dong M, Tepp WH, Liu H, Johnson EA, et al. Mechanism of botulinum neurotoxin B and G entry into hippocampal neurons. J Cell Biol 2007;179(7):1511–1522.

19 Flynn TC, Clark RE 2nd. Botulinum toxin type B (MYOBLOC) versus botulinum toxin type A (BOTOX) frontalis study: rate of onset and radius of diffusion. Dermatol Surg 2003;29(5):519–522; discussion 522.

20 Oguma K, Fujinaga Y, Inoue K. Structure and function of Clostridium botulinum toxins. Microbiol Immunol 1995;39(3): 161–168.

21 Setler P. The biochemistry of botulinum toxin type B. Neurology 2000;55(12 Suppl 5):S22–S28.

22 Simpson LL. Molecular pharmacology of botulinum toxin and tetanus toxin. Annu Rev Pharmacol Toxicol 1986;26:427–453.

23 Atassi MZ, Dolimbek BZ, Jankovic J, et al. Molecular recognition of botulinum neurotoxin B heavy chain by human

antibodies from cervical dystonia patients that develop immunoresistance to toxin treatment. Mol Immunol 2008;45(15): 3878–3888.

24 Berman B, Seeberger L, Kumar R. Long-term safety, efficacy, dosing, and development of resistance with botulinum toxin type B in cervical dystonia. Mov Disord 2005;20(2):233–237.

25 Jankovic J, Hunter C, Dolimbek BZ, *et al.* Clinico-immunologic aspects of botulinum toxin type B treatment of cervical dystonia. Neurology 2006;67(12):2233–2235.

26 Callaway JE. Botulinum toxin type B (Myobloc): pharmacology and biochemistry. Clin Dermatol 2004;22(1): 23–28.

27 Carruthers A, Carruthers J, Flynn TC, Leong MS. Dose-finding, safety, and tolerability study of botulinum toxin type B for the treatment of hyperfunctional glabellar lines. Dermatol Surg 2007;33(1 Spec No.):S60–S68.

28 Gilsdorf J, Gul N, Smith LA. Expression, purification, and characterization of *Clostridium botulinum* type B light chain. Protein Expr Purif 2006;46(2):256–267.

29 Kranz G, Paul A, Voller B, *et al.* Long-term efficacy and respective potencies of botulinum toxin A and B: a randomized, double-blind study. Br J Dermatol 2011;164(1):176–181.

30 Sadick NS. Prospective open-label study of botulinum toxin type B (Myobloc) at doses of 2,400 and 3,000 U for the treatment of glabellar wrinkles. Dermatol Surg 2003; 29(5):501–507; discussion 507.

31 Ramirez AL, Reeck J, Maas CS. Botulinum toxin type B (MyoBloc) in the management of hyperkinetic facial lines. Otolaryngol Head Neck Surg 2002;126(5):459–467.

32 Lowe PL, Lowe NJ. Botulinum toxin type B: pH change reduces injection pain, retains efficacy. Dermatol Surg 2014;40(12): 1328–1333.

33 Lowe NJ, Yamauchi PS, Lask GP, *et al.* Botulinum toxins types A and B for brow furrows: preliminary experiences with type

B toxin dosing. J Cosmet Laser Ther 2002;4(1):15–18.

34 Kim EJ, Ramirez AL Reeck JB, Maas CS. The role of botulinum toxin type B (Myobloc) in the treatment of hyperkinetic facial lines. Plast Reconstr Surg 2003;112 (5 Suppl):88S–93S; discussion 94S–97S.

35 Sadick NS, Herman AR. Comparison of botulinum toxins A and B in the aesthetic treatment of facial rhytides. Dermatol Surg 2003;29(4):340–347.

36 Patel S, Martino D. Cervical dystonia: from pathophysiology to pharmacotherapy. Behav Neurol 2013;26(4):275–282.

37 Pappert EJ, Germanson T, Myobloc/ Neurobloc European Cervical Dystonia Study. Botulinum toxin type B vs. type A in toxin-naive patients with cervical dystonia: Randomized, double-blind, noninferiority trial. Mov Disord 2008;23(4):510–17.

38 Chapman MA, Barron R, Tanis DC, *et al.*, Comparison of botulinum neurotoxin preparations for the treatment of cervical dystonia. Clin Ther 2007;29(7): 1325–1337.

39 Ascher B, Zakine B, Kestemont P, Baspeyras M, *et al.* A multicenter, randomized, double-blind, placebo-controlled study of efficacy and safety of 3 doses of botulinum toxin A in the treatment of glabellar lines. J Am Acad Dermatol 2004;51(2):223–233.

40 Baumann L, Slezinger A, Vujevich J, Halem M, *et al.* A double-blinded, randomized, placebo-controlled pilot study of the safety and efficacy of Myobloc (botulinum toxin type B)-purified neurotoxin complex for the treatment of crow's feet: a double-blinded, placebo-controlled trial. Dermatol Surg 2003;29(5):508–515.

41 Blitzer A, Binder WJ, Aviv JE, *et al.* The management of hyperfunctional facial lines with botulinum toxin. A collaborative study of 210 injection sites in 162 patients. Arch Otolaryngol Head Neck Surg 1997;123(4): 389–392.

42 Carruthers JA, Lowe NJ, Menter MA, *et al.* A multicenter, double-blind, randomized, placebo-controlled study of the efficacy and

safety of botulinum toxin type A in the treatment of glabellar lines. J Am Acad Dermatol 2002;46(6):840–849.

43 Erickson BP, Lee WW, Cohen J, Grunebaum LD. The role of neurotoxins in the periorbital and midfacial areas. Facial Plast Surg Clin North Am 2015;23(2): 243–255.

44 Fagien S, Brandt FS. Primary and adjunctive use of botulinum toxin type A (Botox) in facial aesthetic surgery: beyond the glabella. Clin Plast Surg 2001;28(1): 127–148.

45 Flynn TC, Carruthers JA, Carruthers JA. Botulinum-A toxin treatment of the lower eyelid improves infraorbital rhytides and widens the eye. Dermatol Surg 2001;27(8): 703–708.

46 Foster JA, Barnhorst D, Papay F, *et al.* The use of botulinum A toxin to ameliorate facial kinetic frown lines. Ophthalmology 1996;103(4):618–622.

47 Hankins CL, Strimling R, Rogers GS. Botulinum A toxin for glabellar wrinkles. Dose and response. Dermatol Surg 1998;24(11):1181–1183.

48 Huilgol SC, Carruthers A, Carruthers JD. Raising eyebrows with botulinum toxin. Dermatol Surg 1999;25(5):373–375; discussion 376.

49 Lew MF, Adornato BT, Duane DD, *et al.* Botulinum toxin type B: a double-blind, placebo-controlled, safety and efficacy study in cervical dystonia. Neurology 1997;49(3):701–707.

50 Lowe NJ, Maxwell A, Harper H. Botulinum A exotoxin for glabellar folds: a double-blind, placebo-controlled study with an electromyographic injection technique. J Am Acad Dermatol 1996;35(4): 569–572.

51 Spencer JM, Gordon M, Goldberg DJ. Botulinum B treatment of the glabellar and frontalis regions: a dose response analysis. J Cosmet Laser Ther 2002;4(1): 19–23.

52 Vecchione TR. Glabellar frown lines: direct excision, an evaluation of the scars. Plast Reconstr Surg 1990;86(1):46–52.

53 Knize DM. Muscles that act on glabellar skin: a closer look. Plast Reconstr Surg 2000;105(1):350–361.

54 Dubow J, Kim A, Leikin J, *et al.* Visual system side effects caused by parasympathetic dysfunction after botulinum toxin type B injections. Mov Disord 2005;20(7):877–880.

55 Francisco GE. Botulinum toxin: dosing and dilution. Am J Phys Med Rehabil 2004;83(10 Suppl):S30–S37.

5

Abobotulinumtoxin: Development and Aesthetic Usage

Gary D. Monheit, MD

Total Skin and Beauty Dermatology Center, PC Private Practice,
Associate Clinical Professor, Department of Dermatology, Department of Ophthalmology, University of Alabama at Birmingham, Birmingham, USA

Clinical studies

Since the muscle-paralyzing activity of botulinum toxin (BoNT) was first noted in the nineteenth century, the clinical usefulness of this "most poisonous of all poisons" [1] has evolved into a diversity of therapeutic uses. Currently, several commercial preparations of botulinum toxin serotype A (BoNTA) are available for the treatment of strabismus, blepharospasm, cervical dystonia, migraine, laryngeal spasms, and other disorders of muscle contraction. Since Carruthers and Carruthers first published their sentinel article on the relationship of muscle activity with wrinkles and its correlation with BoNTA, the aesthetic uses have expanded greatly [2].

Onabotulinumtoxin (Botox®, Allergan, Irvine, California) was first FDA approved in 2002 for glabellar lines, but since then it has been applied off-label for other facial dynamic wrinkles and other aesthetic indications [3].

Abobotulinumtoxin (Dysport®; Ipsen, Medicis US and Azzalure®, Galderma, Europe) was first licensed for medical usage in Europe in 1990[4]. Clinical studies for aesthetic indications were first performed in Europe 2002 and 2003, followed by US FDA studies until 2009. FDA approval for treatment of glabellar frown lines occurred May 2009.

All the preparations are BONTA molecules, but there are some technical differences in the formulations. Though most clinical properties seem to act the same, there may be some subtle differences the clinician must understand. It is thus important to review the science of the molecule, its formulations, and its physiologic action to use each of the preparations correctly.

To use this new product correctly it is necessary to understand the following points:

1. The science of the BoNTA molecule and its differences.
2. The clinical studies demonstrating efficacy and safety.
3. Differences in the products.
4. Experience in worldwide usage.

The three most widely used products – obobotulinumtoxin (Botox®), abobotulinumtoxin (Dysport®/Azzalure®) and incobotulinumtoxin (Xeomin®) – are produced from different strains of bacteria, purified using different methods, and therefore they have distinct properties; however, the toxins are all derived from the BoNTA molecule, which is a polypeptide with a light and a heavy chain activated by "nicking' at the junction of the disulfide bond. The BoNTA cleaves SNAP-25 (synaptosomal associated protein, 25 kDa), blocking the neuromuscular junctions, thus interrupting neurotransmission of acetylcholine [5].

The units of Azzalure/Dysport and Vistable/Botox are not interchangeable, as different bioassays were used for measuring their activities [6, 7]. Azzalure and Dysport are quantified in Speywood Units (s.U.) and are therefore collectively referred to as BoNTA (Speywood Unit) [8]. It is important to understand this concept as the assays used to compare these products unit by unit are not reliable, thus putting question into most direct comparisons of other products. This includes efficacy and safety as these are directly related to dosage and dilution.

The BoNTA (Speywood unit) toxin exists as a complex with a surrounding coat of protective proteins: the hemagglutinin and nontoxin nonhemagglutinin proteins. The surrounding complex protein can serve to protect the neurotoxin from its potential destruction by the low pH of stomach acid. On absorption as the pH becomes physiologic, the outer protein coat releases the neurotoxin [9]. Similarly, the full complex found in the vial prior to injection (750 or 900 kDa) dissociates upon injection to the naked 150 kDa neurotoxin molecule [10].

Though both the Botox and Dysport neurotoxin molecules are the same weight (150 kDa), the complexes are different sizes due to variations in production. Botox is 900 kDa and Dysport is approximately 750 kDa [11]. The influence of the complexes once injected is unknown, especially since dissociation occurs at physiologic pH. Questions concerning field of effect, diffusion, and onset of action of each toxin are not fully answered. We do know that each has different units of potency (Botox units versus Dysport units) and this has a major impact on its clinical significance.

Technical differences in the two products are less than the similarities. The complex size is as follows:

1. OnabotulinumtoxinA: 900 kDa
2. AbobotulinumtoxinA: 500–700 kDa

Thus, the relevance of the accessory proteins as well as the molecular weight is under question [10]. Other differences are in the composition of the product, which is summarized in Table 5.1. Protein content is slightly greater in onabotulinumtoxinA with more serum albumin, but the carriers – NaCl and lactose – do differ; it is unknown if this makes a clinical difference. Note that dissociation of the 150 kDa molecule from its accessory proteins does occur rapidly, in the vial

Table 5.1 Constituents of botulinum toxin.

	Dysport [4]	Botox cosmetic [3]
Vial size	300 U	100 U[a]
Composition	*Clostridium botulinum* toxin type A hemagglutinin complex	*Clostridium botulinum* toxin type A hemagglutinin complex
	125 µg (0.125 mg) human serum albumin	500 µg (0.5 mg) human serum albumin
	2.5 mg lactose	0.9 mg sodium chloride
Molecular weight (neurotoxin)	150 kDa	150 kDa
Bulk active substance (total protein content)	~3 ng	~5 ng
Storage (post-reconstitution)	2–8°C/until vial expiration (2–8°C / use within 4 h)	2–8°C / 36 months (2–8°C / use within 4 h)

[a]BOTOX Cosmetic is also available in a 50 U vial. The 100 U vial is referenced in this comparison.

with reconstitution or in the needle prior to injection, but definitely upon injection when pH returns to physiologic status. Eisele has shown that this takes place in less than a minute [12]. This gives further evidence that molecular weights of the different toxins do not influence their behavior *in vivo*. The argument that spread or diffusion is based on molecular weight of the toxin is thus not relevant.

Aesthetic studies for abobotulinumtoxin (Dysport) followed a similar pattern as those performed for Botox by Carruthers and Carruthers a few years earlier. The first European studies for aesthetic usage of Dysport were performed by Ascher in the later 1990s and again by Ascher and Rzany in 2004 and 2006 [13]. A "dose-finding" study was first performed on 119 patients using placebo, 25, 50 and 75 U in a double-blinded control. The subjects were measured for efficacy as a responder at 1 month and then assessed for safety and duration. A responder rate of over 80% was found for all three groups, and at 6 months two-thirds of the treated patients were still responders. There was a favorable safety profile of 7% mild adverse events, with headache the most common. There were no reported cases of blepharoptosis or a diplopia. The result suggested 50 Speywood units was the optimal dosage for the glabella with 10 units injected into each of five glabellar sites [14].

This was followed by the US studies beginning in 2003 and extending to the present. The Inamed, Ipsen and Medicis studies included phase II, phase III single and repeat dosage studies with a total of 2,300 patients assessed for efficacy and safety. All studies evaluated efficacy and safety of glabellar frown lines with rating scales at rest and at maximal frown. The US studies used the same injection points as the US onabotulinumtoxinA trials and were evaluated at maximal frown as its end points. In Europe, end points for response were determined at rest for efficacy and the lateral corrugator injection points were placed 0.5 cm more medial; however, the results for efficacy and safety for both studies were similar.

Phase II trials involved a dosage-ranging study including placebo, 20, 50 and 75 U. There was a 90% responder rate at both 50 U and 75 U. All doses were well tolerated with only minor side effects including headache, needle pricks, and bruising. Blepharoptosis was observed in only three patients, of which only one demonstrated to the investigator a true clinical ptosis. Ptosis had been reported in other product studies but not in other studies involving abobotulinumtoxinA [15].

Antibody production has always been of concern with clinical usage of BoNTA, but has only been studied with cervical dystonia [16]. None of the patients in this study showed any evidence of neutralizing antibodies either at baseline or on follow-up evaluations. From these observations, the 50 U dosage was recommended as the optimal dose for safety and efficacy. The lower dosage of 50 U was chosen for all of the phase III trials [17].

The initial single-dosage, placebo-controlled, double-blinded, randomized trial of glabellar frown lines for FDA Phase III included over 400 subjects followed for 150 days [18]. The patients were then enrolled in a repeat dosage trial for 23 months including four cycles of repeat dosage when the patient's frown lines returned to baseline. The patients were evaluated for efficacy (i.e., number of responders at 30 days and duration of response) and safety. Over 90% responder rate was recorded at 30 days, with duration at 4 months of 40% responders and at 5 months 25% were still full responders [19]. This produced a very similar efficacy case for responders and duration as onabotulinumtoxinA.

One factor reported by the subjects was an onset of action within 1–2 days. Subsequent studies have included a diary that the patient recorded when an onset of effect was first noted. In three of the studies the onset was recorded: 50% of subjects noted an onset within 2 days and 80% noted it within 3 days [20]. Onset studies were to follow with onabotulinumtoxinA and incobotulinumtoxinA toxins which were performed in a similar manner and with results that were comparable. Re-injection treatment studies were performed to ensure that repeated exposure to the toxin did not influence efficacy or duration.

The repeat administration studies involved 768 individuals from phase III clinical trials who received up to six repeated treatments over 17 months. A patient was reinjected when glabellar wrinkle lines returned to baseline. The patients were followed for efficacy and safety including adverse effects and assessment of serum-neutralizing antibodies to abobotulinumtoxinA. Results confirmed continued effectiveness throughout the study with no increase of active events and no patients developed neutralizing antibodies.

The possibility of blocking antibodies influencing efficacy and toxin action has been noted with large therapeutic doses given over years for treatment of spastic torticolis and cerebral palsy. Antibody blocking effect, as of this time, has not been recorded with the cosmetic use of abobotulinumtoxinA [21].

As the data of these initial trials were reviewed, it was noted that efficacy and duration of action for men was less than that for women on a 50 U dosage for treating the glabella. This observation stimulated a variable-dose study which stratified patients by race/ethnicity, sex, and randomized by muscle mass. The muscle mass groups were to receive a single treatment of various doses of abobotulinumtoxinA. AbobotulinumtoxinA was administered as a single dose of 50, 60 or 70 U for women and 60, 70, or 80 U for men based on glabellar muscle mass. This is based on procerus/corrugator muscle mass, small, medium or large. This was determined by the observation of an active frown, noted individual muscle bulging, length of the infrabrow space, and brow depression. Efficacy and duration was evaluated during a 5 month period. The results indicated that 87% of men and women had full efficacy at 30 days with a mean duration of 109 days for both men and women with no difference in ethnicity or gender [22]. Duration of action was found to be increased with the greater doses for larger muscle mass.

Though clinicians have individualized abobotulinumtoxinA glabellar treatment for sex, ethnicity, and muscle mass in clinical practice, this was the first controlled clinical study to verify this common practice.

Dysport was first licensed for medical usage in Europe in 1990. Clinical studies for aesthetic indications were first performed in Europe in 2002 and 2003, followed by US FDA studies in 2009. FDA approval for treatment of glabellar frown lines occurred May 2009. Table 5.2 summarizes the differences between the two formulations of BoNTA. While variations in progenitor complex size as described earlier may exist and the excipients differ, it must be stressed that the "active" ingredient is thought to be identical and as such the clinical properties of the two agents are largely similar. Purported variations in clinical behavior are likely to be subtle when controlled for volume, toxin concentration, and injection technique.

The most important difference between onabotulinumtoxinA and abobotulinumtoxinA is in the activity units employed by their respective manufacturers: Botox units (b.U.) for onabotulinumtoxinA and Speywood units (s.U.) for abobotulinumtoxinA. Both define one unit as the quantity necessary to kill 50% of mice (LD50) with an intraperitoneal injection. Because of differences in the experimental design of their murine assays, however, the units are not equivalent. The Dysport assay is undeniably more sensitive, that is, less toxin is required to kill a mouse when toxin of any formulation is tested in this assay versus the Botox assay [23]. Indeed, in a small study it was shown that, when tested in the Dysport assay, the LD50 of Botox is achieved with 0.32 b.U. (68% less product than that required for LD50 in the Botox assay) [23]. Therefore, a Speywood unit corresponds to a smaller quantity of active toxin than does a Botox

Table 5.2 Overview of product composition for the FDA approved Botulinum toxin serotype A agents. IncobotulinumtoxinA (Xeomin) is only approved for therapeutic use [35–40].

Product	Botox	Dysport	Xeomin
Manufacturer	Ipsen (Europe) Medicis (USA)	Allergan	Merz Pharmaceuticals
Units per vial	100 b.U.	300 s.U. (for cosmetic use)	50 or 100 U
Active ingredient (molecular weight)	Botulinum toxin serotype A complex (900 kDa)	Botulinum toxin serotype A complex (500–900 kDa)^a	Uncomplexed Botulinum toxin serotype A (150 kDa)
Total toxin protein per vial (active toxin + NAPs^b)	5 ng	2.61 ng	0.6 ng (in 100 U)
Excipients	Human serum albumin 500 µg NaCl 0.9 mg	Human serum albumin 125 µg Lactose 2.5 mg	Human serum albumin 1 mg Sucrose 4.7 mg
Bacterial source	*Clostridium botulinum,* Hall strain^c	*Clostridium botulinum,* Hall strain^c	*Clostridium botulinum,* Hall strain^c
Storage conditions	2–8°C	2–8°C	Up to 25°C
Purification process	Dialysis and acid precipitation then vacuum dried	Column chromatography then freeze-dried (lyophilized)	Column chromatography then freeze-dried (lyophilized)

^{a}Molecular weight of AboA is not firmly established –See discussion in text.
^{b}Neurotoxin-associated proteins
^{c}There are numerous "Hall strains" and the manufacturers do not necessarily use identical bacteria.

unit. The exact potency ratio between s.U. and b.U. remains an open question. Since, in any competitive marketplace, product interchangeability is not a desirable attribute, the BoNTA manufacturers have predictably emphasized the uniqueness of their formulations and have discouraged the use of any unit conversion factors. Nevertheless, practitioners have sought to define a conversion factor to guide the novice injector when transitioning from one toxin to the other for a given application.

Numerous *in vivo* and *in vitro* studies have attempted to define this conversion factor with conflicting results. For a comprehensive review of this literature, please refer to the recently published review by Karsai *et al.* [24]. Only a brief summary of the pertinent human studies follows. A 2004 meta-analysis, using Cochrane review methodology,

identified four high-quality comparative clinical studies all examining neurologic indications, two employed a 1:4 (OnaA:AboA) dose ratio, one a 1:3 ratio, and the last used 1:3 and 1:4 in separate arms [25]. This analysis concluded that a 1:4 ratio was too high, and a 1:3 ratio approached bioequivalence although the included studies suggested that an even lower ratio might be more appropriate. An independently funded, double-blind study of Dysport versus Botox for the treatment of glabellar lines found a longer duration of action as assessed by electromyographic studies with Dysport used at a 1:3 ratio. This led the authors to conclude that the bioequivalent ratio was less than 1:3 [26]. Lowe *et al.* examined the relative effects of a 1:2.5 dose ratio on glabellar lines assessed by blinded investigator rating and found greater longevity with Botox [27]. Therefore, while the preponderance of current evidence supports a dose ratio of no more than 1 : 3, a more precise definition awaits additional controlled, head-to-head comparisons with ideally objective measurements of muscle activity. The authors recommend a conversion factor of 1 : 2.5, which has become the most commonly quoted unit dose ratio among experienced injectors. The multiple studies that underpinned the FDA approved dosages for glabellar lines (50 s.U. of Dysport and 20 b.U. of Botox) demonstrated comparable efficacy with the two BoNTA products, further supporting the 1 : 2.5 ratio as a starting point for cosmetic applications.

The perception that an increased capacity for a toxin to diffuse from the site of injection translates into increased side effects has encouraged a lively debate among the manufacturers of the BoNTA products. The question of diffusion has mostly been investigated in humans by measuring anhidrotic haloes after injecting equal volumes of each agent into the forehead. Some comparative studies of Botox and Dysport have demonstrated that anhidrotic haloes are significantly larger for Dysport [28, 29]. The only double-blind randomized study utilized a Botox : Dysport unit ratio of 1 : 3, and one could argue that the increased anhidrotic haloes observed in this study with Dysport is a consequence of not using equipotent dosages. In other words, diffusion is primarily driven by concentration gradients, and it would be expected that a higher injected concentration of neurotoxin would result in greater diffusion. In an unblinded study, Trindade De Almeida *et al.* [29] examined three different dose ratios: 1 : 2.5, 1 : 3, and 1 : 4. They found significantly increased anhidrotic haloes with all dose ratios (the mean absolute increase in area of the anhidrotic halo was 1.2 cm^2 with the lowest Dysport dosage). These results were challenged by a similarly designed comparative trial conducted by Hexsel *et al.* which found no significant difference in the field of anhidrosis using only the more widely accepted equipotent dose ratio of 1 : 2.5 [30]. Hexsel *et al.* reported taking great care to

standardize injection technique, which would certainly influence results. Of note, the first two described studies [28,29] were sponsored by Allergan and the third [30] by Ipsen. A definitive answer to this question will await an impartial, double-blind study comparing truly equipotent injections of neurotoxins.

In conclusion, it must be emphasized that subtle differences in the properties of the BoNTA formulations may exist. Extant data on product composition, diffusion properties, and relative clinical potencies remains inconclusive. Indeed, the number and types of NAPs probably differ between BoNTA products. NAPs have known biologic relevance in the pathogenesis of food-borne botulism [31]. One recent study demonstrated that a hemagglutinin protein binds E-cadherin to facilitate passage of toxin through epithelial tight junctions within the alimentary canal [32]. This raises the unexplored and previously discounted possibility that NAPs could have other specific biologic functions, some of which might impinge on the neuromuscular activity of injected BoNTA. Until we possess a better understanding of these various issues, the injector is advised to think and treat independently with each BoNTA product – as one learns a foreign language – and avoid converting for usage.

AbobotulinumtoxinA has been used worldwide for aesthetic needs for over 10 years. Those clinicians who have the greatest experience have defined injection points, minimal dosage, and a range of doses for each of the facial areas.

Both glabella and crow's feet have been well studied by Asher with results comparable to onabotulinumtoxinA [33]. Forehead, eyebrows and full upper face are successfully treated with abobotulinumtoxinA in a similar fashion to onabotulinumtoxinA.

AbobotulinumtoxinA has been used in clinical cosmetic practice worldwide over the past decade with similar injection points and techniques as onabotulinumtoxinA, but with different dosages. A full understanding of anatomy and product effect on distinctive facial muscles is essential for ensuring optimal treatment results and should be acquired through proper training. Since there are only a few clinical studies concerning off-label indications, one of the original consensus conferences was held in Paris in January, 2009, which provided general guidelines for effective and safe use of abobotulinumtoxinA on the generally useful yet off-label sites for injection. This focused on the European experience and served as one of the initial guides for therapy in the United States. These have included the common upper face sites – the glabella, forehead, brow, crows' feet, and eyelid – and other less common facial sites including bunny lines, depressor angularis oris, obicularis oris, mentalis, and platysma. These recommendations gave guidelines to starting dosage and range for each site as well as injection points and technique.

On January 12–13, 2009, an International Board of Botulinum Toxin was assembled in Paris to develop a consensus of dosage recommendation for the use of abobotulinumtoxin. The following physicians were part of the board giving a consensus of recommendations for common treatment sites.

The site-specific recommendations were given as shown in Table 5.3.

Treatment of the Upper Face

Glabellar lines

Injection of the glabella is the original and by far most common cosmetic usage of BoNTA. Numerous randomized, placebo-controlled trials have demonstrated the efficacy of abobotulinumtoxinA for this indication.

The standard five-injection point approach is appropriate for most patients with two

Table 5.3 Recommended Dysport® dosage for upper face.

Indications	Total usual dose (Dysport® units)	Dose range (Dysport® units)
Glabella	50	30–70
Forehead	40–50	40–70
Crows' feet	30×2	$20–50 \times 2$
Lateral eyebrow lift	20×2	$20–40 \times 2$
Glabella & forehead	90–100	70–140
Glabella & lateral eyebrow lift	90	50–110
Complete upper third face	150	110–240

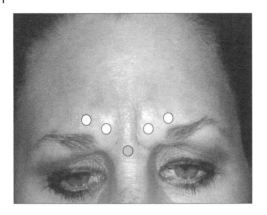

Figure 5.1 Injection sites for glabellar line treatment. Blue dots, corrugator insertion/orbicularis oculi fibers; yellow dots, corrugator body; green dot, procerus.

injections in each corrugator and one injection in the procerus as shown in Figure 5.1. The procerus and medial corrugators are injected deeply and directly into the bodies of the muscles, which are easily identified at maximal frown in most patients. The lateral corrugator is injected slightly more superficially where it inserts into the dermis and medial to the midpupillary line. These lateral injections also target fibers of the orbicularis oculi. All injections should be 1.0 cm (approximately one finger's breadth) above the orbital rim to limit the risk of eyelid ptosis from the spread of toxin to the levator palpebrae muscle. The measurement should be made from the orbital rim and from the brow itself as a dropped brow may mislead the physician to inject the toxin below the orbital rim. This can cause toxin penetration through the orbital septum and weaken the levator muscle. Injecting too high on the forehead – above 1 cm at the lateral glabellar site – can also cause ptosis in those individuals who recruit eyelid elevation from the frontalis muscle.

The on-label total dose of abobotulinumtoxinA is 50 s.U., divided evenly among the five injections, in women and those with small to medium muscle mass with moderate frown. As always, doses must be adjusted for the strength of individual muscles and the

patient's desired outcome. The authors do use a higher dose of toxin in men and may add two additional injection points at the midpupillary line in patients with bulky corrugators; however, we rarely exceed a total dose of 80 s.U. in any patient.

In the initial clinical trials with abobotulinumtoxinA, men did not have as robust a response to the 50 s.U. dose as did women, presumably due to increased muscle mass. This inspired a further study which varied abobotulinumtoxinA dosage with corrugator/procerus volume. Men with mild frown (small muscle mass) received 60 s.U., moderate 70 s.U., and severe 80 s.U. Correlating the dose with muscle mass raised the response rate of men to that of women and increased the longevity of response in all subjects [34].

Forehead Lines

Although an off-label usage, BoNTA provides excellent smoothing of forehead rhytides and is, in general, a very gratifying procedure for patients when performed properly. However, the more severe forms of forehead wrinkles cannot be corrected by BoNTA denervation alone and may need soft tissue augmentation.

The goal for the treatment of forehead wrinkles is to soften the undesirable lines without causing brow ptosis or eliminating all expressiveness on the upper face. A conservative approach is preferred, informing the patient preoperatively that more than one treatment may be needed to reach the desired level of wrinkle reduction while avoiding undesirable side effects. The patient is asked to forcefully raise his/her eyebrows and the strength of the frontalis is assessed. Any discrepancy in brow position at baseline and at maximal contraction is noted and brought to the attention of the patient. It is especially important to note brow asymmetry, photograph it and bring it to the patient's attention prior to treatment. Using appropriate doses, it can be corrected by using appropriate forehead dosage and injection points. A compensatory downward dose adjustment should be made on the side with the "higher" eyebrow.

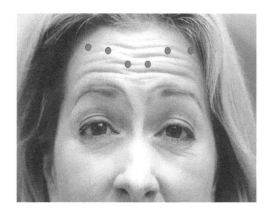

Figure 5.2 Forehead line treatment in women. Variation favored by authors to accentuate the lateral arching of the feminine brow pattern.

In the "average" brow, 5–10 s.U. are injected in four to six sites at least 2.5–3.0 cm above the orbital rim. Administration more inferiorly greatly increases the risk of brow ptosis as can be seen with onabotulinumtoxin.

The authors commonly use a V-shaped configuration for injections in women (Figure 5.2). While often desirable in females, this should be avoided in male patients. This approach can also produce an excessively arched brow (the mephisto sign or "Dr. Spock look"). This is prevented with a high lateral forehead injection above the tail of the brow. If an excessive arched brow occurs, it

can be corrected with a small dose of additional toxin 1–2 cm superior to the apex of the arched brow.

Unless no significant glabellar lines are present, the authors commonly inject the glabella simultaneously whenever treating forehead wrinkles. This generally produces better overall aesthetic results and the concomitant paralysis of the brow depressors reduces the incidence of brow ptosis.

Lateral Eyebrow Lift

The paresis of muscles of facial expression not only smooths dynamic wrinkles but can also influence the resting position of various facial elements. This property has been successfully exploited to lift the eyebrow, correcting mild brow ptosis, restoring a youthful brow arch, and giving the eye a more "open" appearance.

The vertical fibers of the lateral orbicularis oculi function to depress the lateral brow. For this chemical brow lift, the authors typically inject 5 U of onabotulinumtoxinA or 10 U of abobotulinumtoxinA intradermally at the lateral tail of the eyebrow 5–7 mm superolateral to the orbital rim (Figure 5.3a). If performed only for brow lift and not to correct frown lines, an additional injection into each

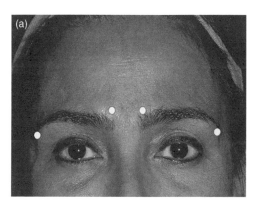
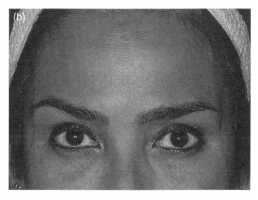

Figure 5.3 The chemical brow lift: (a) Injection sites for a chemical brow lift if performed alone are shown (5–10 s.U. or 3–5 b.U. per injection site). This patient had a male pattern eyebrow without perceptible arching. She received abobotulinumtoxinA treatment to the lateral tail of each eyebrow (10 s.U. per side), into the corrugators bodies (total 20 s.U.), and to the frontalis (20 s.U.). (b) Posttreatment photo at 33 days reveals an elevated and laterally arched feminine brow.

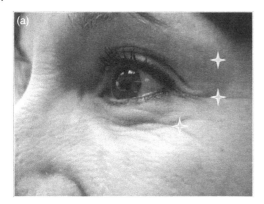 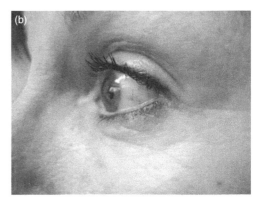

Figure 5.4 Crow's feet injection. (a) Standard three point crow's feet injection. (b) This patient received 5 b.U. at each point and had an excellent response.

corrugator body is typically added to complete the chemical brow lift. More commonly, the lateral brow lift injection is carried out in tandem with other upper face treatments, especially injection of the glabellar complex and forehead. In combination with medial and central frontalis denervation, which tends to lower the medial brow, a pleasingly arched female pattern eyebrow can be shaped (Figure 5.3b).

Crow's Feet

Lateral perioribital wrinkling is one of the earliest signs of aging. Hyperkinetic lateral canthal lines are effectively treated with neurotoxin.

Crow's feet are typically treated with three equal injections of 10–15 s.U. evenly spaced along an arc lying at least 1 cm external to the orbital rim to avoid diffusion to the palpebral portion of the orbicularis oculi or to the levator palpebrae muscle (Figure 5.4a,b). The middle injection is placed in line with the lateral canthus. Injections flanking this point at 8–10 mm are then placed, but their exact positioning depends on the width of the individual's canthal lines. The highest crow's feet injection is inferior to the lateral eyebrow tail injection described earlier for a chemical brow lift.

An additional injection of 2 s.U. microinjections can be judiciously placed in the lower lid at the midpupillary line 2 mm below the tarsal plate (Figure 5.5). This will flatten the bulging muscle and create an image of an "open eye." Overaggressive treatment may, though, create an unwanted ectropion.

Treatment of the Lower Face

Treatment of the lower face should be performed with more precaution as overdosage leads to significant dysfunction of the obicularis oris, creating an asymmetric smile and oral aperture. I would also recommend the more concentrated dilution of 1.5 cm^3 saline per 300 U vial to titrate, the toxin for

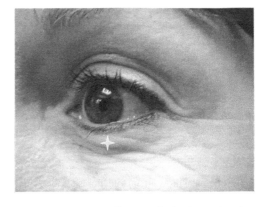

Figure 5.5 Location of lower palpebral injection. A tiny dose of toxin into the lower eyelid can create a more youthful "open" eye (2 s.U. or 0.5–1 b.U.).

Table 5.4 Recommended Dysport® dosage for lower face.

Indications	Total usual dose (Dysport® units)	Dose range (Dysport® units)
Obicularis oris	2.5 per injection point	10–15 total
Depressor angularis oris	5–10 per site	10–20
Mentalis	5–10 per site	10–20
Platysma	5–10 per injection point	20–40
		Maximum total dosage 50/side

contouring within appropriated muscles. Dosage recommendations in the lower face are given in Table 5.4.

As with onabotulinumtoxinA treatment, the physician must have a thorough understanding of facial musculature and the balance between elevator and depressor muscles. It is especially important in the lower face to be familiar with the anatomy and function of the facial muscles. Injections in or near many perioral muscles can cause facial asymmetry with expression. Because the field of effect is influenced by volume, the 1.5 cm^3 dilution is recommended to limit abobotulinumtoxinA effect to the muscles injected.

AbobotulinumtoxinA can be used for elevation of the oral commissure by injecting the depressor angularis oris (DAO) with 10 DUs or units of abobotulinumtoxinA. The mentalis can be treated with 10 U to suppress chin dimpling. Care is taken to keep both injections away from the depressor labialis inferioris. Platysma injections for bands use 5 DUs or units of abobotulinumtoxinA per injection with a total of 20 U per band. This is a superficial injection spaced out at 1-cm intervals along the platysmal band.

As aesthetic physicians have become familiar with this second botulinum toxin and now a third botulinum toxin product in the US, new innovations and techniques have evolved, and new and interesting data have emerged. It is with the large usage numbers that we gain a further understanding of both efficacy and safety.

References

1 Schantz EJ, Johnson EA. Botulinum toxin: the story of its development for the treatment of human disease. Perspect Biol Med 1997 Spring;40(3):317–327.

2 Carruthers JA, Lowe NJ, Menter MA, et al. BOTOX Glabellar Lines I Study Group. A multicenter, double-blind, randomized, placebo-controlled study of the efficacy and safety of botulinum toxin type A in the treatment of glabellar lines. J Am Acad Dermatol 2002 Jun;46(6):840–849.

3 Botox Cosmetic [package insert]. Irvine, Ca: Allergan, Inc; 2008.

4 Dysport [package insert]. Scottsdale, AZ: Medicis Aesthetics Inc; 2009.

5 Simpson LL. Peripheral Actions of the Botulinum Toxins. In LL Simpson (ed.) Botulinum Neurotoxin and Tetanus Toxin. San Diego, CA: Academic Press, 1989: 153–178.

6 Pickett AM, Hambleton P. Dose standardization of botulinum toxin. Lancet 1994; 344:474–475.

7 Karsai S, Raulin C. Current evidence on the unit equivalence of different botulinum neurotoxin A formulations and recommendations for clinical practice in Dermatology. Dermatol Surg 2008;34:1–8.

8 Ascher B, Talarico S, Cassuto D, et al. International consensus recommendations

on the aesthetic usage of botulinum toxin type A (Speywood Unit)—Part II: Wrinkles on the middle and lower face, neck and chest. J Eur Acad Dermatol Venereol 2010 Nov;24(11):1285–1295.

9 Eisele KH, Taylor HV. Dissociation of the 900 kDa neurotoxin complex from c. botulinum under physiological conditions. Poster presented at: Toxins 2008; June 12–14, 2008; Baveno, Lake Maggiore, Italy.

10 Pickett A. Diffusion of Type A Botulinum Toxin. Presented at the International Masters Course on Aging Skin; January 8–11, 2009. Paris, France.

11 Hasegawa K, Watanabe T, Suzuki T, et al. A novel subunit structure of clostridium botulinum serotype D toxin complex with three extended arms. J Biol Chem 2007;282(34):24777–24783.

12 Eisele KH, Fink K, Vey M, Taylor HV. Studies on the dissociation of botulinum neurotoxin type A complexes. Toxicon 2011 Mar 15;57(4):555–565.

13 Ascher B, Zakine B, Kestemont P, et al. A multicenter, randomized, double-blind, placebo-controlled study of efficacy and safety of 3 doses of botulinum toxin type A in the treatment of glabellar lines. J Am Acad Dermatol 2004;51(2):223–233.

14 Vandenbergh PYK, Lison DF. Dose standardization of botulinum toxin. Adv Neurol 1998;78:231–235.

15 Kessler KR, Skutta M, Benecke R. Long-term treatment of cervical dystonia with botulinum toxin A: efficacy, safety, and antibody frequency. German Dystonia Study Group. J Neurol 1999 Apr;246(4):265–274.

16 Carruthers J, Lowe NJ, Mentor MA, Gibson J. Double-blind placebo-controlled study of the safety and efficacy of Botulinum toxin type A for patients with glabellar lines. Plastic Reconstr Surg 2003;112:1089–1098.

17 Monheit G, Carruthers A, Brandt F, Rand R. A Randomized, double blind, placebo controlled study of botulinum toxin A for the treatment of glabellar lines: Determination of optimal dose. Dermatol Surg 2007 January;33:51–59.

18 Carruthers J, Fagien S, Matarasso SL. Consensus recommendations on the use of botulinum toxin type A in facial aesthetics. Plast Reconstr Surg 2004;114 (Suppl 1): S1–S22.

19 Ascher B, Rzany BJ, Grover R. Efficacy and safety of botulinum toxin type A in the treatment of lateral crow's feet: double-blind, placebo-controlled, dose-ranging study. Dermatol Surg 2009;35:1478–1486.

20 Monheit G, Cohen J, Reloxin Investigational Group. Long-term safety of repeated administration of a new formulation of botulinum toxin type A in the treatment of glabellar lines: Interim analysis from an open-label extension study. J Am Acad Derm 2009 Sept;61(3): 421–425.

21 Rubin M, Dover J, Glogau R, et al. The efficacy and safety of a new US botulinum toxin type A in the retreatment of glabellar lines following open-label treatment. J Drugs Dermatol 2009;8(5):439–444.

22 Kane MA, Brandt F, Rohrich RJ, et al.; Reloxin Investigational Group. Evaluation of variable-dose treatment with a new U.S. Botulinum Toxin Type A (Dysport) for correction of moderate to severe glabellar lines: results from a phase III, randomized, double-blind, placebo-controlled study. Plast Reconstr Surg 2009 Nov;124(5): 1619–1629. doi: 10.1097/PRS .0b013e3181b5641b.

23 Hambleton P, Pickett AM. Potency equivalence of botulinum toxin preparations. J R Soc Med 1994 Nov;87(11):719.

24 Karsai S, Raulin C. Current evidence on the unit equivalence of different botulinum neurotoxin A formulations and recommendations for clinical practice in dermatology. Dermatol Surg 2009;35(1): 1–8.

25 Sampaio C, Costa J, Ferreira JJ. Clinical comparability of marketed formulations of botulinum toxin. Mov Disord 2004 Mar;19 Suppl 8:S129–S136.

26 Karsai S, Adrian R, Hammes S, et al. A randomized double-blind study of the

effect of Botox and Dysport/Reloxin on forehead wrinkles and electromyographic activity. Arch Dermatol 2007 Nov;143(11):1447–1449.

27 Lowe P, Patnaik R, Lowe N. Comparison of two formulations of botulinum toxin type A for the treatment of glabellar lines: A double-blind, randomized study. J Am Acad Dermatol 2006;55(6):975–980.

28 Cliff SH, Judodihardjo H, Eltringham E. Different formulations of botulinum toxin type A have different migration characteristics: a double-blind, randomized study. J Cosmet Dermatol. 2008;7(1):50–54.

29 Trindade De Almeida AR, Marques E, et al. Pilot study comparing the diffusion of two formulations of botulinum toxin type A in patients with forehead hyperhidrosis. Dermatol Surg 2007;33:S37–S43.

30 Hexsel D, Dal'Forno T, Hexsel C, et al. A randomized pilot study comparing the action halos of two commercial preparations of botulinum toxin type A. Dermatol Surg 2008;34(1):52–59.

31 Sugawara Y, Fujinaga Y. The botulinum toxin complex meets E-cadherin on the way to its destination. Cell Adh Migr 2011 Jan 8;5(1).

32 Sugawara Y, Matsumura T, Takegahara Y, et al. Botulinum hemagglutinin disrupts the intercellular epithelial barrier by directly binding E-cadherin. J Cell Biol 2010 May 17;189(4):691–700.

33 Ascher B, Zakine B, Kestemont P, et al. A multicenter, randomized, double-blind, placebo-controlled study of efficacy and safety of 3 doses of botulinum toxin type A in the treatment of glabellar lines. J Am Acad Dermatol 2004;51(2):223–233.

34 Kane MA, Brandt F, Rohrich RJ, et al. Evaluation of variable-dose treatment with a new U.S. Botulinum Toxin Type A (Dysport) for correction of moderate to severe glabellar lines: results from a phase III, randomized, double-blind, placebo-controlled study. Plast Reconstr Surg 2009 Nov;124(5):1619–1629.

35 Dysport [package insert]. Scottsdale, Arizona: Medicis Aesthetics Inc.; 2009.

36 Wortzman MS, Pickett A. The science and manufacturing behind botulinum neurotoxin type A-ABO in clinical use. Aesth Surg J 2009;29(6, Suppl 1): S34–S42.

37 Pickett A, Perrow K. Formulation composition of botulinum toxins in clinical use. J Drugs Dermatol 2010 Sep;9(9):1085–1091.

38 Botox cosmetic [package insert]. Irvine, CA: Allergan, Inc; 2002.

39 Xeomin cosmetic [package insert]. Frankfurt, Germany. Merz Pharmaceuticals; 2010.

40 Carruthers A, Carruthers J. Botulinum toxin products overview. Skin Ther Lett 2008 Jul–Aug;13(6):1–4.

6

IncobotulinumtoxinA (Xeomin®/Bocouture®)

Ulrich Kühne, MD (DALM) and Matthias Imhof, MD (DALM)

Board Certified Dermatologist and Allergologist, Aesthetische Dermatologie im Medico Palais, Bad Soden, Germany

Introduction

IncobotulinumtoxinA (Merz Pharmaceuticals GmbH, Germany) is a botulinum neurotoxin type A (BoNTA) preparation, which represents a new development in the rapidly expanding field of botulinum toxin therapies. In contrast to other commercially available preparations, incobotulinumtoxinA is free from complexing proteins. It has shown good efficacy and tolerability in a range of therapeutic and aesthetic applications. It is approved for the treatment of blepharospasm, post-stroke upper-limb spasticity, and cervical dystonia in several countries under the trade name Xeomin® or Xeomeen®. It also received approval in August 2010 from the Food and Drugs Administration (FDA) for treatment of blepharospasm and cervical dystonia in the United States of America. In the aesthetic setting, incobotulinumtoxinA is currently licensed for use in the treatment of glabellar frown lines, lateral periorbital lines (crow's feet) and upper facial lines in Europe under the trade name Bocouture®. The indication glabellar frown lines alone is approved in the USA and Canada as well as in several other countries in Latin America and Asia.

This chapter includes a discussion of the pharmacological properties of incobo-tulinumtoxinA and how being free of complexing proteins could hold clinical relevance. The use of incobotulinumtoxinA in aesthetic applications is also discussed.

Manufacture and production of incobotulinumtoxinA

Free from complexing proteins

IncobotulinumtoxinA is produced from *Clostridium botulinum* type A, Hall strain, which is fermented under anaerobic conditions. This process yields the 150 kDa neurotoxin heavy and light chains, linked by a disulfide bridge, in the context of a large molecular weight complex containing other clostridial proteins. Thereafter, several purification steps are performed to remove nucleic acids, hemagglutinins, and other contaminants, to yield only the 150 kDa active neurotoxin free from complexing proteins (Figure 6.1). OnabotulinumtoxinA (Allergan, Irvine, CA, USA) is produced by repeated cycles of precipitation and redissolution, while abobotulinumtoxinA (Ipsen Ltd, Berkshire, UK) is produced by a column separation method of purification [1]. Both processes yield products with toxin complexes of different sizes [2].

Botulinum Toxins: Cosmetic and Clinical Applications, First Edition. Edited by Joel L. Cohen and David M. Ozog.
© 2017 John Wiley & Sons Ltd. Published 2017 by John Wiley & Sons Ltd.
Companion Website: www.wiley.com/go/cohen/botulinum

(a)

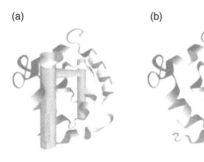

(b)

(c)

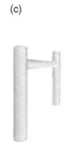

Figure 6.1 Most commercially available BoNTA preparations consist of the neurotoxin and associated complexing proteins (a). The manufacture of incobotulinumtoxinA removes the complexing proteins (b) to leave only the pure active neurotoxin (c) (reproduced with permission of Merz Pharmaceuticals GmbH).

Free from denatured or inactive neurotoxin

In addition to being free from complexing proteins, incobotulinumtoxinA contains the smallest amount of neurotoxin protein. Using rabbit and guinea pig antibodies raised against the 150 kDa neurotoxin purified from *C. botulinum* type A strain ATCC 3502 (Hall strain), a sensitive sandwich ELISA was performed to determine the mean concentration of the 150 kDa neurotoxin present in different batches of onabotulinumtoxinA, abobotulinumtoxinA and incobotulinumtoxinA [3]. The mean concentration was then used to calculate the biological activity (units, U) per ng of neurotoxin protein, which is a measure of the specific neurotoxin potency. The mean concentration of 150 kDa neurotoxin per 100 U was 0.73 ng for onabotulinumtoxinA, 0.65 ng for abobotulinumtoxinA, and 0.44 ng for incobotulinumtoxinA. The resulting specific potency was calculated to be 137, 154, and 227 g/ng for onabotulinumtoxinA, abobotulinumtoxinA, and incobotulinumtoxinA, respectively [3], showing that incobotulinumtoxinA had the highest specific neurotoxin activity. However, it should be noted that the units of abobotulinumtoxinA cannot be directly compared to the units of onabotulinumtoxinA and incobotulinumtoxinA and therefore an assessment of the amount of inactive neurotoxin in abobotulinumtoxinA, compared to onabotulinumtoxinA or incobotulinumtoxinA, cannot be made. The implication of these results, given

that clinical trials show similar efficacy of onabotulinumtoxinA and incobotulinumtoxinA when used at a 1 : 1 dose conversion ratio [4–6], is that the 0.44 ng neurotoxin per 100 U incobotulinumtoxinA has the same potency as the 0.73 ng neurotoxin per 100 U onabotulinumtoxinA, which suggests that onabotulinumtoxinA may contain a considerable amount of inactive or denatured neurotoxin. Any inactive neurotoxin present, while incapable of contributing to the therapeutic or aesthetic effect, could contribute to the stimulation of antibody production [3], which is discussed in detail later. It has been reported that the manufacturing process of incobotulinumtoxinA does not lead to denaturation or inactivation of the active toxin [3].

Implications of Being Free from Complexing Proteins and Inactive Neurotoxin in IncobotulinumtoxinA

In the past, it was suggested that the complexing proteins present in some commercially available formulations of BoNTA played a beneficial role in stabilizing the 150 kDa active neurotoxin and limiting its migration. While evidence suggests that the neurotoxin must remain within the 900 kDa complex to maintain its oral activity [7], when BoNTA preparations are used for therapeutic or cosmetic applications, complexing proteins are

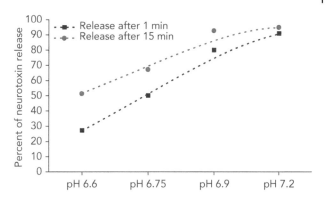

Figure 6.2 Dissociation of the neurotoxin from the complexing proteins occurs in less than a minute at physiological pH (reproduced with permission of Merz Pharmaceuticals GmbH).

Dissociation

The dissociation of the 150 kDa neurotoxin from complexing proteins has been studied by exposing the 900 kDa complex to various pH values prior to elution of the dissociated complex from a chromatographic matrix [8]. The eluted fractions were then analyzed by Western blotting and for toxin activity. At physiological pH, the 150 kDa neurotoxin dissociated from the 900 kDa complex in less than a minute (Figure 6.2). Considering that the dissociation is so rapid, the complexing proteins cannot stabilize the neurotoxin, nor limit its spread. These results call into question the necessity of the complexing proteins in BoNTA formulations used for therapeutic and cosmetic purposes.

Stability

The results described earlier suggest that complexing proteins play little or no role in stabilizing the neurotoxin after injection. Further experiments have shown that complexing proteins are also not required to stabilize the lyophilized neurotoxin during long-term storage at room temperature or short-term storage at temperatures above 40°C, prior to reconstitution [9–11]. IncobotulinumtoxinA was stored at temperatures up to 40°C with no significant reduction in the quality

of the product, as tested using standardized analytical methods for the batch-release testing of incobotulinumtoxinA. The results of these experiments have shown that incobotulinumtoxinA can be stored unopened at room temperature for 3 years [10,12,13]. Furthermore, no negative effects on the quality of incobotulinumtoxinA were detected following a temperature stress test, during which vials of incobotulinumtoxinA were stored at temperatures between 40°C and 60°C for up to 1 month [10]. The efficacy of freshly constituted and room-temperature-stored incobotulinumtoxinA has been compared in a split-face study in which 10 U was injected into the crow's feet of 21 subjects [11]. Over 4 months of follow-up, there was no statistically significant difference in either efficacy or longevity between the fresh and stored products. So not only are complexing proteins unnecessary to maintain the stability of the neurotoxin at room temperature and higher, but incobotulinumtoxinA can be stored without refrigeration, unlike other BoNTA preparations [14–16], a property that is of practical benefit to physicians.

Onset and duration of effect

The possibility that some BoNTA preparations contain denatured or inactive neurotoxin in addition to active neurotoxin may result in a slower onset of effect as these components may compete with the active neurotoxin for binding sites on the surface of nerve terminals at the neuromuscular junction. The onset and duration of effect of BoNTA preparations have been compared in a study of 180 subjects treated for glabellar frown lines who were randomized to treatment with incobotulinumtoxinA (21 U), onabotulinumtoxinA (21 U) or abobotulinumtoxinA (63 U) [17]. For both men and women, a significantly earlier time to onset of treatment effect as well as a longer duration of effect was seen for incobotulinumtoxinA compared with the other BoNTA preparations.

Neurotoxin spread

Migration of neurotoxin into untargeted muscles can cause unwanted effects and adverse events, especially in cosmetic applications of botulinum toxins where muscles are in close proximity [18]. The dissociation of active neurotoxin from the complexing proteins is very rapid at physiological pH, so the complexing proteins are unlikely to have an impact on the spread of the toxin [8], although this remains a controversial topic [19]. This is supported by studies demonstrating that the mean anhidrotic areas induced by preparations with complexing proteins compared with those without are not statistically significantly different sizes, indicating that the migratory potential of the neurotoxin is independent of the presence or absence of complexing proteins [20].

This is supported by data from a histological assessment of diffusion, which examined neural cell adhesion molecule (N-CAM) expression following injection of onabotulinumtoxinA, abobotulinumtoxinA, or incobotulinumtoxinA into the mouse leg [21]. N-CAM is expressed after denervation and therefore its appearance is an indication of BoNTA activity. All three products displayed modest diffusion into nearby muscles and abobotulinumtoxinA showed a wider spread than onabotulinumtoxinA or incobotulinumtoxinA [21]; however, the ratio of onabotulinumtoxinA: incobotulinumtoxinA: abobotulinumtoxinA used was 1:1:4. There is some evidence to suggest that this was too high for abobotulinumtoxinA and

could have accounted for the wider spread of abobotulinumtoxinA in this study. Varying conversion ratios could also explain the contradictory results concerning the relative spread of BoNTA preparations with complexing proteins seen in various other studies [22–26]. One study recommended using an onabotulinumtoxinA: abobotulinumtoxinA conversion ratio of not more than 1:2 [24], although a ratio of 1:2.5 is commonly used in clinical practice.

Several studies indicate that the absence of complexing proteins in incobotulinumtoxinA has no influence on the spread of neurotoxin to adjacent muscles. A double-blind, randomized, single-center trial in 32 healthy male volunteers measured the contraction of muscles adjacent to those targeted by injection after treatment with incobotulinumtoxinA and onabotulinumtoxinA in an intra-individual comparison design where equivalent doses of the toxins (either 2, 4, 16 or 32 Units) were injected into the extensor digitorum brevis (EDB) muscles of contralateral feet [27]. Local diffusion was assessed by measuring the compound muscle action potential (CMAP) M-wave amplitude in two muscles adjacent to the EDB – the abductor digiti quinti (ADQ) and the abductor hallucis (AH) muscle – 4 weeks postinjection relative to baseline. The results showed that, for all dose groups, the CMAP M-wave amplitude was more than 80% the baseline value in both ADQ and AH muscles at week 4 and all subsequent postinjection visits, despite a marked paretic effect on the injected EDB muscle. There were no statistically significant differences between the mean CMAP M-wave amplitudes obtained after incobotulinumtoxinA and onabotulinumtoxinA treatment in any dose group [27].

A comparison of incobotulinumtoxinA and abobotulinumtoxinA in the forehead of 80 subjects using a conversion ratio of 1.0:2.5 U found a larger field of anhidrotic effects with abobotulinumtoxinA, but similar results for fields of muscular effects [28].

The influence of injection volume on neurotoxin diffusion was investigated in a

onabotulinumtoxinA have been tested in product-specific mouse LD50 assays, leading to discussion of whether differences in potency may exist between the two products. Using the batch-release mouse LD50 assay for incobotulinumtoxinA, five unopened batches of incobotulinumtoxinA and onabotulinumtoxinA were compared. The results showed that the potencies of incobotulinumtoxinA (103.0 ± 5.7) and onabotulinumtoxinA (101.7 ± 6.2) were not statistically significantly different ($p = 0.734$) [44]. The authors concluded that the biological potencies of incobotulinumtoxinA and onabotulinumtoxinA are equivalent and that a $1:1$ dose conversion ratio is appropriate in clinical practice [44]. As required by governmental agencies, the LD50 assay is being replaced by more humane, cell-based assays, which must be cross-validated against the LD50 assay to provide the same potency result. Each manufacturer is developing their own proprietary cell-based assay [45, 46].

The dose conversion ratio established in the earlier biological potency study has been borne out in clinical studies published to date. A randomized, controlled phase I study compared the efficacy and tolerability of equal doses of incobotulinumtoxinA and onabotulinumtoxinA injected into the EDB muscle of 14 healthy volunteers [47]. Based on the EDB test, no statistically significant differences were found between incobotulinumtoxinA and onabotulinumtoxinA for time to onset of action, response rate, CMAP ratios, and tolerability [47]. The between-treatment comparison showed that incobotulinumtoxinA was at least as effective as onabotulinumtoxinA in paralyzing EDB muscle activity over the study period.

In comparative phase III studies in therapeutic indications using a $1:1$ dose conversion ratio of incobotulinumtoxinA : onabotulinumtoxinA, incobotulinumtoxinA demonstrated comparable efficacy and safety to onabotulinumtoxinA, further supporting the preclinical equipotency data. In a large, randomized, actively controlled study in 463 patients with cervical dystonia, the average improvement on the Toronto Western

Spasmodic Toricollis Rating Scale at day 28 posttreatment compared with baseline was −6.6 for incobotulinumtoxinA and −6.4 for onabotulinumtoxinA [4]. Similarly, in a double-blind phase III trial in 304 patients with blepharospasm comparing the effect of incobotulinumtoxinA with that of onabotulinumtoxinA, there were no statistically significant differences found between incobotulinumtoxinA and onabotulinumtoxinA for any efficacy or safety variable [5]. In aesthetics, the efficacy of incobotulinumtoxinA has been compared to that of onabotulinumtoxinA in several head-to-head trials using a $1:1$ dose conversion ratio and showed comparable efficacy [6, 48, 49].

A French consensus, based on a biological, bibliographic, and clinical analysis of incobotulinumtoxinA and onabotulinumtoxinA, concluded that the two toxins are clinically equivalent for efficacy and safety, and that a switch from one drug to the other can be made using a simple $1:1$ conversion ratio [50]. A German retrospective analysis of clinical practice also confirmed the results of prospective clinical trials by demonstrating that, in daily practice, incobotulinumtoxinA and onabotulinumtoxinA are used at a $1:1$ dose ratio and display comparable efficacy and safety [51]. A meta-analysis of clinical studies that directly compared incobotulinumtoxinA and onabotulinumtoxinA for aesthetic indications also concluded that there was no difference in relative potency of the two products [52]. In summary, evidence from clinical trials supports the preclinical data that incobotulinumtoxinA and onabotulinumtoxinA have equal biological potency and a $1:1$ dose conversion ratio is appropriate.

Aesthetic Applications of IncobotulinumtoxinA

Glabellar Frown Lines

IncobotulinumtoxinA was approved by The Federal Institute for Drugs and Medical

Devices (Bundesinstitut für Arzneimittel und Medizinprodukte [BfArM]) in 2009 for the temporary improvement in the appearance of moderate to severe glabellar lines seen at frown in adults <65 years, when the severity of these lines has an important psychological impact for the patient. The recommended injection volume is 0.1 ml (4 U) injected into each of five injection sites: two in each corrugator muscle and one in procerus muscle for a total dose of 20 U. FDA approval was received in July 2011 based on the results of two pivotal placebo-controlled trials that used the new more stringent FDA responder definition of an improvement of at least 2 points from baseline as assessed by both investigator and subject on separate 4-point scales. In both studies, the primary composite efficacy endpoint at maximum frown on Day 30 was achieved in a significantly higher number of patients treated with incobotulinumtoxinA (47.8% and 60.3%) than placebo, none of whom achieved the composite endpoint [53, 54]. To allow comparisons with earlier studies, a recent post hoc study has pooled the data from these two trials and analyzed them using the previous FDA responder definition: subject with at least a 1-point improvement on the Facial Wrinkle Scale (FWS). Responder rates were significantly greater for incobotulinumtoxinA than placebo at all follow-up visits ($p < 0.0001$) [55]. IncobotulinumtoxinA achieved a maximum responder rate of 93.1% at 30 days and a long duration of treatment effect: 45.7% of subjects showed efficacy at 4 months.

Various other placebo-controlled, open-label and head-to-head phase III studies have evaluated the efficacy and safety of incobotulinumtoxinA for the treatment of glabellar frown lines [6, 56–61].

In a head-to-head study that used unmatched doses of each product, the authors concluded that 20 U onabotulinumtoxinA was as effective as 30 U of incobotulinumtoxinA in reducing the severity of glabellar frown lines at 28 days postinjection, despite the 50% difference in unit doses administered [58]. Using a similar study

design, the reverse has also been shown to be true [59]. Active comparator should be given at the optimal dose. It had already been established and reflected in the SPCs that the correct starting dose for incobotulinumtoxinA (and onabotulinumtoxinA) in the treatment of moderate to severe glabellar frown lines is 20 U [12, 13, 15]. There is little or no incremental clinical benefit in start doses >20 U for either product [62, 63].

The efficacy of two treatments for the same indication can only be directly compared in head-to-head comparative randomized studies using optimal doses. A large, European head-to-head study investigated the non-inferiority of incobotulinumtoxinA to onabotulinumtoxinA, when a 1:1 dose ratio was used [6]. Female subjects with moderate to severe glabellar frown lines (severity score of 2–3 on FWS, as assessed by the investigator) were randomized to receive 24 U of incobotulinumtoxinA ($n = 284$) or onabotulinumtoxinA ($n = 97$). At week 4 postinjection, response at maximum frown – defined as an improvement of at least 1 point on the FWS compared with baseline – was 96.4% and 95.7% in the incobotulinumtoxinA and onabotulinumtoxinA groups, respectively, as assessed by an independent assessor from standardized clinical photographs (Figure 6.3a and Figure 6.4a,b). Therapeutic effect was maintained at week 12, with 80.1% of subjects in the incobotulinumtoxinA group and 78.5% of subjects in the onabotulinumtoxinA group defined as responders at maximum frown (Figure 6.3a). Similar results were observed by the investigator (Figure 6.3b). Importantly, the subjects themselves rated their treatment highly on the patient's global assessment and the incidence of adverse events throughout the study was low. This study confirmed that incobotulinumtoxinA is non-inferior to onabotulinumtoxinA for the treatment of glabellar frown lines and is well tolerated [6].

To extend and confirm the results of this non-inferiority trial, a new US head-to-head study, this time powered to test equivalence, randomized 250 subjects in a

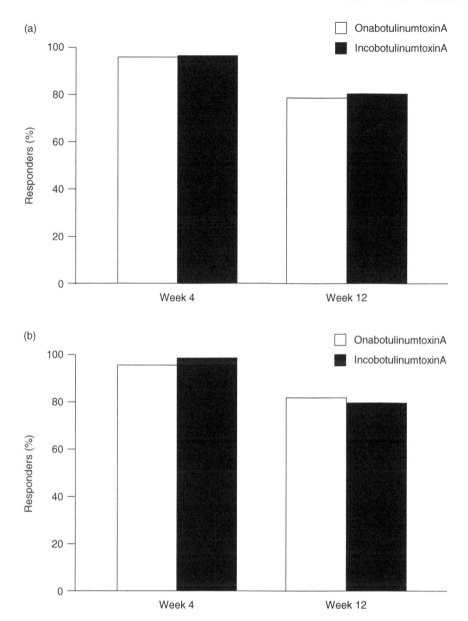

Figure 6.3 Percentage of responders at maximum frown at weeks 4 and 12 according to the facial wrinkle scale for the per protocol set. (a) Independent rater assessment based on digital photographs. (b) Investigator assessment based on the live patient. *Source:* Sattler 2010 [6]. Reproduced with permission of Wolters Kluwer Health, Inc.

1 : 1 ratio to incobotulinumtoxinA or onabo-tulinumtoxinA, with both treatments given at their optimal dose of 20 U for the treatment of moderate-to-severe glabellar frown lines [49]. Primary efficacy analysis showed a very high and statistically equivalent response rate for incobotulinumtoxinA and onabotulinum-toxinA at 1 month (95.7% and 99.2%, respec-tively). Similar efficacy profiles were demon-strated at 1, 2, 3, and 4 months whether assessed by independent raters or treating physicians. In the US head-to-head study,

(a) Baseline   Week 4

(b) Baseline   Week 4

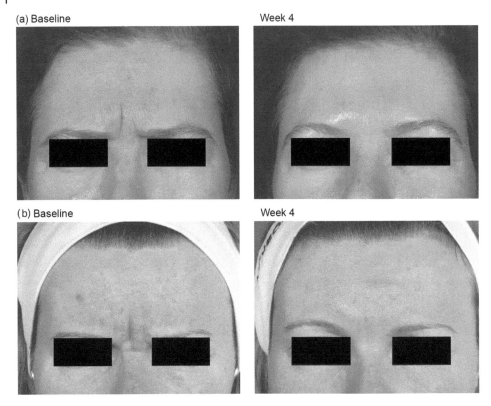

Figure 6.4   Clinical photographs taken at maximum frown in patients treated with (a) incobotulinumtoxinA and (b) onabotulinumtoxinA. *Source:* Sattler 2010 [6]. Reproduced with permission of Wolters Kluwer Health, Inc.

subject assessments of treatment satisfaction with incobotulinumtoxinA were over 90% throughout the study and similar to onabotulinumtoxinA at all timepoints, thus confirming results from the European study.

In an open-label study of 105 patients with moderate or severe glabellar frown lines, patients received 20 U incobotulinumtoxinA (0.1 ml to each of five injection sites) and were assessed at week 4 and week 12 postinjection. Response at maximum frown was 98.1% at week 4 and 80.0% at week 12. Adverse events were low and no patients developed neutralizing antibodies. The authors concluded that incobotulinumtoxinA is effective and well tolerated in the treatment of glabellar frown lines [57].

Men typically have a stronger glabellar muscle mass than women and require higher doses. In a small study of 12 men,

the effectiveness of BoNTA preparations for hyperdynamic forehead lines was similar when administered at a dose ratio of $1:1:3$ onabotulinumtoxinA: incobotulinumtoxinA: abobotulinumtoxinA [64]. A study of 29 subjects with Fitzpatrick skin types IV to VI has confirmed that the efficacy and safety of incobotulinumtoxinA for the correction of glabellar lines is similar to that among individuals with fairer skin [61].

A prospective, open-label, multicenter, repeat-dose, phase III trial has investigated the long-term safety and efficacy of incobotulinumtoxinA for the treatment of glabellar frown lines over 2 years and up to 8 injection cycles in 796 subjects [60]. Efficacy was assessed by percentage of responders at maximum frown (score of 0 [none] or 1 [mild]) on the FWS at day 30 of each treatment cycle. Responder rates remained stable during cycles 1–7 at approximately 80% (range 79.1–82.7%), and were higher in cycle 8 (89.6%). Results from the subject assessment on a 4-point scale at maximum frown (subjects with ≥1-point improvement) also showed a maintained response to repeat doses over time [60].

Crow's Feet

Two head-to-head studies have compared the efficacy of incobotulinumtoxinA and onabotulinumtoxinA in the treatment of crow's feet [48, 65]. In the first study, 21 patients with a score of 2 or 3 on the FWS (moderate or severe) received treatment for crow's feet with 12 U of either onabotulinumtoxinA or incobotulinumtoxinA in an intra-individual split-face, double-blind, proof-of-concept study. At 1 month postinjection, the response rates were 95% for the side of the face treated with incobotulinumtoxinA and 90% for the onabotulinumtoxinA-treated side. The study showed that there were no statistically significant differences in response rates between the two products over the entire observation period of 4 months, supporting the theory that the two products are equipotent and that the commonly used 1 : 1 dose conversion ratio is appropriate. Tolerability was also rated as 'very good' by most patients over the entire study period, leading the authors to conclude that both products are well-tolerated and effective treatments for periorbital wrinkles [48].

The second study used a split-face, crossover design to compare incobotulinumtoxinA and onabotulinumtoxinA at a 1 : 1 dose conversion ratio in two consecutive treatment cycles, each of 3 months, separated by 6 months [65]. The study recruited 14 women with symmetrical crow's feet with a score of 1 to 4 on the Merz 5-point scale at maximum contraction. Using the same injection sites and techniques, 12 U of incobotulinumtoxinA or onabotulinumtoxinA were injected into the lateral periorbital region of each eye. Both treatments

were similarly effective in reducing the severity of crow's feet at rest and at maximum contraction, in both treatment cycles, and on both sides of the face.

A randomized, split-face study has also compared the safety and efficacy of incobotulinumtoxinA and abobotulinumtoxinA for the treatment of crow's feet at a dose conversion ratio of 1 : 3 [66]. Twenty women with moderate-to-severe crow's feet at rest according to the Merz Aesthetics scale received 9 U incobotulinumtoxinA or 27 U abobotulinumtoxinA to the lateral periorbital region. Both products demonstrated comparable efficacy with responder rates (≥1-point improvement from baseline) of 100% and 83% at 2 weeks and 4 months posttreatment, respectively. At 6 months posttreatment, responder rates were 67% and 61% for incobotulinumtoxinA and abobotulinumtoxinA, respectively. In this study the clinical data were supported by electromyography findings, which showed that both treatments induced similar levels of neuromuscular blockade. In addition, the electromyographic values recorded 6 months posttreatment, although higher when compared with the 4-month data, were still lower than baseline values, indicating a partial persistence of the therapeutic effect at 6 months posttreatment.

Upper Facial Lines

The efficacy and safety of incobotulinumtoxinA for upper facial lines, a combination of glabellar frown lines (GFL), horizontal forehead lines (HFL), and lateral periorbital lines (LPL) has been assessed in two studies [67, 68]. In a placebo-controlled, double-blind study, 156 subjects with moderate-to-severe upper facial lines on the Merz Aesthetics scales were randomized to incobotulinumtoxinA ($n = 105$) or placebo ($n = 51$). IncobotulinumtoxinA was administered as doses of 54–64 U as follows: GFL 20 U, HFL 10–20 U, and LPL 24 U. Compared with placebo, incobotulinumtoxinA demonstrated significantly greater efficacy in treating upper facial lines separately and combined. Investigator-assessed scores of 0 (no lines) and 1 (mild) on day 30 at maximum contraction for incobotulinumtoxinA versus placebo were: GFL (84.5% versus 0.0%), HFL (70.9% versus 2.1%), LPL (64.1% versus 2.1%) and upper facial lines combination (55.3% versus 0.0%), all ($p \leq 0.0001$).

In the second study, 27 women were treated for upper facial lines as follows: GFL 10–30 U, LPL 10–30 U, and HFL 6–15 U [68]. Wrinkle severity was assessed at days 0 (baseline), 2, 7, 14, 28, and 112 using the Merz Aesthetics scales. Responders were defined as those with an improvement from baseline of at least 1 point. IncobotulinumtoxinA had a rapid onset of action with a noticeable decrease in the mean wrinkle severity score from day 2. Responder rates for the different indications generally peaked at days 7 to 14. At 112 days, mean wrinkle severity scores remained significantly lower than baseline ($p < 0.05$). Patients' self-perception was greatly improved after treatment, with beneficial effects lasting up to 4 months after treatment.

Platysmal Bands

Two studies have evaluated the efficacy of incobotulinumtoxinA in the treatment of platysmal bands. In the first study, 25 subjects with platysmal bands scoring 2 or 3 on the validated 5-point Merz dynamic platysmal bands scale [69] received a total of 60 U incobotulinumtoxinA divided between four platysmal bands (20 U in both medial bands and 10 U in both lateral bands) [70]. In the second study, 23 subjects with 2 to 4 platysmal bands scoring ≥1 on the Merz platysmal band scale received 15 U incobotulinumtoxinA in each band [71]. In both studies, a responder was defined as a subject with at least a 1-point improvement from baseline on the dynamic platysmal bands scale. Response rates at maximum contraction of 100% were achieved at day 14 in the first study and day 8 in the second study. Response rates remained high at the end of follow-up and treatment

was well tolerated in both trials. Further studies investigating the use of incobotulinumtoxinA in a range of aesthetic applications are ongoing.

Personal Experience

In our practice for aesthetic dermatology, we have been using incobotulinumtoxinA for aesthetic indications since 2005, after having mainly used onabotulinumtoxinA before. We could not observe any difference in efficacy, tolerability, and patient satisfaction between the two products. Besides the standard indications such as glabellar lines, horizontal frown lines, crow's feet, and more advanced indications such as brow lift, perioral lines, cobblestone chin, lifting of oral commissures, and softening platysmal bands, we also use incobotulinumtoxinA in formerly forbidden zones such as the lower lateral forehead, lower eyelids, and over the zygoma. In these areas, we use an intradermal injection technique with multiple injection points and very small aliquots (0.3–0.5 U of incobotulinumtoxinA) (Figure 6.5) [72].

Summary

In conclusion, incobotulinumtoxinA is an effective and well-tolerated formulation of BoNTA. In clinical trials, incobotulinumtoxinA displays comparable efficacy and safety to onabotulinumtoxinA and abobotulinumtoxinA when administered at dose conversion ratios of 1:1 and 1:3, respectively. It is not only free from complexing proteins, but also inactivated or denatured neurotoxin, bringing the foreign protein load to a minimum. In this respect, incobotulinumtoxinA represents a novel advance in BoNTA formulations that have now been used in aesthetic applications for over 20 years. This development has yielded a product that is also stable at room temperature for long-term storage, giving it a practical advantage. As the

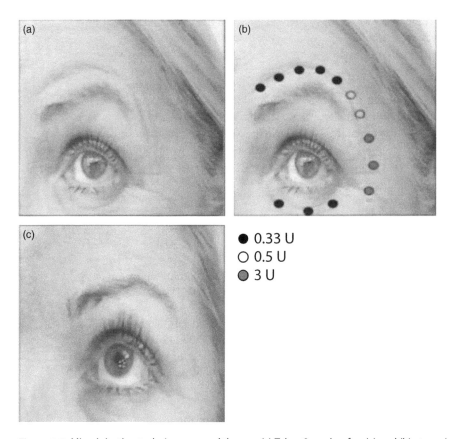

● 0.33 U
○ 0.5 U
◉ 3 U

Figure 6.5 Microinjection technique around the eye. (c) Taken 2 weeks after (a) and (b) at maximum eyebrow elevation. Note smoothing of periorbital wrinkling above eyebrow and at lower lid without losing significant eyebrow height.

use of BoNTA in cosmetic medicine continues to grow and long-term comparative studies are published, evidence will accumulate to resolve the controversial issue of complexing proteins and their role in antibody-induced secondary treatment failure.

References

1 Carruthers A, Carruthers J. Botulinum toxin products overview. Skin Ther Lett 2008;13:1–4.
2 Bigalke H. Properties of pharmaceutical products of botulinum neurotoxins. In Jankovic J, Albane A, Atassi MZ, et al., eds. Botulinum Toxin. Philadelphia: Saunders; 2009:389–397.
3 Frevert J. Content of botulinum neurotoxin in Botox®/Vistabel®, Dysport®/Azzalure®, and Xeomin®/Bocouture®. Drugs R D 2010;10:67–73.
4 Benecke R, Jost WH, Kanovsky P, et al. A new botulinum toxin type A free of complexing proteins for treatment of cervical dystonia. Neurology 2005;64: 1949–1951.
5 Roggenkämper P, Jost WH, Bihari K, et al. Efficacy and safety of a new botulinum toxin type A free of complexing proteins in the treatment of blepharospasm. J Neural Transm 2006;113:303–312.
6 Sattler G, Callander M, Grablowitz D, et al. Non-inferiority of NT201, free from

complexing proteins, compared with another botulinum toxin type A in the treatment of glabellar frown lines. Dermatol Surg 2010;36(Suppl 4): 2146–2154.

7 Chen F, Kuziemko GM, Stevens RC. Biophysical characterization of the stability of the 150-kilodalton botulinum toxin, the nontoxic component, and the 900-kilodalton botulinum toxin complex species. Infect Immun 1998;66: 2420–2425.

8 Eisele KH, Fink K, Vey M, Taylor HV. Studies on the dissociation of botulinum neurotoxin type A complexes. Toxicon 2011;57:555–565.

9 Grein S, Mander GJ, Taylor HV. Xeomin® is stable without refrigeration and is not affected by short-term temperature stress. Mov Disord 2008;23(Suppl. 1):S24.

10 Grein S, Mander GJ, Taylor HV. Xeomin® is stable without refrigeration: Complexing proteins are not required for stability of botulinum neurotoxin type A preparations. Toxicon 2008;51:13 (Abstr. 36).

11 Soares DJ, Dejoseph LM, Zuliani GF, Liebertz DJ, Patel VS. Impact of postreconstitution room temperature storage on the efficacy of incobotulinumtoxinA treatment of dynamic lateral canthus lines. Dermatol Surg 2015;41:712–717.

12 Merz Pharmaceuticals GmbH. BOCOUTURE Summary of Product Characteristics; Frankfurt am Main, Germany: Merz Pharmaceuticals GmbH; 2016.

13 Merz Pharmaceuticals GmbH. XEOMIN Summary of Product Characteristics; Frankfurt am Main, Germany: Merz Pharmaceuticals GmbH; 2015.

14 Dysport. Dysport Summary of Product Characteristics. Slough: Ipsen Ltd. 2007.

15 Botox. Botox (botulinum toxin type A) Summary of Product Characteristics. Allergan, Inc, Irvine, CA. 2009.

16 Neurobloc. Neurobloc Summary of Product Characteristic. Eisai, Hertfordshire, UK. 2009.

17 Rappl T, Parvizi D, Friedl H, et al. Onset and duration of effect of incobotulinum-toxinA, onabotulinumtoxinA, and abobotulinumtoxinA in the treatment of glabellar frown lines: a randomized, double-blind study. Clin Cosmet Investig Dermatol 2013;6:211–219.

18 Klein AW. Complications and adverse reactions with the use of botulinum toxin. Dis Mon 2002;48:336–356.

19 de Boulle K, de Almeida AT. Addressing recent concerns in comparative studies of botulinum toxin type A. J Cosmet Laser Ther 2010;12:181–183.

20 Kerscher M, Roll S, Becker A, Wigger-Alberti W. Comparison of the spread of three botulinum toxin type A preparations. Arch Dermatol Res 2012;304: 155–161.

21 Carli L, Montecucco C, Rossetto O. Assay of diffusion of different botulinum neurotoxin type A formulations injected in the mouse leg. Muscle Nerve 2009;40: 374–380.

22 Cliff SH, Judodihardjo H, Eltringham E. Different formulations of botulinum toxin type A have different migration characteristics: a double-blind, randomized study. J Cosmet Dermatol 2008;7:50–54.

23 Hexsel D, Dal'Forno T, Hexsel C, et al. A randomized pilot study comparing the action halos of two commercial preparations of botulinum toxin type A. Dermatol Surg 2008;34:52–59.

24 Kranz G, Haubenberger D, Voller B, et al. Respective potencies of Botox and Dysport in a human skin model: a randomized, double-blind study. Mov Disord 2009;24: 231–236.

25 Wohlfarth K, Schwandt I, Wegner F, et al. Biological activity of two botulinum toxin type A complexes (Dysport and Botox) in volunteers: a double-blind, randomized, dose-ranging study. J Neurol 2008;255: 1932–1939.

26 Trindade de Almeida AR, Marques E, de Almeida J, et al. Pilot study comparing the diffusion of two formulations of botulinum toxin type A in patients with forehead

hyperhidrosis. Dermatol Surg 2007;33: S37–S43.

27 Wohlfarth K, Muller C, Sassin I, *et al.* Neurophysiological double-blind trial of a botulinum neurotoxin type a free of complexing proteins. Clin Neuropharmacol 2007;30:86–89.

28 Hexsel D, Soirefmann M, Porto MD, *et al.* Fields of muscular and anhidrotic effects of 2 botulinum toxin-A commercial preparations: a prospective, double-blind, randomized, multicenter study. Dermatol Surg 2015;41(Suppl 1): S110–S118.

29 Hsu TS, Dover JS, Arndt KA. Effect of volume and concentration on the diffusion of botulinum exotoxin A. Arch Dermatol 2004;140:1351–1354.

30 Lee JC, Yokota K, Arimitsu H, *et al.* Production of anti-neurotoxin antibody is enhanced by two subcomponents, HA1 and HA3b, of Clostridium botulinum type B 16S toxin-haemagglutinin. Microbiology 2005;151:3739–3747.

31 Jankovic J, Vuong KD, Ahsan J. Comparison of efficacy and immunogenicity of original versus current botulinum toxin in cervical dystonia. Neurology 2003;60:1186–1188.

32 Greene P, Fahn S, Diamond B. Development of resistance to botulinum toxin type A in patients with torticollis. Mov Disord 1994;9:213–217.

33 Borodic G. Botulinum toxin, immunologic considerations with long-term repeated use, with emphasis on cosmetic applications. Facial Plast Surg Clin North Am 2007;15:11–16.

34 Torres S, Hamilton M, Sanches E, *et al.* Neutralizing antibodies to botulinum neurotoxin type A in aesthetic medicine: five case reports. Clin Cosmet Investig Dermatol 2013;7:11–17.

35 Aoki KR, Merlino G, Spanoyannis AF, Wheeler LA. BOTOX (botulinum toxin type A) purified neurotoxin complex prepared from the new bulk toxin retains the same preclinical efficacy as the original but with reduced antigenicity. Neurology 1999;52(Suppl 2):A521–A522.

36 Borodic G. Immunologic resistance after repeated botulinum toxin type A injections for facial rhytides. Ophthal Plast Reconstr Surg 2006;22:239–240.

37 Lee S-K. Antibody-induced failure of botulinum toxin type A therapy in a patient with masseteric hypertrophy. Dermatol Surg 2007;33:S105–S110.

38 Kamm C, Schümann F, Mix E, Benecke R. Secondary antibody-induced treatment failure under therapy with incobotulinumtoxinA (Xeomin®) in a patient with segmental dystonia pretreated with abobotulinumtoxinA (Dysport®). J Neurol Sci 2015;350(1–2):110–111.

39 Jochim A, Castrop F, Jochim B, Haslinger B. Secondary treatment failure in cervical dystonia after treatment with inco- and abobotulinumtoxinA. Parkinsonism Relat Disord 2015;21:663–664.

40 Dressler D. New formulation of BOTOX. Complete antibody-induced therapy failure in hemifacial spasm. J Neurol 2004;251: 360.

41 Blümel J, Frevert J, Schwaier A. Comparative antigenicity of three preparations of botulinum neurotoxin A in the rabbit. Neurotox Res 2006;9:238.

42 Jost WH, Blumel J, Grafe S. Botulinum neurotoxin type A free of complexing proteins (XEOMIN) in focal dystonia. Drugs 2007;67:669–683.

43 Kanovsky P, Platz T, Comes G, Grafe S, Sassin I. NT 201, botulinum neurotoxin free from complexing proteins (Xeomin®) provided sustained efficacy and was safe in spasticity: 89 weeks long-term data. J Neurol Sci 2009;285:S75–S76.

44 Dressler D. Equivalent potency of Xeomin and Botox. Mov Disord 2008;23:S20–S21.

45 Fernández-Salas E, Wang J, Molina Y, *et al.* Botulinum neurotoxin serotype A specific cell-based potency assay to replace the mouse bioassay. PloS One 2012;7:e49516.

46 Mander G. Potency assay for botulinum neurotoxin type A based on neuronal cells as a replacement for the mouse bioassay. Poster presented at Toxins 2015: Basic Science and Clinical Aspects of Botulinum

and Other Neurotoxins, Lisbon, Portugal, Jan 14–17, 2015.

47 Jost WH, Kohl A, Brinkmann S, *et al.* Efficacy and tolerability of a botulinum toxin type A free of complexing proteins (NT 201) compared with commercially available botulinum toxin type A (BOTOX) in healthy volunteers. J Neural Transm 2005;112:905–913.

48 Prager W, Wissmüller E, Kollhorst B, Williams S, Zschocke I. Comparison of two botulinum toxin type A preparations for treating crow's feet: a split-face, double-blind, proof-of-concept study. Dermatol Surg 2010;36(Suppl 4):2155–2160.

49 Kane MA, Gold MH, Coleman WP, *et al.* A randomized, double-blind trial to investigate the equivalence of incobotulinumtoxinA and onabotulinumtoxinA for glabellar frown lines. Dermatol Surg 2015;41:1310–1319.

50 Poulain B, Trevidic P, Clave M, *et al.* Clinical equivalence of conventional OnabotulinumtoxinA (900 KDa) and IncobotulinumtoxinA (neurotoxin free from complexing proteins—150 KDa): 2012 multidisciplinary French consensus in aesthetics. J Drugs Dermatol 2013;12: 1434–1446.

51 Prager W, Huber-Vorländer J, Taufig AZ, *et al.* Botulinum toxin type A treatment to the upper face: retrospective analysis of daily practice. Clin Cosmet Investig Dermatol 2012;5:53–58.

52 Jandhyala R. Relative potencyf incobotulinumtoxinA vs onabotulinumtoxinA a meta-analysis of key evidence. J Drugs Dermatol 2012;11: 731–736.

53 Hanke CW, Narins RS, Brandt F, *et al.* A randomized, placebo-controlled, double-blind phase III trial investigating the efficacy and safety of incobotulinumtoxinA in the treatment of glabellar frown lines using a stringent composite endpoint. Dermatol Surg 2013;39:891–899.

54 Carruthers A, Carruthers J, Coleman WP 3rd, *et al.* Multicenter, randomized,

phase III study of a single dose of incobotulinumtoxinA, free from complexing proteins, in the treatment of glabellar frown lines. Dermatol Surg 2013;39:551–558.

55 Jones D, Carruthers J, Narins RS, *et al.* Efficacy of incobotulinumtoxinA for treatment of glabellar frown lines: a post hoc pooled analysis of 2 randomized, placebo-controlled, phase 3 trials. Dermatol Surg 2014;40:776–785.

56 Prager W, Bee EK, Havermann I, Zschocke I. Onset, longevity, and patient satisfaction with incobotulinumtoxinA for the treatment of glabellar frown lines: a single-arm, prospective clinical study. Clin Interv Aging 2013;8:449–456.

57 Imhof M, Kühne U. A phase III study of incobotulinumtoxinA in the treatment of glabellar frown lines. J Clin Aesthet Dermatol 2011;4:28–34.

58 Moers-Carpi M, Dirschka T, Feller-Heppt G, *et al.* A randomised, double-blind comparison of 20 units of onabotulinumtoxinA with 30 units of incobotulinumtoxinA for glabellar lines. J Cosmet Laser Ther 2012;14:296–303.

59 Prager W, Rappl T. Phase IV study comparing incobotulinumtoxinA and onabotulinumtoxinA using a 1:1.5 dose-conversion ratio for the treatment of glabellar frown lines. J Cosmet Dermatol 2012;11:267–271.

60 Rzany B, Flynn TC, Schlöbe A, Heinz M, Harrington L. Long-term results for incobotulinumtoxinA in the treatment of glabellar frown lines. Dermatol Surg 2013;39(1 Pt 1):95–103.

61 Jackson BA, Vogel MR. Efficacy and safety of incobotulinumtoxin A for the correction of glabellar lines among patients with skin types IV to VI. J Drugs Dermatol 2015;14: 350–353.

62 Carruthers A, Carruthers J, Said S. Dose-ranging study of botulinum toxin type A in the treatment of glabellar rhytids in females. Dermatol Surg 2005;31: 414–422.

63 Dressler D, Rothwell JC. Electromyographic quantification of the paralysing effect of botulinum toxin. Eur Neurol 2000;43:13–16.

64 Oliveira de Morais O, Matos Reis-Filho E, Vilela Pereira L, Martins Gomes C, Alves G. Comparison of four botulinum neurotoxin type A preparations in the treatment of hyperdynamic forehead lines in men: a pilot study. J Drugs Dermatol 2012;11:216–219.

65 Muti G, Harrington L. A prospective rater- and subject-blinded study comparing the efficacy of incobotulinumtoxinA and onabotulinumtoxinA to treat crow's feet: a clinical crossover evaluation. Dermatol Surg 2015;41(Suppl 1):S39–S46.

66 Saybel A, Artemenko A, Nikitin S, Kurenkov A. A prospective, neurophysiologic comparative study to assess the efficacy and duration of effect of incobotulinumtoxinA and abobotulinumtoxinA in the treatment of crow's feet. J Drugs Dermatol 2015;14: 1291–1296.

67 Kerscher M, Rzany B, Prager W, et al. Efficacy and safety of incobotulinumtoxinA in the treatment of upper facial lines: results from a randomized, double-blind, placebo-controlled, phase III study. Dermatol Surg 2015;41(10):1149–1157.

68 Streker M, Luebberding S, Krueger N, et al. Patient-reported outcomes after incobotulinumtoxinA treatment for upper facial wrinkles. Dermatol Surg 2015;41 (Suppl 1):S29–S38.

69 Geister TL, Bleßmann-Gurk B, Rzany B, et al. Validated assessment scale for platysmal bands. Dermatol Surg 2013;39: 1217–1225.

70 Gubanova EI, Panova OS, Sanchez EA, Rodina MY, Starovatova PA. Efficacy and safety of IncobotulinumtoxinA for the treatment of platysmal bands of the aging neck: an open-label, prospective pilot study. J Drugs Dermatol 2013;12: 1461–1466.

71 Prager W, Bee EK, Havermann I, Zschocke I. IncobotulinumtoxinA for the treatment of platysmal bands: a single-arm, prospective proof-of-concept clinical study. Dermatol Surg 2015;41(Suppl 1):S88–S92.

72 Imhof M, Kuhne U. Introduction of the microdroplet technique with incobotulinumtoxin A for the treatment of crow's feet. J Clin Aesthet Dermatol 2013;6: 40–44.

7

Future Injectable Toxins
Michael H. Gold, MD

Medical Director, Gold Skin Care Center, Nashville, USA

Introduction

The world of aesthetic surgery changed dramatically with the advent of Botox Cosmetic® (Allergan Inc., Irvine CA) for the improvement of glabellar lines and furrows. From the advent of Botox Cosmetic, doors for many cosmetic surgeons have opened beyond what many of us expected, with its approval in the early 2000s. The increase in its use can be directly related to the surge in other cosmetic procedures that are now performed as more and more individuals seek our services and learn more about the cosmetic procedures we perform routinely in our daily practice. This has led to the global increase in what is now known simply as noninvasive or minimally invasive cosmetic surgery.

Since the advent and marketing successes of Botox Cosmetic, several other pharmaceutical companies have developed and have hoped that their botulinum toxins would find the same or similar success in the marketplace. These companies have either marketed their toxins or are on the verge of finalizing their clinical trials, hoping to bring them into the market in the near future. It is with these new toxins in mind that this manuscript is being prepared. Unfortunately, with new toxins being evaluated in US Food and Drug Administration (FDA) clinical trials, not all the data for these US clinical studies is in the public domain, so only information that is in the public domain is presented here. It

is hoped that in future editions of *Botulinum Toxins: Principles and Practice*, that more updated information can be provided, that several if not all these toxins may be available in the US, and that clinicians will have more choice and a reason to choose one toxin over another. But let us always remember that it has been the success of Botox Cosmetic which has fueled the flames of this minimally invasive cosmetic world.

Botox Cosmetic and Dysport® (Galderma Laboratories, Lausanne, Switzerland) will not be reviewed here as they have been covered extensively in this textbook. Xeomin® will be reviewed in some detail even though it also has received a prominent place here. PurTox® will be described in this manuscript, although this toxin is not expected to be brought to market. During the first draft of this manuscript there was much interest in the phase III US FDA clinical trials for PurTox. For reasons unclear to many, the drug never made it past its promising phase III results and we will not have this toxin in our armentarium. But what is interesting – and why it is being included – is that we can show how diligent the FDA trials were for this drug and what is needed for any company in today's world to bring a toxin into the US market and through the FDA process.

As well, several newer toxins which are in or just finished their clinical trials in the US will also be mentioned here. These include a botulinum toxin from Daewoong

Botulinum Toxins: Cosmetic and Clinical Applications, First Edition. Edited by Joel L. Cohen and David M. Ozog.
© 2017 John Wiley & Sons Ltd. Published 2017 by John Wiley & Sons Ltd.
Companion Website: www.wiley.com/go/cohen/botulinum

Pharmaceutical Company (South Korea) with North American and other country rights being held now by Alphaeon Pharmaceuticals (Irvine, CA). The drug is currently known as Nabota outside the United States, and just as DWP-450 in the United States. Clinical trials outside of the United States show Nabota to be useful and effective. The US clinical trials for DWP-450 showed positive results in the treatment of glabellar lines and furrows.

In addition, another Korean company, Hugel, has expanded its botulinum toxin footprint by selling the rights to its Botulax product – which is currently undergoing phase III clinical trials in the United States – to Croma Pharma (Austria). Once again, two parallel multicenter, randomized, placebo-controlled studies are ongoing here in the United States and we hope to know the data later in 2016 or early in 2017.

Other toxins in the world of interest include Neuronox, made by MediTox (Korea) and currently with US rights owned by Allergan and a Chinese toxin which has been typically called ChinaTox. Other toxins exist beyond those that will be covered in this chapter. Hopefully, in future editions of this textbook, more toxins will be described and perhaps used in everyday practice.

Xeomin

Xeomin, known generically as incobotulinumA, is manufactured by Merz Pharmaceuticals, Frankfurt, Germany. In some parts of Europe, Xeomin is also known as Bo-Couture. It is known as a "pure" neurotoxin. A pure neurotoxin is a toxin without the associated hemagglutinin complexes found with Botox and Dysport, and thus has the advantage of being void from the potential of antigenicity, which theoretically makes the product safer than those toxins with hemagglutinin complexes. Whether this is important from a clinical point of view is still the subject of debate, as antibody formation to Botox or Dysport is not a common occurrence and has not been a major concern in

everyday clinical practice. But Xeomin is the first "pure" toxin that has been produced and released into the US market, making it an important entry in the toxin field.

Xeomin is cleared in the European Union and in Mexico and Argentina for the treatment of blepharospasm and spasmodic torticollis. It also received US FDA approval for the treatment of blepharospasm and for cervical dystonia in 2010 [1]. This was the twentieth country in which Xeomin was approved and in December, 2013, Xeomin received its US FDA approval for treatment of glabellar lines and furrows, making it the third botulinum toxin A approved in the United States [2].

As far as cosmetic indications for Xeomin, in both Europe and the United States, Xeomin is approved for the treatment of glabellar lines and furrows. In Europe in 2016, Xeomin received approval from the European Union officials to use the toxin on all areas of the face – making it the first toxin to receive this indication – based on the results of a pivotal randomized, double-blind, placebo-controlled phase 3 study with 156 patients from France, Germany, and the United Kingdom receiving treatment of upper facial lines with Xeomin. Clinical trial data demonstrates that Xeomin has a favorable safety and efficacy profile in treating upper facial lines, both combined and separately, with treatment effects maintained for up to 4 months.

The main question asked by those using Xeomin in clinical practice is what is the proper dose ratio to Botox Cosmetic when comparing the two toxins. Much has been written about this, with many studies being industry sponsored with possible associated built-in biases. But we have the data and need to use the data appropriately [3].

Most of the European literature indicates a dilution ratio for Xeomin and Botox of 1 : 1. In one recent report, Fritsch [4] reported an equivalent duration of action when each of the products were injected into the lateral orbicular lines, more commonly known as the crow's feet area. The Botox group had a duration of effect of 3.5 months while the Xeomin group had a duration of effect of 3.7 months. Patient acceptance and adverse event profiles were similar for both groups – showing the effectiveness of Xeomin in cosmetic indications and showing that there is no real difference between Xeomin and Botox in the cosmetic arena. Several other clinical trials confirmed these findings and most clinicians agree that there is a 1:1 ratio for the two products [5,6].

A full listing of the European clinical trials concerning cosmetic indications for Xeomin are shown in Table 7.1 [7].

In the United States, two parallel, randomized, placebo-controlled, double-blinded studies were performed with over 270 patients enrolled into each trial to study the effects on Xeomin on glabellar lines and furrows. The results from the trials, with more stringent primary endpoints needed by the FDA were all positive. In the trials that were performed, both the physician and the patient had to give the treatment a two-point patient improvement for it to be considered a success. This was different from some other toxin trials that only required a one-point clinical improvement. Even with the two-point change, there was statistical significance, which then led to its FDA approval. Figure 7.1 and Figure 7.2 are clinical examples from the clinical trial that were put into the public domain early from the

Table 7.1 Xeomin European Clinical Trials – Published.

1.	Efficacy and Safety of IncobotulinumtoxinA for the Treatment of Platysmal Bands of the Aging Neck An Open-Label, Prospective Pilot Study. Elena I Gubanova MD, Olga S. Panova MD, Elena A Sanchez MD, Maria Y Rodina MD, and Polina A Starovatova	J Drugs Dermatol. 2013;12(12):146–1466
2.	A Phase III Study of IncobotulinumtoxinA in the Treatment of Glabellar Frown Lines. Matthias Imhof MD, and Ulrich Kuhun MD	J Clin Aesthet Dermatol, 2011;4(10):28–34
3.	Efficacy and Safety of IncobotulinumtoxinA in the Treatment of Upper Facial Lines: Results from a Randomized, Double-Blind, Placebo-Controlled, Phase III Study. Martina Kerscher MD, Berthold Rzany MD, Welf Prager MD, Catriona Turnbull PhD, Patrick Trevidic MD, and Christopher Inglefield BSc, MBBS	Dermatol Surg 2015;41:1149–1157
4.	A Randomised, Double-Blind Comparison of 20 Units of OnabotulinumtoxinA with 30 Units of IncobotulinumtoxinA for Glabellar Lines. Marion Moers-Carpi, Thomas Dirschka, Gabrielle Feller-Heppt, Said Hilton, Klaus Hoffmann, Wolfgang G. Philipp-Dormston, Antia Rutter, Kelvin Tan, Aary Ann Chapman, Anthony Fulford-Smith	J Cosmet Laser Ther. 2012 Dec; 14(6):296–303
5.	A prospective Rater – and Subject-Blinded Study Comparing the Efficacy of IncobotulinumtoxinA and OnabotulinumtoxinA to Treat Crow's Feet A Clinical Crossover Evaluation. Gabriele Muti MD, and Laura Harrington PhD	Dermatol Surg 2015;41:S39–S46
6.	IncobotulinumtoxinA Use in Aesthetic Indications in Daily Practice: A European Multicenter, Noninterventional, Retrospective Study. Tatjana Pavicic, Welf Prager, Markus Kloppel, Simon Ravichandran, and Olivier Galatoire	Clinical, Cosmetic and Investigational Dermatology 2015;8: 135–142
7.	Botulinum Toxin Type A Treatment to the Upper Face: Retrospective Analysis of Daily Practice. Welf Prager, Jurgen Huber-Vorlander, A Ziah Taufig, Matthias Imhof, Ulrich Kuhne, Ruth Weissberg, Lars-Peter Kuhr, Volker Rippmann, Wolfgang G Philipp-Dormston, Thomas M Proebstls, Claudia Roth, Martina Kerscher, Claudius Ulmann, and Tatjana Pavicic	Clinical, Cosmetic and Investigational Dermatology 2012;5: 53–58

(continued)

Table 7.1 (Continued)

8.	Onset, Longevity, and Patient Satisfaction with IncobotulinumtoxinA for the Treatment of Glabellar Frown Lines: A Single-arm, Prospective Clinical Study. Welf Prager, Eva K Bee, Isabel Havermann and Ina Zschocke	Clinical Interventions in Aging, 2013;8:449–456
9.	Comparison of Two Botulinum Toxin Type A Preparations for Treating Crow's Feet: A Split-Face, Double-Blind, Proof-of-Concept Study. Welf Prager MD, Esther Wissmuller MD, Bianca Kollhorst MSc, Stefanie William MD, and Ina Zschocke PhD	Dermatol Surg 2010;36:2155–2160
10.	Quantitative Evaluation of the Onset and Longevity of the Action of IncobotulinumtoxinA by Skin Displacement Analysis in the Treatment of Glabellar Frown Lines. Thomas M. Proebstle MD, Gary Chung MS, Ruth Weissberg MD and Tatajana Pavicic MD,	J Drugs Dermatol. 2014;13(9):1067–1072
11.	Onset and Duration of Effect of IncobotulinumtoxinA, OnabotulinumtoxinA, and AbobotulinumtoxinA in the Treatment of Glabellar Frown Lines: A Randomized, Double-Blind Study. Thomas Rapp, Daryousch Parviz, Herwig Friedl, Maria Wiedner, Simone May, Bettina Kranzelbiner, Paul Qurzer, Bengt Hellbom	Clinical, Cosmetic and Investigational Dermatology 2016;6: 211–219
12.	Long-Term Results for IncobotulinumtoxinA in the Treatment of Glabellar Frown Lines. Berthold Rzany MD, Timothy Corcoran Flynn MD, Andrea Schlobe MD, Moritz Heinz and Laura Harrington PhD	Dermatol Surg 2012;1–9
13.	Noninferiority of IncobotulinumtoxinA, Free from Complexing Proteins, Compared with Another Botulinum Toxin Type A in Treatment of Glabellar Frown Lines. Gerhard Sattler MD, Michael J. Callander MD, Doris Grablowitz MD, Torsten Walker MD, Eva K. Bee MD, Berthold Rzany MD, Timothy Corcoran Flynn MD, and Alastair Carruthers MD	Dermatol Surg 2010;36:2146–2154
14.	Patient-Reported Outcomes After IncobotulinumtoxinA Treatment for Upper Facial Wrinkles. Meike Streker PhD, Stefanie Luebberding PhD, Nils Krueger PhD, Laura Harrington PhD, and Martina Kerscher MD	Dermatol Surg 2015;41:S29–S38

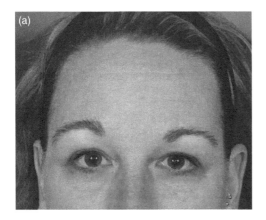
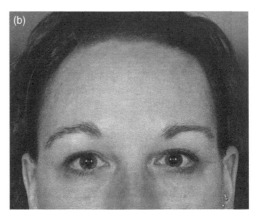

Figure 7.1 Xeomin clinical examples: (a) day 0; (b) 180 days posttreatment. Photos courtesy of Michael H. Gold, MD.

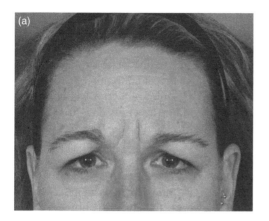
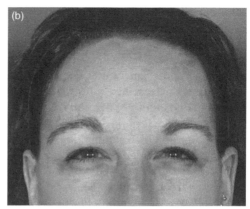

Figure 7.2 **Xeomin clinical examples: (a) day 0; (b) 180 days posttreatment. Photos courtesy of Michael H. Gold, MD.**

phase III Xeomin trials [8, 9]. These are photographs at rest and maximum frown for one of my patients comparing day 0 and day 180.

Of further interest, in one of the largest clinical trials comparing Xeomin and Botox Cosmetic ever performed in the United States, a Xeomin–Botox Cosmetic trial was performed to look closely at all the parameters we judge when evaluating a toxin. Xeomin was found to be as effective as Botox Cosmetic for duration of affect, time to maximum benefit, and duration of treatment effect. In over 250 adult women, Xeomin performed as well as Botox Cosmetic in every category studied [10]. To many, this showed that Xeomin is interchangeable with Botox Cosmetic when FDA dosing is used.

PurTox

PurTox was being developed by Mentor Corporation, Santa Barbara, CA. Mentor is now a subsidiary of Johnson & Johnson Inc., New Brunswick, NJ. PurTox, as its name implies, is also a "pure" toxin, as described earlier. It is also a product that currently has negligible data in the public domain; therefore, we will describe what is known from the initial clinical trials and what is in the public domain thus far. We also can report that Mentor has decided not to pursue the development of

PurTox further, but this author considers it important to show the work that was carried out with this product, and reflect on why the product has never come to market.

Whereas Xeomin was initially studied in Europe and much of this initial data guided the US clinical trial program, the Mentor PurTox program was solely performed in the United States. The US FDA phase I clinical trial was entitled "To Determine the Dose Range for Safety and Efficacy of Mentor's Purified Botulinum Toxin for the Treatment of Glabellar Rhytides." This was a single-center, dose escalation study of 40 subjects; it was open-label, randomized, double-blind, and placebo-controlled. Each subject received five injections into the glabella area at preset injection sites, which have been the same for every toxin study. For evaluations, subjects used a static subjective global assessment (SGA) scale of 1–100 mm, the physician used a validated photoscale of 0–3, and photo documentation was maintained throughout the study. The summary data from the phase I clinical trial was that there was no premature discontinuation from the study due to adverse events (AEs); no serious AEs or deaths on this clinical trial; no ptosis or diplopia were observed; there were five AEs (13.9%), which were moderate in intensity, and none were thought to be related to the study drug; the majority (86.1%) of AEs were mild in intensity; mild events included injection site pain in two subjects (considered mild by the subjects), a slight headache in one subject, and a taste perversion in three subjects; higher response rates were seen at higher doses; and higher response rates were sustained at higher doses of PurTox. PurTox to Botox ratio has been determined to also be a 1 : 1 ratio, the same as with Xeomin [7].

The phase I clinical trial led to the development of a phase II US-based clinical trial. Its title was "To Determine the Optimal Dose for Efficacy of Mentor's Purified Botulinum Toxin for the Treatment of Glabellar Rhytides." In this clinical trial, 136 subjects were enrolled at two clinical research sites; it was double-blind, placebo-controlled, and randomized and four dose ranges of the toxin were evaluated. Each subject received five injections as in previous clinical trials in the glabella area. The subjects and physicians used the same scales throughout the study as those used in the phase I clinical trials. A summary of the findings from the phase II clinical trial showed that a dose-dependent increase in the response rate was observed for primary and secondary efficacy endpoints in the clinical trial.

The highest dose tested consistently resulted in the highest response rate, which was statistically significantly different from that of the placebo. The duration of effect was dose dependent with trends of increasing duration with increasing dose levels of toxin. Many subjects reported the onset of a change in appearance within 2 days of toxin administration [7].

These positive results led to the development of a phase III clinical trial program which is described below. This phase III program consisted of three distinct clinical trials:

Phase IIIa, entitled "A MultiCenter, Randomized, Double-Blind, Placebo-Controlled, Two-Arm, Single-Dose Pivotal Trial to Demonstrate the Safety and Efficacy of Repeat Treatment with PurTox for the Treatment of Glabellar Rhytides ("Frown Lines")" consisted of 402 patients enrolled at 10 clinical sites. Each injection session utilized 30 units of PurTox injected into the glabellar area. This phase involved a 6-month follow-up period. The primary endpoint for this clinical endpoint was to achieve at least a 2-point reduction in line severity at maximum frown at day 30 as scored by the subject and by the investigator. Secondary endpoints included investigator rating of 1 or 0 at maximum frown at day 30; a 2-point reduction at day 30 from baseline maximum frown by an independent reviewer; a 1-point reduction at day 3 from baseline maximum frown by the investigator; a 1-point reduction at day 7 from baseline maximum frown by the investigator; a 2-point reduction at day 30 from baseline maximum frown by the investigator; and a 2-point reduction at day 3 from baseline maximum frown by the subject.

Phase IIIb, entitled "A Multi-Center Trial to Demonstrate the Safety and Efficacy of Repeat Treatment with PurTox for the Treatment of Glabellar Rhytides ("Frown Lines")" was also commenced. It enrolled 699 subjects at 12 clinical sites and looked at repeat injections and long-term safety effects of PurTox.

Phase IIIc, entitled "A Multi-Center, Long-Term, Repeat-Treatment, Open-Label, Single-Arm Trial to Demonstrate the Safety of Repeat Treatment with PurTox for the Treatment of Glabellar Rhytides ("Frown Lines")" was also performed in 576 subjects at 12 clinical sites, also looking at the safety and efficacy of repeated injections of PurTox [7].

From the clinical trials, with data not yet in the public domain, several clinical photographs are now available and will be shared here. Figure 7.3 and Figure 7.4 show PurTox effects at day 0, 3, and 7 at maximum frown, whereas Figure 7.5 and Figure 7.6 show PurTox results at days 0 and day 180 at maximum frown. Again, this product is not available despite much exemplary research

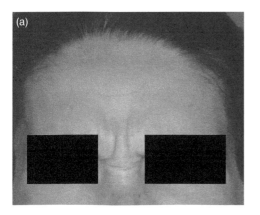
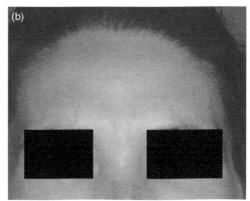
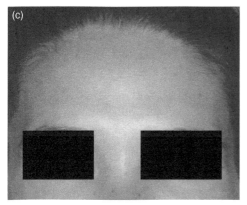

Figure 7.3 PurTox clinical examples, effects seen as: (a) day 0; (b) day 3; (c) day 7.

being performed on it, with public results all being positive.

Nabota – DWP-450

Recently, Nabota, a botulinum toxin from Daewoong Pharmaceuticals in South Korea, developed a strategic alliance with Alphaeon Pharmaceuticals (Irvine, CA) here in the United States. With positive results from the Korean trials and a marketed drug in Asia [11], the US FDA clinical trials began with a large phase III program. This was set up as two randomized clinical trials similar to that seen with the Xeomin clinical trial program. Again, a 2-point improvement by both the physician and the patient. The results from these two clinical trials were recently released and they showed statistical significance over

that of placebo, and very acceptable 2-point improvement scores. More clinical results will be brought out at a later time and this toxin may be on the market by early 2017.

Hugel Botulax – Croma Pharma

Also a Korean toxin, approved in Asia, Croma Pharma has recently begun its phase III US clinical trials in a manner similar to that carried out for both Xeomin and DWP-450. Results from this will be expected later in 2016 or 2017.

Neuronox

Neuronox is made by the Korean company MedyTox. It is also being marketed by Ranbaxy Pharmaceuticals in India and is

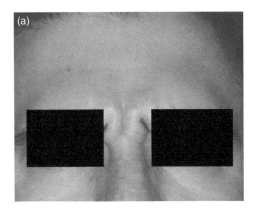
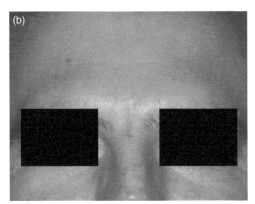
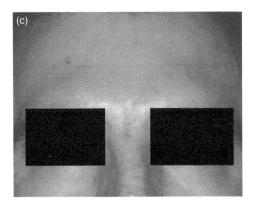

Figure 7.4 PurTox clinical examples, effects seen as: (a) day 0; (b) day 3; (c) day 7.

commercially available in South America where it is known as Siax. In 2014, the US rights to this product was purchased by Allergan (Irvine, CA).

At the time of writing, there are no current US clinical trials pending for this neurotoxin, and we may not see this toxin in the United States for many years to come or

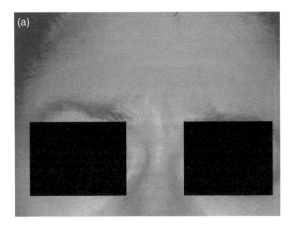
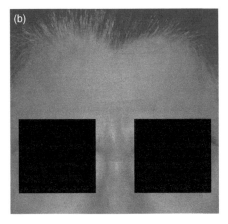

Figure 7.5 PurTox clinical examples, effects seen as: (a) day 0; (b) day 180.

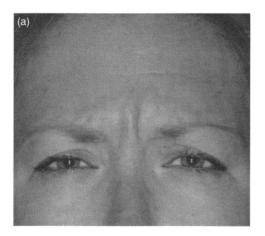 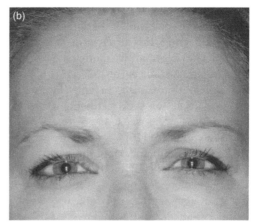

Figure 7.6 PurTox clinical examples, effects seen as: (a) day 0; (b) day 180.

not at all. There is also a limited amount of data available for the cosmetic uses of Neuronox, although there are photographs on the website from MedyTox regarding its cosmetic indications.

In one clinical trial in which Neuronox and Botox were compared in a double-blind study in the treatment of hemifacial spasm, 173 individuals received either Neuronox or Botox. The results showed the equivalence in efficacy amongst the two products, and that the Botox to Neuronox dilution ratio was 1 : 1 [12].

Clinical trials with Neuronox for cosmetic indications are not easily accessible. Siax is the same product as that available from Medy-Tox, although, once again clinical trials for cosmetic indications are not readily available.

ChinaTox

There are also botulinum toxins that are manufactured in China and routinely referred to as ChinaTox. Many clinicians are attempting to find out more about the development of these toxins. There appears to be two main manufacturers of toxins in China: Lanzhou Biological Products Institute, and Nanfeng Medical Science and Tech Co.

The only published clinical trial which is accessible, was an open-label clinical trial that enrolled 785 patients with focal spasm and dystonia: 192 patients received Botox; 593 ChinaTox. It was found that the ChinaTox was less powerful than Botox – higher doses were required to achieve similar effects and five cases of skin rashes were seen in the ChinaTox group, which was not evident in the Botox group [13].

Further clinical information regarding ChinaTox is not currently readily available.

Other Toxins

It should be noted that there are several other toxins that have been evaluated and may have an impact in the future. Galderma has brought to the forefront a "liquid" toxin and phase II US clinical trials have been completed [14]. The results have been promising although no other data from the clinical trials are currently in the public domain. We hope to learn more in the near future.

Another company that will be bringing both an injectable and a topical toxin to market is Revance Therapeutics (Newark, CA). They have been actively working on a topical neurotoxin and have had some significant results thus far. Their drug, known as daxibotulinumtoxinA Topical Gel (RT001) has shown positive results in several phase II clinical trials for the treatment of lateral canthal lines. Currently, this drug is in its phase III clinical trials and we anticipate more results in late 2016 or early 2017 [15]. This topical preparation is also currently in phase II clinical trials for the treatment of axillary hyperhidrosis. At week 4, positive results have been obtained [16]. Again, more results will be forthcoming. Daxibotulinum-toxinA for injection (RT002) is also being evaluated by Revance. Its phase 2 active comparator study assesses the safety, efficacy, and duration of effect of three doses of RT002 versus placebo and Botox Cosmetic. The topline interim data presented thus far showed that RT002 achieved its primary efficacy measurement for all three doses at 4 weeks. The study demonstrated 6-month RT002 median duration of effect based upon at least 1-point improvement in glabellar lines at maximum frown on the Investigator Global Assessment-Facial Wrinkle Severity (IGA-FWS) scale [17]. More studies and more results are expected with this drug shortly.

And finally, another topical neurotoxin, by Anterios (New York, NY) was developed for the treatment of hyperhidrosis [18]. Phase II clinical data showed positive results and Anterios was purchased by Allergan. Further investigations with this drug are expected in the near future.

Conclusions

There are some exciting recent developments for "Future Toxins." In the United States we now have Xeomin, whereas PurTox has been removed from its potential place in our toxin armamentarium. We have two more toxins in development – one just finished its phase III studies and one just in the midst of its phase III studies. Other topical toxins are being developed and that discussion is beyond the scope of this manuscript. We also look forward to other toxins potentially developed – perhaps longer lasting, perhaps liquid in nature, and perhaps with other virtues that will improve things even more. But as noted in the beginning, we owe all of this to Botox Cosmetic, which changed the aesthetic landscape for many of us.

Only FDA approved toxins are to be injected in the United States – Period! Never waver or flinch in your desire to use toxins from other countries or from other sources – it is not allowed here. We will continue to follow the toxin development process and report on any new medications as they become available.

References

1 Cervical Dystonia and Blepharospasm: U.S. Food and Drug Administration. Xeomin (incobotulinumtoxinA) Injection Label and Approval History. July 20, 2010. Available at http://www.accessdata.fda.gov/drugsatfda_docs/appletter/2010/125360s000,s001ltr.pdf. Accessed February 22, 2017.

2 Glabellar Lines: U.S. Food and Drug Administration. Xeomin (incobotulinumtoxinA) Injection Label and Approval History. July 20, 2011. Available at http://www.accessdata.fda.gov/scripts/cder/drugsatfda/index.cfm?fuseaction=Search. Label_ApprovalHistory#apphist. Accessed February 22, 2017.

3 Merz Announces European Approval of Bocouture for the Treatment of Upper Facial Lines, Franfurt am Main, March 17, 2016, http://www.fda.gov/downloads/Drugs/DrugSafety/UCM222360.pdf

4 Fritsch C. Efficacy of the new Botulinum toxin (Xeomin®) free of complexing proteins in the therapy of mimical smile lines. Kosmet Med 2006;27(3):124–129.

5 Sattler G, Callander M, Grablowiz D, et al. Noninferiority of incobotulinumtoxinA,

free from complexing proteins, compared with another botulinum toxin type A in the treatment of glabellar frown lines. Dermatol Surg 2010;36:2146–2154.

6 Prager W, Wissmuller E, Kollhorst B, *et al.* Comparison of two botulinum toxin type A preparations for treating crow's feet: a split-face, double-blind, proof-of-concept study. Dermatol Surg. 2010;36: 2155–2160.

7 Personal communication, Mentor Corp.

8 Hanke CW, Narins RS, Brandt F, *et al.* A randomized, placebo-controlled, double-blind phase iii trial investigating the efficacy and safety of incobotulinumtoxinA in the treatment of glabellar frown lines using a stringent composite endpoint. Dermatol Surg 2013;39(6):891–899.

9 Carruthers A, Carruthers J, Coleman W, *et al.* Multicenter, randomized, phase iii study of a single dose of incobotulinumtoxinA, free from complexing proteins, in the treatment of glabellar frown lines. Dermatol Surg 2013; 39 (4):551–558.

10 Kane MA, Gold MH, Coleman WP, *et al.* A randomized, double-blind trial to investigate the equivalence of incobotulinumtoxinA and onabotulinumtoxinA for glabellar frown lines. Dermatol Surg 2015;41:1310–1319

11 Won Ch, Kim HK, Kim BJ, *et al.* Comparative trial of a novel botulinum neurotoxin type A versus onabotulinumtoxinA in the treatment of glabellar lines: A multicenter, randomized, double-blind, active-controlled study. Int J Dermatol 2015;54(2):227–234.

12 Walker TJ, Dayan S. Comparison and overview of currently available neurotoxins. J Clin Aesthet Dermatol February 2014;7(2):31–39.

13 Jiang HY, Chen S, Zhou J, *et al.* Diffusion of two botulinum toxins type A on the forehead: double-blinded, randomized, controlled study. Dermatol Surg 2014; 40(2):184–192.

14 Liquid toxin and Phase II US clinical trials. October 6, 2014. Available at http://www .galderma.com/News/articleType/Article View/articleId/70/Galderma-Initiates-US-Study-of-Novel-Muscle-Relaxant-for-Aesthetic-Dermatology-and-Cosmetic-Surgery. Accessed July 21, 2016.

15 Revance Report Results for RT001 Topical Phase 3 Trial. June 13, 2016. Available at http://investors.revance.com/releasedetail .cfm?ReleaseID=975537. Accessed July 21, 2016.

16 Revance Positive Phase 2 Results for RT002. December 23, 2015. Available at http://investors.revance.com/releasedetail .cfm?ReleaseID=948101. Accessed February 22, 2017.

17 Revance 6-Month duration results for BELMONT Phase 2 Active Comparator Study for Injectable RT002. March 5, 2016. Available at http://investors.revance.com/ releasedetail.cfm?ReleaseID=958981. Accessed February 22, 2017.

18 Topical neurotoxin by Anterios. January 7, 2016. Available at http://www.allergan .com/news/news/thomson-reuters/ allergan-acquires-medical-dermatology-and-aestheti. Accessed on February 22, 2017.

8

Reconstitution, Dilution, Diffusion, and Migration of Botulinum Toxin

Murad Alam, MD (MSCI, MBA),[1] Hayes B. Gladstone, MD,[2] and David M. Ozog, MD (FAAD, FACMS)[3]

[1] Professor and Vice-Chair, Department of Dermatology, Section of Cutaneous and Aesthetic Surgery, Departments of Dermatology, Otolaryngology, and Surgery, Northwestern University, Chicago, USA
[2] Gladstone Clinic, San Ramon, USA
[3] Chair, Department of Dermatology; C.S. Livingood Chair in Dermatology; Director of Cosmetic Dermatology, Henry Ford Hospital, Detroit, MI, USA

Introduction

When applied to the preparation and usage of botulinum toxin, dilution, reconstitution, and diffusion of botulinum toxin are controversial concepts, the clarity of which is further clouded by a lack of consensus regarding their definitions. Nonetheless, these are important variables that have therapeutic implications. In this section, we will put forth working definitions for dilution, reconstitution, and diffusion, and review the clinical evidence pertaining to safety and efficacy when these parameters are varied. For simplicity, we will focus primarily on aesthetic use of botulinum toxin A.

Definitions

Reconstitution

Needless to say, dictionary definitions are too vague, and even medical dictionary definitions are insufficiently targeted to botulinum toxin. For the purposes of this discussion, we take reconstitution to denote the addition of diluent, specifically some form of sterile saline, to prepackaged sterile solid botulinum toxin provided in a sealed glass vial. Reconstitution may be with various forms of saline, including saline with or without benzyl alcohol preservative. Additionally, the method of reconstitution need not be specific beyond this definition: for instance, it may or may not include defeating of the vacuum in the vial prior to fluid injection, and similarly may or may not include full removal of the rubber vial stopper prior to fluid addition.

Dilution

Dilution, in colloquial usage when referring to botulinum toxin preparation, is often considered synonymous with reconstitution. This, however, is clearly contrary to the primary meaning of the word since dilution implies further reduction or variation in the concentration of a solution, while the preparation of botulinum toxin for clinical use commences not with a solution but with a solid, which cannot be "diluted." Moreover there is no need to use the term dilution if it means exactly the same as reconstitution. For the purposes of discussion, dilution can thus be redefined as a measure of the volume in milliliters (ml) of saline that is used to reconstitute one vial of botulinum toxin. An alternative, more precise but less commonly used, construct entails specifying dilution as the number of units per saline volume in ml. Regardless of the method chosen, since multiple botulinum toxin preparations with different numbers of units per vial are now commercially available, the type of toxin and the number of units per vial also need to be listed.

Diffusion, Migration, and Action Halo

Diffusion, in routine usage, is a measure of the maximum distance from the site of a skin injection at which clinical effectiveness is observed. This is at variance of the general meaning of diffusion as a measure of the ability of a gas or liquid to travel through another substance, usually either gas or liquid. In this general definition, the rate of diffusion or the distance to which diffusion occurs in a certain time period may be further clarified. But, in any event, diffusion remains a measure of where a substance is and how it moves, and not of the distance at which pharmacologic efficacy occurs. To explain, as a neurotoxin, botulinum toxin may theoretically affect local nerves, with this effect propagating at a distance, even all the way to the central nervous system, without concomitant movement of the toxin itself; conversely, botulinum toxin may diffuse in very small amounts to a broad radius from the point of injection, but the concentration at the periphery may be below the threshold required to elicit a clinical response.

For the purposes of discussion, we leave diffusion (a true synonym may be "migration") to denote the movement in a unit of time of a standard dilution of a botulinum toxin solution through the skin and subcutaneous tissues. And we suggest the term "action halo," which has been successfully pioneered by others, to mean what "diffusion" is colloquially taken to mean: the maximum distance from the site of injection at which clinical effectiveness, either muscle motion reduction or hypohidrosis, is observed.

Notably, from the point of view of fluid dynamics, the rate of diffusion and the action halo may be related. However, as previously discussed, more than just diffusion can affect the action halo. One such factor is dilution. When botulinum toxin is diluted in a higher volume of saline, an injection of equivalent potency in units may diffuse relatively further due to the higher fluid load. Let us assume for a moment that there are two hypothetical forms of botulinum toxin, one with a narrower action halo than the other. If the type with the smaller action halo is mixed in a much higher volume of saline, the action halo may be modified and become much wider. Thus, by definition, if action halo is used to compare different types of botulinum toxin preparations, the halo must be specified for a particular dilution. So we propose two measures of action halo: (i) action halo$_s$, or static action halo, which is measured for a fixed dilution, and under standard conditions, and can be used to compare and characterize different commercially available formulations of botulinum toxin; and (ii) action halo$_d$, or dynamic action halo, which can vary based on dilution and other patient and physician specific-factors, and measures the utility of a particular injection of botulinum toxin in a particular patient.

Reconstitution

Current FDA guidelines found on package inserts for storage before and after reconstitution of botulinum toxins is as follows:

- Unopened vials of abobotulinumtoxinA must be stored under refrigeration at 2–8°C (36–46°F). Once reconstituted abobotulinumtoxinA should be stored in the original container in a refrigerator (2–8°C) and used within four (4) hours.
- Unopened vials of onabotulinumtoxinA should be stored in a refrigerator (2–8°C). Onabotulinumtoxina should be administered within 24 hours after reconstitution. During this time period, reconstituted onabotulinumtoxinA should be stored in a refrigerator (2–8°C).
- Unopened vials of incobotulinumtoxinA can be stored at room temperature 20–25°C (68–77° F), in a refrigerator at 2–8°C

(36–46°F), or a freezer at −20 to −10°C (−4 to 14°F) for up to 36 months. Reconstituted incobotulinumtoxinA should be stored in a refrigerator at 2–8°C (36–46°F) and administered within 24 hours.

- The recommended storage condition for rimabotulinumtoxinB is refrigeration at 2–8°C. No constitution is required since rimabotulinumtoxinB is provided as a clear and colorless to light-yellow sterile injectable solution. However, rimabotulinumtoxinB may be diluted with normal saline. Once diluted, the product must be used within four (4) hours.
- The FDA approved reconstitution diluent for the three type A toxins is sterile (0.9%) normal saline. However, we will thoroughly discuss common off-label storage and reconstitution practices.

Adverse Events

At present, there is no evidence that modification of the FDA-approved reconstitution regimen (i.e., with sterile saline, and with usage within 4–24 hours) for botulinum toxin A leads to minor or serious adverse events (AEs). Cote and colleagues reviewed all AEs reported to the FDA for therapeutic and cosmetic use of botulinum toxin for December 1989 to May 2003, and did not note any AEs as specifically emanating from reconstitution or dilution decisions [1]. They did report that among the cases of minor (995) or serious (36) adverse events associated with cosmetic use, there were frequent cases of diluent substitutions, including replacement of the standard saline diluent with bupivacaine, lidocaine, water, and previously reconstituted toxin. However, there was no evidence that such substitutions were any more common in the AE group than in the much larger group without AEs, or that there was any casual relationship between substitutions and adverse events. We could find no case control studies that compared the incidence of AEs between standard and nonstandard reconstitution regimens. Beer [2] reported a case in which a small rubber core was displaced into

the reconstituted toxin by the motion of the needle used for diluents injection; he noted that this type of fragmentation posed a potential risk for foreign body emboli, were the particles small enough to be pulled into a syringe with the fluid and inadvertently injected. But no such theoretic risk has materialized, and this risk is not related to the diluent used or the method of reconstitution. United States practitioners should be aware that the Centers for Disease Control (CDC) guidelines insist on strict adherence to single patient use for each vial of toxin based on concern regarding spread of infection [3]. However, their instances of contamination were largely based on unsafe practices including reinserting needles to dispense intravenous medications and anesthetics. Following this, an expert dermatology panel reviewed the data and formed a consensus recommendation determining that a single vial of botulinum toxin can be safely administered to multiple patients, assuming standard safe injection techniques are followed, However, the authors believe that only preserved saline should be used in these instances to further reduce risk of infection [4].

Effectiveness of Stored Solution

Regarding the manufacturer recommendation that storage of reconstituted toxin should not exceed 4–24 hours, there is a preponderance of anecdotal information that this is not necessary for effective and safe usage. Many if not most physicians who use botulinum toxin for cosmetic indications store residual reconstituted toxin for days if not weeks and use the so-called "single-use" vials for treatment of multiple patients, as appropriate. At least four randomized control trials (RCT) have confirmed that clinical effectiveness of botulinum toxin does not decrease for at least several weeks after reconstitution. In a multicenter RCT, four vials of onabotulinumtoxinA were reconstituted for 1–6 weeks, respectively, before their use for treatment of glabella frown lines [5]. Blinded raters could not detect any difference in clinical efficacy among the groups. Another RCT employed a split-face design, with one side of the forehead receiving freshly reconstituted toxin and the other side toxin that had been prepared 2 weeks previously, and then either refrigerated (4°C) or frozen (−20°C) [6]. Again, no difference was detected between the clinical response of the two treatment arms. A third blinded, split-face RCT of onabotulinumtoxinA found no difference in the reduction of dynamic crow's feet lines associated with freshly reconstituted botulinumtoxinA and toxin prepared 1 week earlier and then refrigerated (4°C) before use [7]. An RCT of abobotulinumtoxinA similarly found that toxin samples reconstituted 8 hours, 8 days, and 15 days before use were indistinguishable based on clinical response as evaluated by blinded raters [8]. Very long-term freezing of toxin after reconstitution and before usage also does not appear to render it less effective. In a prospective, nonrandomized, nonblinded split-face study of 80 patients, onabotulinumtoxinA was either reconstituted within 4 hours of use, or reconstituted and immediately frozen (−15°C) for up to 6 months before being thawed at room temperature for use [9]. No significant difference in efficacy or side effects was noted between the frozen and fresh toxin injections.

Safety and Sterility of Stored Solution

Regarding the safety of botulinum toxin vials reconstituted days or weeks before use, and possibly each used for multiple patients, there is evidence that microbial contamination does not occur. In a study of 127 reconstituted vials, these were accessed for extraction of reconstituted toxin by multiple different medical personnel several times each over a mean period of 7 weeks [10]. Subsequent sterility assessment of the vials with thioglycolate broth indicated no evidence of contamination. A follow-on study from the ophthalmology literature similarly demonstrated no microbial growth from botulinum toxin bottles reconstituted per protocol, kept at room temperature for 4 hours, and then stored in a refrigerator (3–5°C) for 5–7 days prior to sampling [11]. A survey of physician members of the American Society for Dermatologic Surgery found no local infections after toxin injection among 322 respondents, most of whom routinely kept reconstituted toxin for 1–4 weeks [4]. The safety of off-label storage time (greater than 4 hours) and multiple patient use for a single vial is dependent on standard safe injection practices and may be enhanced by our recommended use of preservative containing (benzyl alcohol) bacteriostatic saline rather than manufacturers recommendation of preservative-free sterile saline for reconstitution.

Effect of Vigorous Mixing of Solution

Beyond the time elapsed between reconstitution and usage, and the use of each vial for multiple patients, other factors pertaining to the reconstitution method have been investigated with regard to effectiveness and not found to be relevant. For instance, the force with which the toxin is reconstituted is immaterial to clinical response. Kazim and Black [12] in a blinded, split-face RCT, compared gentle mixing in of the diluent during reconstitution, as specified in the package insert, and vigorous reconstitution for 1.5 minutes. Both types of mixing induced similar response of onabotulinumtoxinA injected into forehead lines, and eyebrow excursion was similar after treatment. A similar split-face study compared the clinical effect on crow's feet and glabellar lines of onabotulinumtoxinA reconstituted slowly to avoid foaming, and of toxin reconstituted rapidly and shaken to deliberately produce as many bubbles as possible [13]. Clinical efficacy was similar with and without foaming.

Effect of Diluent Type on Injection Pain

Modification of the botulinum toxin reconstitution regimen has been definitively shown to reduce pain and discomfort on injection.

Specifically, reconstitution with saline containing benzyl alcohol, a preservative and mild anesthetic, can reduce patient self-reported injection pain by a third to a half with 100% of subjects preferring bacteriostatic saline in the prospective arm [14]. This difference has been verified in double-blind RCTs in which glabellar, forehead and crow's feet lines were treated with onabotulinumtoxinA [14] as well as with abobotulinumtoxinA [15]. Additionally, further RCTs have shown the same benefit for injections of the neck and axillary areas [16]. A consensus panel agreed that the use of preserved saline can be used for reconstitution, given its improved clinical tolerability [17]. In the ophthalmology literature, RCT data has revealed similar pain reduction for therapeutic injections, such as those for essential blepharospasm [18]. Given this evidence, almost 78% of surveyed US dermatologists now use bacteriostatic saline with benzyl alcohol as their diluent. At least one split-face, blinded RCT has extended these findings to reconstitution of onabotulinumtoxinA with 2% lidocaine, which has been reported to provide pain relief during injection of axilla for hyperhidrosis [19]. Such pain reduction may be more appropriate during use of botulinum toxin B, which has been shown in side-by-side studies to be more painful on injection when reconstituted with normal saline than either onabotulinumtoxinA or abobotulinumtoxinA [20]. However, this study was performed comparing normal saline reconstitution to 2% lidocaine. Since most surveyed dermatologists now use preservative containing saline, a more clinically relevant comparison would involve preservative (benzyl alcohol) containing saline versus 2% lidocaine.

Dilution Volume

In cosmetic usage, dilution volumes for commercially available botulinum toxins vary from 1 to 10 ml per vial [21]. For onabotulinumtoxinA, this means a dilution of 10–100 U/ml. More commonly, vials are reconstituted with 1–3 ml. The theoretical arguments in favor of concentrated solutions include: (i) greater precision in delivering the dose as there is less migration or diffusion away from the point of injection; (ii) potentially increased effectiveness associated with equivalent dosages delivered in higher concentrations; (iii) fewer side effects like injection pain [22], erythema, edema, visible bumps, bruising, and brow ptosis, which may be associated with injections of larger total volumes; and (iv) ease of administration as fewer syringes are needed. The theoretical arguments proposed in support of more dilute solutions are: (i) greater accuracy in delivering exactly the correct dosage to each injection site as each μl represents a smaller number of units and an inadvertent extra droplet is unlikely to markedly alter dosage; (ii) reduced unit loss in the "hub" of the syringe or during reconstitution or loading of syringes (which the proponents of concentrated injections say can be reduced by use of an insulin syringe with no dead space); (iii) improved efficacy of per unit as each unit migrates further and has a greater total effect; (iv) smooth, continuous (rather than focal) resolution of dynamic creases associated with a wider action halo of dilute solutions. In empirical research and practice, the evidence for these various hypotheses is limited [23]. Differences in technique are predicated on preference rather than hard data. Given that many hard to delineate factors, such as injection pressure, angle of incidence, depth of insertion, needle type, and patient skin type or ethnicity, may also influence injection effectiveness, it may be that everyone is right. Certain dilution methods may indeed be best for some practitioners without necessarily being intrinsically optimal. Also, by maintaining constant technique, practitioners may be able to better predict outcomes precisely, and this too, is a very important consideration when providing an elective, cosmetic intervention designed to effect small changes.

Diffusion and Migration

Two distinct approaches have been used to study diffusion and migration of toxin from the point of injection. Neither relies on tagging of the dissociated molecules or other direct observations of movement. Rather, both are indirect intermediate measures. The first is a clinical assessment of the locus of reduction of dynamic creases of the upper face, and the correspondence of this phenomenon with the likely spread of the toxin; the second is a clinical assessment of the radius of an induced hypohidrotic halo around the point of injection.

Action Halo Measured by Reduction in Facial Rhytides

A split-face randomized control trial of onabotulinumtoxinA injections into forehead lines entailed injecting one side of the forehead with 5 U in 0.25 ml (5 ml per vial dilution volume) of preserved saline, and the other side with 5 U in 0.05 ml (1 ml per vial dilution volume) [24]. At 14 days after injection of 10 subjects, the action halo$_d$ had on average a 50% greater surface area in subjects receiving the high volume injections, with the area of wrinkle reduction being oval with width greater than height. A similar, subsequent study – sponsored by the manufacturer of onabotulinumtoxinA – of 80 patients randomized to 4 dilution groups (1, 3, 5l, and 10 ml per vial dilution volume) studied the effect on glabellar wrinkle severity [25]. No significant differences were found. Notably, the latter study did not study multiple dilutions in the same patients, and it examined glabella rhytides rather than forehead rhytides, so the different results are not necessarily conflictual. Another split-face RCT of 20 subjects (also funded by the company) examined not the forehead or glabella but rather crow's feet rhytides [26]. Half the subjects received a single injection of dilute 5 U (5 ml per vial dilution volume) to the left lateral canthus, and concentrated 5 U (1 ml per vial dilution volume) to the right lateral canthus; the other half were randomized to receive the opposite. No difference in visually estimated action halo$_d$ was detected between the two arms.

Action Halo Measured by Extent of Hypohidrosis

Some have suggested that measurement of hypohidrotic action halos provides a better measure of diffusion [27]. This method requires application of the starch–iodine test once the toxin has taken effect. In comparing different toxin formulations, the greatest challenge is to select an appropriate conversion factor to ensure dosage comparability in units. A method to do this perfectly remains elusive, so there is always the risk that rather than comparing intrinsic diffusion properties of different formulations, investigators are inadvertently confounding this measurement with disparities in total dosage. For comparisons of onabotulinumtoxinA and abobotulinumtoxinA, the commonly used conversions in units are 1 : 2.5 or 1 : 3. In one RCT of forehead hyperhidrosis, subjects received two injections of 3 U each of onabotulinumtoxinA to one side of the forehead and two injections of 7.5, 9, or 12 U each of abobotulinumtoxinA to the contralateral side [28]. This corresponded to onabotulinumtoxinA : abobotulinumtoxinA ratios of 1 : 2.5, 1 : 3, and 1 : 4. Injections volumes were the same for all injections (0.6 ml/injection). For each side, one injection was intradermal and one intramuscular. The anhidrotic halos produced by abobotulinumtoxinA were larger than those with onabotulinumtoxinA at all dilution volumes (Figure 8.1). Significantly, clinical assessment of forehead wrinkles by a blinded rater revealed no superior inhibition of forehead rhytides with abobotulinumtoxinA. Kerscher *et al.* looked at the spread of abobotulinumtoxinA, onabotulinumtoxinA, as well as incobotulinumtoxinA. No difference was seen in the spread of onabotulinumtoxinA (5 U)

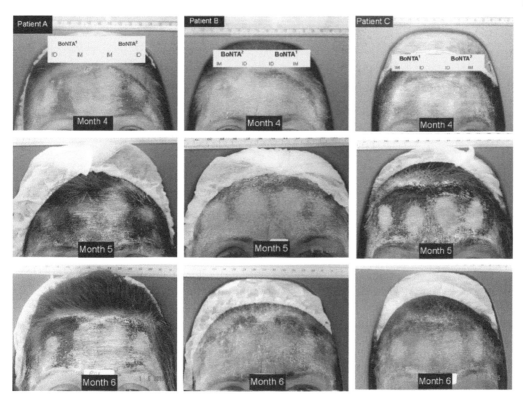

Figure 8.1 Pattern of anhidrosis after BoNTA treatment showing greater area of anhidrosis at the medial injection sites than the lateral injection sites and the greater area of diffusion with BoNTA² than BoNTA¹. The dose ratio was 1 : 2.5 in Patients A and B and 1 : 3 in Patient C. BoNTA, botulinum toxin type A; IM, intramuscular injection; ID, intradermal injection.

compared to incobotulinumtoxinA (5 U). However, once again abobotulinumtoxinA (12.5 U) had statistically larger anhidrotic halos at 6 weeks compared with the other two type A toxins. The injection volumes were identical and the onabotulinumtoxinA : abobotulinumtoxinA and incobotulinumtoxinA : abobotulinumtoxinA ratios were 1 : 2.5 [29]. A similar study by Hexsel *et al.* (and supported by the manufacturer of onabotulinumtoxinA) injected contralateral sides of the forehead with either 2 U onabotulinumtoxinA or 5 U abobotulinumtoxinA (1 : 2.5 ratio), each in 0.02 ml volume (1 ml dilution volume per vial of onabotulinumtoxinA), and detected no difference in the mean size of the hypohidrotic halos [30] (Figures 8.2 and 8.3).

Comparison of Botulinum Toxin A and B

Botulinum toxin A preparations have also been compared to botulinum toxin B formulations. One study compared forehead injections of 5 U of onabotulinumtoxinA to contralateral side injections of 500 U of rimabotulinumtoxinB [31]. The area of diffusion or migration was greater with the latter, as measured by area of wrinkle reduction. A similar study that assessed action halos$_d$ by measuring anhidrotic areas with starch–iodine tests found significantly larger halos with rimabotulinumtoxinB versus onabotulinumtoxinA at 3 weeks after injection with a 75 : 1 dosage ratio [32]. However, the rate of shrinkage of the onabotulinumtoxinA action halo was slower over time, and after week 24,

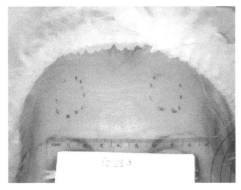 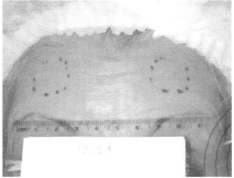

Figure 8.2 Same patient at rest and at the maximum voluntary frowning of the forehead area. On day 28, the border area of muscular weakness around the injected points was demarcated with a marker pen, followed by measurement using a standard ruler.

the mean size of the onabotulinumtoxinA action halos was larger. At least one study compared the hypohidrotic action halos of onabotulinumtoxinA, abobotulinumtoxinA, and rimabotulinumtoxinB side-by-side [33]. When the 3 formulations were reconstituted at a dose per volume of 100 U/ml, the anhidrotic halos were approximately equivalent. This is at variance with the other studies that suggest very large dose conversion factors. Overall, the lowest concentrations, 20 U/ml for onabotulinumtoxinA, and 100 U/ml for the other two formulations, induced the largest mean anhidrotic area per unit. Interestingly, other studies of therapeutic usage of botulinum toxin have indicated that a smaller dose conversion factor may be appropriate for these indications.

For instance, for palmar hyperhidrosis, onabotulinumtoxinA at 100 U/ml was found to be equipotent to abobotulinumtoxinA at 100–150 U/ml [34].

Effect of Additives on Migration and Action Halo

Pharmacologic modifications to standard botulinum toxin formulations may also modify their diffusion and migration. For instance, addition of small quantities of epinephrine, at a final concentration of 1 : 100,000, has been reported to improve local response to toxin and to inhibit the radius of the action halo$_d$ [35]. Hantash and Gladstone performed a split-face study evaluating the addition of epinephrine to botulinum toxin

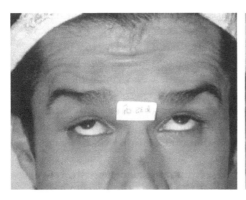 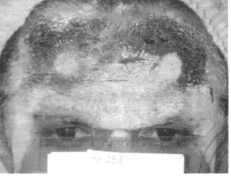

Figure 8.3 Areas of muscular weakness and anhidrosis around the injected points in the frontal area, 28 days later.

on the relaxation of periorbital rhytides [36]. In 14 patients, a single injection of Botox plus epinephrine was compared to Botox alone for the treatment of "crow's feet." The results demonstrated that the addition of epinephrine accelerated the onset of the toxin's effect and improved the short-term efficacy. As with the previous study, the epinephrine most likely enhanced the localization of the toxin.

Conversely, addition of hyaluronidase in small quantities may reduce the need for large quantities of toxin, possibly by improving migration. In a split-body trial of axillary hyperhidrosis, 50 U onabotulinumtoxinA injected had efficacy comparable to 25 U in combination with a small dose of hyaluronidase [37]. The hyaluronidase presumably created channels in the dermis that facilitated migration of the toxin.

Conclusions

In conclusion, it is extremely difficult to generalize regarding comparability of different botulinum toxins. To a large extent, the lack of molecular studies of diffusion, and the consequent well-meaning reliance on imprecise, subjective outcome measures such as visualized area of rhytid relaxation or anhidrotic halo, limits our ability to speak definitively about measures like diffusion and migration. Small but significant differences in study methodology, and because many studies are funded by manufacturers who have specific point of views and reasonably seek to advance these, also make it difficult to compare study results when these are in contradiction. Moreover, even real intrinsic differences in the products are likely minor in magnitude and probably swamped by much larger differences in how various practitioners prepare and use them. Disparate dosages and reconstitution volumes may be effective for specific indications, for certain formulations, in particular patients, and in particular physicians' hands. We recommend reconstitution with bacteriostatic saline containing benzyl alcohol given the preponderance of evidence of improved tolerability and possible improved safety profile, particularly with multiple patients using single-use vials. It is certainly true that botulinum toxin, in all its commercially available forms, is a robust preparation that does not require stringent reconstitution and storage procedures to maintain its effectiveness. Probably the most important message is for every practitioner to have a consistent, rational strategy for preparation and usage, as such consistency is most likely to lead to consistent, predictable results.

References

1 Cote TR, Mohan AK, Polder JA, *et al.* Botulinum toxin type A injections: adverse events reported to the US Food and Drug Administration in therapeutic and cosmetic cases. J Am Acad Dermatol 2005; 53:407–415.

2 Beer K. Case reports: Potential foreign body emboli associated with botulinum toxin A injections. J Drugs Dermatol 2007; 6:220–221.

3 Siegel JD, Rhinehart E, Jackson M, Chiarello L, Health Care Infection Control Practices Advisory Committee. 2007 guideline for isolation precautions: preventing transmission of infectious agents in health care settings. Am J Infect Control 2007;35:S65–S164.

4 Liu A, Carruthers A, Cohen JL, *et al.* Recommendations and current practices for the reconstitution and storage of botulinum toxin type A. J Am Acad Dermatol 2012;67:373–378.

5 Hexsel DM, de Lameida AT, Rutowitsch M, *et al.* Multicenter, double-blind study of the efficacy of injections with botulinum toxin type A reconstituted up to six consecutive

weeks before application. Dermatol Surg 2003;29:523–529.

6 Yang GC, Chiu RJ, Gillman GS. Questioning the need to use Botox within 4 hours of reconstitution. A study of fresh vs 2-week-old Botox. Arch Facial Plast Surg 2008;10:273–279.

7 Lizarralde M, Gutierrez AH, Venegas A. Clinical efficacy of botulinum toxin type A reconstituted and refrigerated 1 week before its application in external canthus dynamic lines. Dermatol Surg 2007;33: 1328–1333.

8 Hexsel D, Rutowitsch MS, de Castro LCM, et al. Blind multicenter study of the efficacy and safety of injections of a commercial preparation of botulinum toxin type A reconstituted up to 15 days before injection. Dermatol Surg 2009;35:933–940.

9 Parsa AA, Lye KD, Parsa FD. Reconstituted botulinum type A neurotoxin: clinical efficacy after long-term freezing before use. Aesth Plast Surg 2007;31:188–191.

10 Alam M, Yoo SS, Wrone DA, et al. Sterility assessment of multiple use botulinum A exotoxin vials: a prospective simulation. J Am Acad Dermatol 2006;55:272–275.

11 Menon J, Murray A. Microbial growth in vials of botulinum toxin following use in clinic. Eye 2007;21:995–997.

12 Kazim NA, Black EH. Botox: shaken, not stirred. Ophthal Plast Reconstr Surg 2008; 24:10–12.

13 de Almeida ART, Kadunc BV, di Chiacchio N, Neto DR. Foam during reconstitution does not affect the potency of botulinum toxin type A. Dermatol Surg 2003;29: 530–532.

14 Alam M, Dover JS, Arndt KA. Pain associated with injection of botulinum A exotoxin reconstituted using saline with and without preservative: a double-blind, randomized controlled trial. Arch Dermatol 2002;38:510–514.

15 Van Laborde S, Dover JS, Moore M, et al. Reduction in injection pain with botulinum toxin type B further diluted using saline with preservative: a double-blind,

randomized control trial. J Am Acad Dermatol 2003;48:875–877.

16 Sarifakioglu N, Sarifakioglu E. Evaluating effects of preservative-containing saline solution on pain perception during botulinum toxin type-A injections at different locations: a prospective, single-blinded, randomized control trial. Aesth Plast Surg 2005;29:113–115.

17 Carruthers J, Fagien S, Matarasso SL, Botox Consensus Group. Consensus recommendations on the use of botulinum toxin type a in facial aesthetics. Plast Reconstr Surg. 2004;114:1S–22S.

18 Kwiat DM, Bersani TA, Bersani A. Increased patient comfort utilizing botulinum toxin type A reconstituted with preserved saline versus nonpreserved saline. Ophthal Plast Reconstr Surg 2004; 20:186–189.

19 Vadoud-Seyedi J, Simonart T. Treatment of axillary hyperhidrosis with botulinum toxin type A reconstituted in lidocaine or in normal saline: a randomized, side-by-side, double-blind study. Br J Dermatol 2007; 156:986–989.

20 Kranz G, Sycha T, Voller B, Gleiss A, Schnider P, Auff E. Pain sensation during intradermal injections of three different botulinum toxin preparations in different doses and dilutions. Dermatol Surg 2006; 32(7):886–890.

21 De Sa Earp AP, Marmur ES. The five D's of botulinum toxin: doses, dilution, diffusion, duration, and dogma. J Cosmet Laser Ther 2008;10:93–102.

22 Boyle MH, McGwin G Jr, Flanagan CE, et al. High versus low concentration botulinum toxin A for benign essential blepharospasm: does dilution make a difference? Ophthal Plast Reconstr Surg 2009;25:81–84.

23 Pickett A, Dodd S, Rzany B. Confusion about diffusion and the art of misinterpreting data when comparing different botulinum toxins used in aesthetic applications. J Cosmet Laser Ther 2008;10: 181–183.

24 Hsu TSJ, Dover JS, Arndt KA. Effect of volume and concentration on the diffusion of botulinum exotoxin A. Arch Dermatol 2004;140:1351–1354.

25 Carruthers A, Carruthers J, Cohen J. Dilution volume of botulinum toxin type A for the treatment of glabellar rhytides: does it matter? Dermatol Surg 2007;33: S97–S104.

26 Carruthers A, Bogle M, Carruthers JDA, *et al.* A randomized, evaluator-blinded, two-center study of the safety and effect of volume on the diffusion and efficacy of botulinum toxin type A in the treatment of lateral orbital rhytides. Dermatol Surg 2007;33:567–571.

27 de Almeida AT, de Boulle K. Diffusion characteristics of botulinum neurotoxin products and their clinical significance in cosmetic applications. J Cosmet Laser Ther 2007;9(Suppl 1):17–22.

28 de Almeida ART, Marques E, de Almeida J, *et al.* Pilot study comparing the diffusion of two formulations of botulinum toxin type A in patients with forehead hyperhidrosis. Dermatol Surg 2007;33: S37–S43.

29 Kerscher M, Roll S, Becker A, Wigger-Alberti W. Comparison of the spread of three botulinum toxin type A preparations. Arch Dermatol Res 2012;304: 155–161.

30 Hexsel D, Dal'Forno T, Hexsel C, *et al.* A randomized pilot study comparing the action halos of two commercial preparations of botulinum toxin type A. Dermatol Surg 2008;34:52–59.

31 Flynn TC, Clark RE II. Botulinum toxin type B (MYOBLOC) versus botulinum toxin type A (BOTOX) frontalis study: rate of onset and radius of diffusion. Dermatol Surg 2003;29:519–522.

32 Kranz G, Paul A, Voller B, *et al.* Long-term efficacy and respective potencies of botulinum toxin A and B: a randomized, double-blind study. Br J Dermatol 2011; 164:176–181.

33 Rystedt A, Swartling C, Naver H. Anhidrotic effect of intradermal injections of botulinum toxin: a comparison of different products and concentrations. Acta Derm Venereol 2008;88:229–233.

34 Rystedt A, Swartling C, Farnstrand C, Naver H. Equipotent concentrations of Botox and Dysport in the treatment of palmar hyperhidrosis. Acta Derm Venereol 2008;88:458–461.

35 Redaelli A, Forte R. Botulinum toxin dilution: our technique. J Cosmet Laser Ther 2003;5:218–219.

36 Hantash BM, Gladstone HB. A pilot study on the effect of epinephrine on botulinum toxin treatment for periorbital rhytides. Dermatol Surg. 2007;33:461–468.

37 Goodman G. Diffusion and short-term efficacy of botulinum toxin A after the addition of hyaluronidase and its possible application for the treatment of axillary hyperhidrosis. Dermatol Surg 2003;29: 533–538.

9

Patient Selection

Ryan M. Greene, MD (PhD, FACS),[1] John P. Arkins, BS,[2] and Steven H. Dayan, MD (FACS)[3]

[1] Director, Plastic Surgery & Laser Center, Fort Lauderdale, USA
[2] DeNova Research, Chicago, USA
[3] Clinical Assistant Professor of Otolaryngology, Chicago Centre for Facial Plastic Surgery, University of Illinois Chicago, Chicago, USA

Since its initial approval by the US Food and Drug Administration (FDA), botulinum toxin type A (BoNTA) has grown to become the most popular cosmetic procedure performed in the United States with almost 4.8 million treatments performed in 2009 [1]. The meteoric rise in popularity and success of BoNTA began with the insightful and pioneering measures of Drs. Jean and Alastair Carruthers in the 1990s. Because of this research, the cosmetic benefits of BoNTA were elucidated. However, BoNTA's history has not always shared its current esteem, and their first cosmetic trial took more than 3 years to enroll 30 patients [2].

Since the cosmetic approval of onabotulinumtoxinA (Botox Cosmetic, Allergan Inc., Irvine, CA) by the US Food and Drug Administration (FDA) in 2002 for dynamic glabella frown lines, the face of cosmetic medicine has been forever changed. With its unit measurements, defined outcomes and reversibility, BoNTA became a treatment that was easier to measure and study in a controlled manner. Measurable outcomes were developed based on standard protocols that could be defined and quantified. Cosmetic medical journals and physicians now expect research with better-defined standards and objective outcomes. It can be argued that BoNTA not only altered the way cosmetic medicine is researched, evaluated, and delivered, but also the demands, expectations, and even the economic background of our patients.

Cosmetic medicine has experienced a shift towards more minimally invasive procedures with less downtime and quicker actualization of results to better meet our patients' demands. Prior to cosmetic use of BoNTA, to gain a meaningful aesthetic improvement, patients were resigned to a surgical procedure often associated with prolonged downtime. Additionally, best practices and procedures were often based on the anecdotal beliefs of the master physicians at the time.

Much changed with the emergence of BoNTA. Aesthetic results could be achieved relatively quickly with no downtime and without the noticeable stigma associated with more invasive forms of cosmetic surgery. The goal of cosmetic medicine and all new devices and procedures shifted to the delivery of treatments that can provide maximum results with the least amount of downtime.

Just as there has been a shift towards more minimally invasive procedures, the relative affordability of BoNTA injections compared to the cost of surgical procedures resulted in a shift in the economic status of patients. Previously, procedures were often expensive and relegated to the realm of the privileged. Results from aesthetic treatments were often noticeable and became a status symbol,

Botulinum Toxins: Cosmetic and Clinical Applications, First Edition. Edited by Joel L. Cohen and David M. Ozog.
© 2017 John Wiley & Sons Ltd. Published 2017 by John Wiley & Sons Ltd.
Companion Website: www.wiley.com/go/cohen/botulinum

defining a generation of aristocracy to those who could afford it. However, with the lower price-point of BoNTA, cosmetic medicine was no longer relegated to one socioeconomic class; cosmetic medical treatments were now available for the masses. This has resulted in a paradigm shift in cosmetic procedures that has seen the advent of fillers and other devices targeting a more price conscious patient.

As our experience with BoNTA progresses, so too has the expected goal for both injectors and patients. While initial focus of the treatment addressed treating individual dynamic lines, the paradigm has shifted toward using BoNTA to contour and sculpt the face.

At the second convening of the BoNTA consensus conference [3], recommended treatment doses were much lower than those reported at the first consensus conferences [4].This revealed that the initial enthusiasm for eliminating all of the dynamic lines of the upper face shifted toward a new emphasis of using BoNTA strategically to shape the face, creating a subtle, yet effective improvement in the way patients appear and project themselves.

With the addition of new BoNTAs into the marketplace, patient confusion has the potential to increase. In 2009, the second BoNTA, abobotulinumtoxinA (Dysport®, Galderma Pharma S.A., Lausanne, Switzerland), was FDA approved for the cosmetic treatment of glabellar rhytids. While the effects of both onabotulinumtoxinA and abobotulinumtoxinA products are secondary to the botulinum toxin purified protein, they are slightly different in molecular composition with abobotulinumtoxinA having fewer complexing proteins surrounding the consistent 150 kDa protein neurotoxin and having a lower molecular weight. The clinical differences between the two products are still being crystallized in the marketplace, but they do seem to have different effects and can be used differently based on the individual patient's preexisting condition and desired goals.

On July 21, 2011, a third option became available with the FDA approval of incobotulinumtoxinA (Xeomin®, Merz Pharmaceuticals, Frankfurt, Germany) for the cosmetic treatment of glabellar rhytids. IncobotulinumtoxinA is considered to be a purer form of the 150 kDa protein neurotoxin, as there are no complexing proteins. While the ultimate effect of incobotulinumtoxinA is identical to that of onabotulinumtoxinA and abobutulinumtoxinA, the absence of any complexing proteins may theoretically lower the risk of neutralizing antibody development. This also increases the stability of the product, allowing its storage at room temperature and eliminating the need for refrigeration. Although there may be subtle differences between the two products, standard clinical practice is to use incobotulinumtoxinA and onabotulinumtoxinA in a 1:1 ratio. Investigation is ongoing concerning the differentiation of these three products [5].

Patients must also be aware of all potential side effects associated with all BoNTAs. In 2009, a black box warning was placed on all BoNTA, mandating that all patients seeking cosmetic treatments with BoNTA be provided with an appropriate informed consent at every visit. However, there has never been a death reported from a cosmetic botulinum toxin treatment [6,7].

Selecting the Right Patient for BoNTA

To optimize patient satisfaction following BoNTA injections, careful patient selection is critical. During the initial consultation, the patient is informed of the likely outcome with a thorough discussion of possible complications and adverse effects (Figure 9.1). Informed consent that confirms the patient is aware of the black box warning is provided at each visit. As BoNTA injections are a medical procedure, it is important to conduct a comprehensive history and physical examination on all new patients. Established patients returning for another BoNTA treatment should have their history and

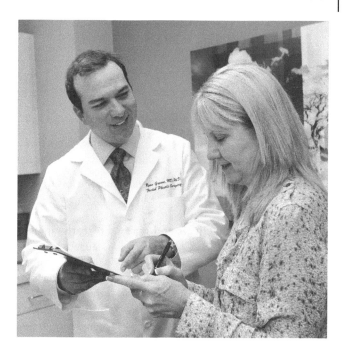

Figure 9.1 During the initial consultation and prior to obtaining an informed consent, the patient is informed of the likely outcome with a thorough discussion of possible complications and adverse effects.

focused physical exam repeated to assure no new contraindicating medical conditions have arisen.

The physical examination involves a thorough evaluation of the facial symmetry at rest and during animation. The patient should be examined with complete relaxation of the facial musculature and then with forced animation. It is important to identify preexisting asymmetry in facial animation, as it is not uncommon to have one brow elevate more than another. It is also extremely important to identify patients with preexisting eyelid ptosis and/or brow ptosis, which can be accentuated following BoNTA treatment. The asymmetry and the potential outcomes should be discussed and demonstrated to the patient prior to treatment.

After the consultation, the patient's expectations should be evaluated to ensure that patient satisfaction can be obtained following treatment. During the consultation, note that the primary goal of BoNTA is not to eradicate all wrinkles, but to weaken the muscle activity contributing to wrinkle formation and the aging characteristics of the face. Occasionally, the intended result is not achieved and

undesirable muscle activity persists, and a touch-up treatment 1–2 weeks following the primary treatment may be necessary.

A secondary touch-up injection may also be required if an asymmetry occurs following BoNTA injection. Minor asymmetries sometimes occur after treatment with BoNTA, and patients should be aware of this possibility. If a patient does not have realistic expectations and expects absolute symmetry following injection, this may be a relative contraindication to treatment.

Contraindications

The safety record of cosmetic BoNTA stands for itself and despite its black box warning, severe adverse events are rare [6]. However, there are a few contraindications, most of which are relative. A known allergy or hypersensitivity to the ingredients in the formulation is an absolute contraindication. The use of BoNTA is not recommended in patients with neuromuscular disorders, such as myasthenia gravis, Eaton–Lambert syndrome or amyotrophic lateral sclerosis, which

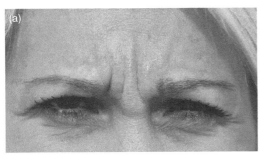
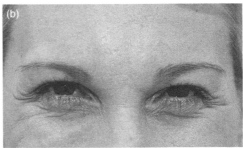

Figure 9.2 Glabellar region with frowning action: (a) before and (b) 1 week after treatment with BoNTA. *Source:* Courtesy of Ryan Greene, MD (PhD, FACS).

may exaggerate its paralytic effects and may have unpredictable results [8, 9].

There are various pharmaceutical agents that interact with the neuromuscular junction as well. Examples include aminoglycoside antibiotics, cyclosporine, chloroquine, and d-penicilinamine. Use of these medications may alter the effect of BoNTA [10–13], so caution should be exercised.

There is very limited information regarding the side effects of BoNTA during pregnancy or breast-feeding, so its use is not advised. However, there are no known teratogenic effects in humans.

Patients who use their facial muscles extensively in their jobs, such as actors, should be counseled that they might have limited expression after injection. Similarly, singers or patients who play wind instruments should be warned that injection of the perioral muscles might alter their performance capabilities.

Glabellar Rhytids

The most widely researched area of the face treated with BoNTA, and for which it has its cosmetic FDA approval, is the glabella, which can form deep vertical creases between the eyebrows. Treatment of the glabellar region with onabotulinumtoxinA received FDA approval on April 15, 2002. Creases in this area can impart a false impression of anger or an aggressive demeanor. It is also one of the first areas of the face to exhibit signs of early aging. These furrows are primarily caused by action of the paired corrugator supercilii muscles. The frontalis, orbicularis, and procerus muscles can also contribute to these wrinkles. After treatment of this area, most patients report that they look more pleasant, rested, and amiable (Figure 9.2). Additionally, patients who are treated with BoNTA in this area have proven to be perceived by unknowing observers as more successful at dating and athletics, and appear more attractive [14].

The glabellar creases are best evaluated while the patient is frowning or squeezing their eyebrows together. During this motion, the corrugator muscles should be palpated to determine their location, size, and strength. This can aid in determining their contribution to the vertical creases. Additionally, the dose of toxin needed to achieve a significant result is dependent on the size and thickness of the paired corrugator muscles [15]. If the glabellar crease does not improve with spreading the skin surrounding the crease apart, then complete correction of the crease should not be expected with BoNTA treatment alone. In these cases, a soft tissue filler in combination with BoNTA should be considered for an optimal treatment. It is also important to evaluate the superior-medial orbicularis muscles, which may also contribute to the deep creases. Finally, the procerus muscle should be examined and palpated as well. Contraction of the procerus can result in the horizontal creases located over the root of the nose.

It is essential to evaluate brow position in any patient considering treatment of their glabellar creases with BoNTA. The ideal female brow position is above the superior orbital rim, with the apex of the arch located on a vertical tangent above the lateral limbus. The tail of the brow should lie on a horizontal plane 1–2 mm above the medial brow head. The ideal male brow has a flatter, more horizontal orientation and is positioned lower on the forehead, approximately at the level of the superior orbital rim [16].

In addition to the brows, the upper eyelids should also be evaluated for asymmetry or ptosis. If this is present, it should be demonstrated to the patient. The position and symmetry of the brows and eyelids affect the technique employed during treatment. Patients who are noted to have an appropriate brow position during the pretreatment assessment receive 3 U 1 cm above the orbital rim in the midpupillary line, to address the contribution of the underlying orbicularis muscle. This orbicularis contribution can be clearly seen when the patient squeezes their eyebrows together. Care is taken when injecting to remain at least 1 cm above the brow at, or lateral to, the midpupillary line, to avoid BoNTA migration into the orbit and a resulting eyelid ptosis.

If a patient has low-set brows, injections over the brow may also lead to mild brow ptosis and a flat, unattractive brow appearance. To prevent an aggressive, low brow appearance, conservative doses above the brow are used. It is important for patients to understand that achievement of a complete reduction in the glabellar creases often requires an amount and placement of BoNTA that will often result in a lowered brow position. Men and women with low-set brows should be treated above the brows more cautiously and counseled about the possibility of a slight brow ptosis if full correction of glabellar creases is desired.

Whether onabotulinumtoxinA, abobotulinumtoxinA, or incobotulinumtoxinA is used, the physical evaluation is systematically the same. While a detailed dose comparison evaluation among the three products is beyond the scope of this chapter, it has been the authors' experience that abobotulinumtoxinA provides for more "spread" or a smoother effect, especially when treating the forehead. Some have believed that abobotulinumtoxinA diffuses more [17–20], but the difference in effect is likely more due to differences in the doses and the pharmokinetics of the products [21]. While similar accuracy and predictability can be achieved with either product in most patients, the products are used in specific indications slightly differently in the authors' hands. For the patient with significant frontalis activity over the lateral forehead, abobotulinumtoxinA seems to provide a smoother effect by effectively reducing frontalis activity over the lateral brow without causing brow ptosis when the injections are inserted over the medial forehead and glabellar area. Although abobotulinumtoxinA often requires injections over the lateral brow to prevent the quizzical wandering brow, these injections may result in a lateral brow ptosis and hooding if not performed judiciously.

Forehead

Patients who have heavy horizontal forehead creases are good candidates for treatment with BoNTA (Figure 9.3). After treatment of these creases, patients have an open, relaxed and friendlier appearance. Patients who have yet to develop deep creases may benefit from the smoother appearance and the possible wrinkle preventative benefits that are achieved.

Patients are first evaluated for the depth and lateral extent of the forehead creases. The lowest crease should be identified and marked, and its distance from the orbital rim and brow should be noted. As in the evaluation before treating glabellar creases, it is important to note the position and symmetry of the brows. Any brow asymmetry should be brought to the patient's attention. Some patients may not seek correction of a

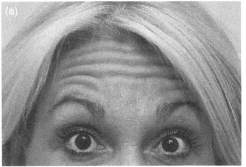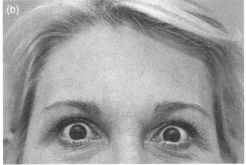

Figure 9.3 Activity of the frontalis muscle (a) before and (b) 1 week after treatment with BoNTA. *Source: Courtesy of Ryan Greene, MD (PhD, FACS).*

brow asymmetry, instead believing it to be a uniquely identifying feature.

An important diagnostic consideration is the relationship of the temporal portion of the frontalis muscle involvement to the brow position. Failure to recognize the patient with prominent lateral brow elevation can result in an overexaggerated lateral brow elevation and a "sinister" look following treatment of the forehead creases and undertreatment of the lateral frontalis muscle [22]; treatment with abobotulinumtoxinA may better suit these patients. Conversely, some patients desire elevation of their lateral brow. In these patients, the temporal area of the frontalis muscle is not treated, which allows the brow elevators to remain intact and contribute to brow elevation.

Women with low-set brows and most men are treated conservatively in the forehead to prevent brow ptosis; however, if patients desire a motionless forehead, they must be counseled that it will likely come at the expense of a lower brow position.

Crow's Feet

Signs of aging that occur lateral to the eye are often referred to as "crow's feet." These are the result of the lateral orbicularis muscle, which is very responsive to BoNTA treatments. Most patients report a softened look to their eyes and a more awake appearance following treatment. Treatment of the lateral

canthal lines with onabotulinumtoxinA (Botox®) was approved by the FDA on September 11, 2013.

Examination should first begin with evaluation of the medial and lateral extents of the wrinkles. Due to the heterogeneity of crow's feet line patterns, better outcomes may be achieved by tailoring treatment depending on the pattern encountered [23]. These should be assessed and discussed with the patient prior to injection. The relationship to the orbital rim and zygomatic arch position should also be assessed. The area should be inspected carefully for superficial venous structures, commonly prominent in this region. Lower eyelid resiliency can be tested with a snap test.

Injections are made into the dermis or subdermally, with avoidance of the identified vessels. In some patients, especially those with dark or tanned skin, it is difficult to identify subcutaneous vessels. If a blood vessel is punctured, immediate application of pressure can avoid an expanding hematoma throughout the loose areolar tissues of the periorbital region.

Superficial injections also can help to avoid placing BoNTA deep to the orbital septum, which could migrate to the ocular muscles and cause diplopia. Injections should be limited to an area superior to the zygomatic arch and lateral to the origin of the zygomaticus major muscle. This will help avoid inadvertent paralysis of this muscle, which would result in a noticeable upper lip ptosis.

OnabotulinumtoxinA has been the authors' preference, as it seems to provide a more localized, accurate effect. Abobotulinumtoxin A, if performed in excessively high doses of more than 20 U, may lead to a weakness in the smile that has not been favorable to our patients. Interestingly, there is evidence that abobotulinumtoxinA may act sooner in the crow's feet area and have more efficacious results [24, 25].

Eyelids

Initially cosmetic BoNTA of the lower eyelid was avoided for fear that postseptal migration to the ocular muscles could occur, causing diplopia. However, this consequence is unlikely if the BoNTA is injected pretarsally. For patients who have fine wrinkles under their eyes or a thickened subciliary muscle ridge, treatment with onabotulinumtoxinA can result in a relaxed appearance. Studies performed on Asian patients indicate patient satisfaction with a widened palpebral aperture and a more desirable appearance [26].

The lower eyelids are evaluated for significant wrinkling or a hypertrophic muscular ridge just below the ciliary margin. If thin, crepe-like skin is present, the patient is counseled that this will not improve after treatment and could possibly worsen. A snap test and lower eyelid retraction test should be performed to evaluate lower eyelid tone. The extent of pseudoherniating orbital fat is also noted.

While careful and effective treatment can produce a very desirable result, the undesirable side effects with pretarsal eyelid injections can be quite noticeable. Caution is advised in all patients being treated. Patients with a lax lower eyelid are at risk of developing lower lid malposition and dry eye and are not treated pretarsally.

Patients with prominent postseptal orbital fat pads should be treated conservatively. Lower eyelid "puffy pockets" may appear to be worse following BoNTA treatment in this region, secondary to weakening of the pretarsal muscle that serves as a supportive sling. Weakening of this sling can allow the fat to pseudoherniate even further.

Temporal Lift

Elevation of the lateral aspect of the eyebrow can have a subtle, but desirable improvement in facial appearance; 4–6 U placed just inferior and lateral to the tail of the brow can expect at least a 1-point reduction in brow severity in 32–47% of patients, respectively [27]. Most patients can expect a 2–3 mm elevation of the lateral brow; however, this may come at the expense of incomplete reduction of the glabellar or forehead creases. In patients with hyperactive lateral brow elevators, an overcorrection and excessive elevation of the lateral brow can occur, resulting in an undesirable sinister appearance [28].

Prior to injection, the lateral portion of the brow should be evaluated in relation to the medial third of the brow. The activity of the temporal portion of the frontalis muscle and the position and force of elevation of the lateral brow should also be assessed. In patients who are at risk for overcorrection and a sinister appearance following treatment, a small injection of BoNTA can be performed above the lateral brow to still achieve a subtle, natural, and desirable elevation. This requires experience and proper evaluation to carefully select these patients.

Perioral Region

Deep-etched vertical creases in the vermillion border can be caused by excessive sun exposure, smoking, and a genetic disposition. This can be disconcerting for those who wear lipstick, which can migrate vertically into the fine lines. These fine lines and creases in the upper and lower lip can be softened when onabotulinumtoxinA is placed periorally [29]; however, the deep ridges and mounds that are accentuated with puckering are what respond best to BoNTA treatments. Unlike many filler injections, BoNTA treatment will not lead to a lumpy, beady look. Caution is advised when treating patients who cannot tolerate any perioral weakness, such as vocalists or wind instrument players.

Evaluation of the extent and depth of the creases should be carried out at rest and during motion. Prior to injection, the patient should purse their lips to allow marking of usually four or five prominent creases. Any pre-existing asymmetry of the lips should be pointed out to the patient, as correction may exaggerate it.

It is important to inject low doses in the perioral area to prevent noticeable weakness and asymmetry. Otherwise, patients can potentially develop difficulty with mastication and articulation, and they might drool. Even therapeutic doses can lead to a subclinical weakness that is not noticeable with regular activity, but may become evident when attempting motions such as whistling [29].

Chin

The irregularly textured area overlying the mentalis muscle of the chin has been described as the peau d'orange appearance. This chin appearance can be softened by placing a small dose of Botox into the inferior-medial chin pad [29].

The chin pad should be palpated at rest and with contraction to evaluate its texture and firmness. Symmetry should be assessed, and any asymmetries should be pointed out to the patient. During injection, care should be taken to stay medial and avoid migration of BoNTA into the depressor labii inferioris muscles. Inadvertent paralysis of these muscles can result in lip weakness with the potential for lip biting, difficulty articulating, and drooling.

Angle of Mouth

Deepening and downward rotation of the creases at the mouth corners can result in an appearance of anger or sadness. The muscle responsible for this downward pull, the depressor anguli oris, can be treated to turn up the corners of the mouth with a subtle elevation.

Symmetry of the lips and the corners of the mouth should first be evaluated at rest and in motion. The patient should be asked to "grit their teeth," and the depressor anguli oris is palpated at its mandibular origin. Its contribution to any depression of the corner of the mouth can be assessed by inspection and palpation during patient contraction. Care is taken to inject into the depressor muscle, rather than the more medial levator labii muscle, which can lead to lip asymmetry, difficulty articulating, lip biting, and drooling [30].

Jaw/Masseter

Hypertrophic masseter muscles can lead to a square-appearing jaw line that is more consistent with a masculine appearance than a feminine one. Often those with enlarged masseters are also afflicted with bruxism and dental sequalae. A thorough history will often reveal this and confirm the indication for masseteric BoNTA treatments.

Hypertrophic masseter muscles can easily be identified and palpated while the patient clenches their teeth. Frequently, the masseters are powerfully projected and protruding. By grasping the muscle between your thumb and index finger, the belly of the muscle can easily be treated with 20–30 U BoNTA. Care is taken to inject laterally. If injections are performed too medially, the lateral extent of the smile will be truncated and the cheeks will appear round and chipmunk-like. However, for most patients who are treated with BoNTA in the masseter muscles, patient satisfaction is very high. Generally, results are not appreciated for 4–6 weeks, but the effects of treatment seem to last longer, up to 6 months. A 2-week touch-up treatment of an extra 10–20 U BoNTA may be needed to achieve full correction.

Mastication should not be affected by masseter treatments as there are four paired muscle groups necessary for mastication, and the weakening of the masseters will not make a significant or clinically recognizable deficit in mastication.

Neck

Prominent cord-like vertically oriented neck-bands secondary to the underlying platysmal muscle can be treated with BoNTA to soften and reduce the bands. For patients who display persistent neckbands despite surgical correction, treatment with onabotulinumtoxinA is an ideal alternative [31].

The neck should be evaluated by inspection and palpation at rest and in motion. By "gritting their teeth," the bands become more prominent. A vertical midline band may be present if the patient has had a previous rhytidectomy or submentoplasty. Depending on the extent of neck banding, the injection amount can vary significantly among patients. However, routinely 10–20 U per band is recommended. The main risks of injection are dysphagia and airway compromise, which are highly unlikely if injections are performed correctly.

Summary

Patient expectations of BoNTA treatments can vary considerably and need to be managed depending on the needs and desires of the patient. It is imperative to understand that each patient is unique, and results may vary from those of their peers. Underlying facial anatomy may also hinder or prevent the desired result. Patient individuality prevents treating each patient in the same manner. An understanding of the preprocedural analysis, BoNTA dosages, patient expectations, potential adverse outcomes, and preventative techniques allows the physician to select patients appropriately to optimize patient outcomes and ultimately assure their satisfaction.

References

1 American Society of Plastic Surgerons. 2010 Report of the 2009 Statistics: National Clearinghouse of Plastic Surgrey Statistics. 2010 [cited 2010 November 5]; Available from: https://www.plasticsurgery.org/news/plastic-surgery-statistics?sub=2009+Plastic+Surgery+Statistics.

2 Carruthers J, Carruthers A. The evolution of botulinum neurotoxin type A for cosmetic applications. J Cosmet Laser Ther 2007 Sep;9(3):186–192.

3 Carruthers JD, Glogau RG, Blitzer A. Advances in facial rejuvenation: botulinum toxin type A, hyaluronic acid dermal fillers, and combination therapies – consensus recommendations. Plast Reconstr Surg. 2008 May;121(5 Suppl):5S–30S; quiz 1S–6S.

4 Carruthers J, Fagien S, Matarasso SL. Consensus recommendations on the use of botulinum toxin type a in facial aesthetics. Plast Reconstr Surg. 2004 Nov;114(6 Suppl):1S–22S.

5 Kane MA, Gold MH, Coleman WP 3rd, J et al. A randomized, double-blind trial to investigate the equivalence of incobotulinumtoxinA and onabotulinumtoxinA for glabellar frown lines. Dermatol Surg 2015 Nov;41(11): 1310–1319.

6 Carruthers J, Carruthers A. Botulinum toxin in facial rejuvenation: an update. Dermatol Clin 2009 Oct;27(4):417–425, v.

7 Kuehn BM. FDA requires black box warnings on labeling for botulinum toxin products. JAMA 2009 Jun 10;301(22):2316.

8 Cote TR, Mohan AK, Polder JA, et al. Botulinum toxin type A injections: adverse

events reported to the US Food and Drug Administration in therapeutic and cosmetic cases. J Am Acad Dermatol 2005 Sep;53(3):407–415.

9 Matarasso SL, Matarasso A. Treatment guidelines for botulinum toxin type A for the periocular region and a report on partial upper lip ptosis following injections to the lateral canthal rhytids. Plast Reconstr Surg 2001 Jul;108(1):208–214; discussion 15–17.

10 Blitzer A, Binder WJ. Current practices in the use of botulinum toxin A in the management of facial lines and wrinkles. Facial Plast Surg Clin North Am 2001 Aug;9(3):395–404.

11 Wang YC, Burr DH, Korthals GJ, Sugiyama H. Acute toxicity of aminoglycoside antibiotics as an aid in detecting botulism. Appl Environ Microbiol. 1984 Nov;48(5): 951–955.

12 *Physicians Desk Reference*. 62nd ed. Montvale (NJ): Thompson Medical Economics; 2008.

13 *Mosby's Drug Consult*. 13th ed. St. Louis (MO): Mosby; 2003.

14 Dayan SH, Lieberman ED, Thakkar NN, *et al.* Botulinum toxin a can positively impact first impression. Dermatol Surg 2008 Jun;34(Suppl 1):S40–S47.

15 Kane MA, Brandt F, Rohrich RJ, *et al.* Evaluation of variable-dose treatment with a new U.S. Botulinum Toxin Type A (Dysport) for correction of moderate to severe glabellar lines: results from a phase III, randomized, double-blind, placebo-controlled study. Plast Reconstr Surg 2009 Nov;124(5):1619–1629.

16 Wieder JM, Moy RL. Understanding botulinum toxin. Surgical anatomy of the frown, forehead, and periocular region. Dermatol Surg 1998 Nov;24(11): 1172–1174.

17 Nussgens Z, Roggenkamper P. Comparison of two botulinum-toxin preparations in the treatment of essential blepharospasm. Graefes Arch Clin Exp Ophthalmol 1997 Apr;235(4):197–199.

18 Marchetti A, Magar R, Findley L, *et al.* Retrospective evaluation of the dose of Dysport and BOTOX in the management of cervical dystonia and blepharospasm: the REAL DOSE study. Mov Disord 2005 Aug;20(8):937–944.

19 Rosales RL, Bigalke H, Dressler D. Pharmacology of botulinum toxin: differences between type A preparations. Eur J Neurol 2006 Feb;13(Suppl 1):2–10.

20 Bihari K. Safety, effectiveness, and duration of effect of BOTOX after switching from Dysport for blepharospasm, cervical dystonia, and hemifacial spasm dystonia, and hemifacial spasm. Curr Med Res Opin 2005 Mar;21(3):433–438.

21 Kranz G, Haubenberger D, Voller B, *et al.* Respective potencies of Botox and Dysport in a human skin model: a randomized, double-blind study. Mov Disord 2009 Jan 30;24(2):231–236.

22 Spencer JM, Gordon M, Goldberg DJ. Botulinum B treatment of the glabellar and frontalis regions: a dose response analysis. J Cosmet Laser Ther 2002 Mar;4(1): 19–23.

23 Kane MA, Cox SE, Jones D, *et al.* Heterogeneity of crow's feet line patterns in clinical trial subjects. Dermatol Surg 2015 Apr;41(4):447–456.

24 Kenneth Y, Sumit B, Maas C, editors. Comparison of Onset of Action of Botox Cosmetic and Dysport in the Treatment of Crow's feet. AAFPRS Fall Meeting 2010; September 23–26, 2010; Boston, MA.

25 Kenneth Y, Sumit B, Maas C, editors. Comparison of Efficacy of Action of Botox Cosmetic and Dysport in the Treatment of Crow's Feet. AAFPRS Fall Meeting 2010; September 23–26, 2010; Boston, MA.

26 Klein AW. Cosmetic therapy with botulinum toxin, Anecdotal memoirs. Dermatol Surg 1996 Sep;22(9):757–759.

27 Cohen JL, Dayan SH. Botulinum toxin type A in the treatment of dermatochalasis: an open-label, randomized, dose-comparison study. J Drugs Dermatol 2006 Jul–Aug;5(7): 596–601.

28 Flynn TC, Carruthers JA. Botulinum-A
toxin treatment of the lower eyelid
improves infraorbital rhytides and widens
the eye. Dermatol Surg 2001 Aug;27(8):
703–708.

29 Dayan SH, Maas CS. Botulinum toxins for
facial wrinkles: beyond glabellar lines.
Facial Plast Surg Clin North Am 2007
Feb;15(1):41–49, vi.

30 Papel ID, Capone RB. Botulinum toxin A
for mentalis muscle dysfunction. Arch
Facial Plast Surg 2001 Oct–Dec;3(4):
268–269.

31 Carruthers J, Carruthers A. BOTOX use in
the mid and lower face and neck. Semin
Cutan Med Surg 2001 Jun;20(2):
85–92.

10

Treatment of the Glabella

Neal D. Varughese, MD (MBA)[1] and David J. Goldberg, MD (JD)[1,2]

[1]*Skin Laser and Surgery Specialists of New York and New Jersey, New York, USA*
[2]*Clinical Professor of Dermatology, Department of Dermatology, Icahn School of Medicine at Mount Sinai, New York, USA*

Introduction

According to statistics released by the American Society for Aesthetic Plastic Surgery, almost 13 million cosmetic surgical and nonsurgical procedures were performed in the United States in 2015. Over the past 5 years, surgical procedures have increased 17% while nonsurgical procedures have increased 44%. This trend towards minimally invasive procedures has led to an increasing popularity of botulinum toxin with an estimated 6.7 million procedures in the United States in the year 2015 [1] (Table 10.1).

In 1992, Carruthers *et al.* introduced the use of botulinum toxin as a therapeutic agent for treating glabellar frown lines [2]. Since then, three formulations have been approved by the US Food and Drug Administration (FDA) for glabellar rhytides: onabotulinumA (Botox®, Cosmetic; Allergan Inc., Irvine, CA), abobotulinumtoxinA (Dysport®, Ipsen Biopharmaceuticals, Inc., Basking Ridge, NJ), and incobotulinumtoxinA (Xeomin®; Merz Aesthetics, Frankfurt, Germany).

General Information

Before administering Botox injections, it is wise to first learn about the different products, procedures, and the possible side effects. Let's go through the procedure step by step.

Botulinum Toxin

There are eight known distinct serotypes of botulinum toxin (A, B, C1, D, E, F, G, and H) produced by different *Clostridium* bacterium strains that affect neural function [3,4]. At the present time only types A and B are used as medical treatments. BoNTA is the most commonly toxin used for cosmetic purposes. The term BoNTA will be used to refer to the general class and serotype of this toxin for the remainder of the chapter.

BoNTA naturally exists as a high-molecular-weight protein complex, containing neurotoxin and nonactive complexing proteins. The three FDA approved BoNTA are produced from the same wild-type strain of *Clostridium botulinum* but differ in their purification procedures. The manufacturing process for the final drug incobotulinumtoxinA (Xeomin®) involves a series of purification steps yielding exclusively active neurotoxin, free from complexing proteins present in onabotulinumtoxinA (Botox® Cosmetic) and abobotulinumtoxinA (Dysport®) [5].

As the individual potencies of the different types of botulinum toxins do vary immensely, it is an absolute necessity to be well aware

Table 10.1 Top surgical and nonsurgical cosmetic procedures among men and women in 2015.

Surgical	Number of procedures	Nonsurgical	Number of procedures
Breast augmentation	279,143	Botulinum toxin type A (Botox®, Dysport®)	6,757,198
Liposuction	222,051	Hyaluronic acid (Hylaform, Restylane, Juvederm)	1,951,692
Eyelid surgery	203,934	Chemical peel	1,310,252
Abdominoplasty	127,967	Laser hair removal	1,116,708
Facelift	125,711	Microdermabrasion	800,340

of which commercial preparation the dosing is referring to, when reading dosage data in the literature. The unit of the different types of toxins is a proprietary measurement of each manufacturer. The dosage is based on the biologic potency of the toxin and is measured on the median lethal dose (LD_{50}) of the toxin when injected intraperitoneally in the rat. The unit of measurement for onabotulinumtoxinA and abobotulinumtoxinA are not interchangeable.

! Clinically, 1 unit of onabotulinumtoxinA (Botox® Cosmetic) and incobotulinumtoxinA (Xeomin®) is approximately equivalent to 2.5–3 U abobotulinumtoxinA (Dysport®).

Mechanism of Action

Botulinum toxin acts by binding irreversibly to the presynaptic surface of cholinergic nerve and decreasing the release of acetylcholine, causing a neuromuscular blocking effect. As the botulinum toxins also block the acetylcholine release from parts of the autonomic nervous system, side effects such as a dry mouth and reduced sweating can be observed.

The recovery from the paralysis induced by botulinum toxin occurs through proximal axonal sprouting and muscle re-innervation by formation of a new neuromuscular junction.

Systemic Effects and Immunogenicity

Electromyographic findings revealed minor variations in nontargeted, nontreated muscles, suggesting that low amounts of botulinum toxin enter the systemic circulation, without exerting a clinically relevant effect [4, 6].

Antigenicity: About 5–10% of the patients treated for nonaesthetic indications develop a clinical resistance to botulinum toxin after repeated injections. The frequency of occurrence seems to be serotype dependent, with more resistance apparently occurring with type B than with type A toxin [7]. Botulinum toxin consists of foreign proteins. The injection of the toxin in the human body can lead to antibody formation against botulinum toxin and its complexing proteins. A postulated relationship between the presence of these neutralizing antibodies and clinical resistance has not been proven yet. Cases of responsive patients who had circulating antibodies and resistant patients who did not have neutralizing antibodies have been reported [8–10]. In practice, it seems that frequent injection intervals and injections at high dosage predispose people to a higher likelihood of antibody development [11]. The dose used for cosmetic treatments is much lower than the dose used for common therapeutic applications. Therefore, cosmetic treatments are less at risk of inducing the formation of neutralizing antibodies. The actual rate of cases with formation of neutralizing antibodies in patients receiving botulinum toxin for cosmetic treatments is thought to be low and infrequently leads to loss of efficacy [12]. Unlike any of the conventional botulinum neurotoxin preparations, incobotulinumtoxinA is free from complexing proteins, which may confer clinical benefits in terms of reduced potential for immunostim-ulating activity [13].

Today, the variety of uses of Botox includes cervical dystonia, blepharospasm, strabis-mus, severe primary axillary hyperhidro-sis, upper limb spasticity, achalasia, and migraine. Other, not yet FDA approved (off-label) uses of botulinum toxin type A include the treatment of incontinence due to overac-tive bladder, anal fissure, vaginismus, spastic disorders associated with injury or disease of the central nervous system including trauma, stroke, multiple sclerosis, Parkinson's dis-ease, or cerebral palsy, focal dystonias affecting the limbs, face, jaw, or vocal cords, temporomandibular join disorders, dia-betic neuropathy, wound healing, excessive salivation, vocal cord dysfunction including spasmodic dysphonia and tremor, and benign prostatic hyperplasia.

OnabotulinumtoxinA (Botox® Cosmetic), abobotulinumtoxinA (Dysport®), and incobotulinumtoxinA (Xeomin®) have been approved for the temporary improvement in the appearance of moderate to severe glabellar lines associated with procerus and corrugator muscle activity in adult patients less than 65 years of age.

Botulinum toxin should not be used in the presence of preexisting neuromuscular transmission disorders, myasthenia gravis or Eaton–Lambert syndrome. It may lead to an increased risk of severe dysphagia and respi-ratory compromise in those patients. Patients with dysphagia should not be treated either.

Botulinum toxin should not be used in patients who have had an allergic reaction to any other botulinum toxin products before.

Although no studies concerning drug inter-action have been carried out, concomitant use of aminoglycosides, cyclosporine or other agents interfering with neuromuscular trans-mission (e.g. cholinesterase inhibitors and calcium channel blockers) should be avoided because these drugs may potentiate the effect of the toxin.

Botulinum toxin should not be injected when there is an active skin infection at the planned injection site, chronic drug or alcohol abuse, clinically diagnosed anxiety or depression, or current facial palsy.

Relative contraindications are coagulation disorders and anticoagulant therapy (e.g., aspirin, ibuprofen, clopidogrel bisulfate or warfarin), resulting in an increased chance of bruising after treatment.

Pregnancy and lactation (Category C): Because of a limited experience in the field, botulinum toxin therapy is not recommended during pregnancy and lactation, even though there are anecdotal reports about it not being harmful when given in early pregnancy.

Depending on what product is being used, the volume of reconstitution has to be adapted according to the physician's prefer-ence and the patient's needs (Table 10.2). It is recommended to dilute the product with preservative-free 0.9% sodium chloride solu-tion. Therefore, the solution is drawn up with a syringe, attached to a 21G-40 mm needle for reconstitution.

The diluent should gently be injected into the vial to avoid the formation of foam in the complex, which could result in toxin denat-uration [14]. However, no difference in effi-cacy between botulinum toxin not shaken and shaken or foamed during reconstitu-tion has been report [15]. Some authors add epinephrine to reduce the diffusion of the drug in the tissues [16]. The solution should be clear, colorless, and free of particulate matter.

A high concentration (low dilution) and low volume injection allows a more precise placement of the product and scarce diffu-sion of the toxin, whereas low concentrations (high dilutions) may be helpful when a cer-tain grade of diffusion in the tissue is needed.

Table 10.2 Reconstitution of onabotulinumtoxinA (Botox® Cosmetic), abobotulinumtoxinA (Dysport®), and incobotulinumtoxinA (Xeomin®).

Type of botulinum toxin Volume of reconstitution	Concentration (U/ml)
Dysport® 300 U vial	
1 ml	15/0.05
1.5 ml	10/0.05
2.5 ml	10/0.08
3 ml	10/0.1
Botox® Cosmetic 100 U vial	
2 ml	5/0.1
2.5 ml	4/0.1
4 ml	2.5/0.1
Botox® Cosmetic 50 U vial	
1 ml	5/0.1
2 ml	2.5/0.1
Xeomin® Cosmetic 100 U vial	
2 ml	5/0.1
2.5 ml	4/0.1
4 ml	2.5/0.1
Xeomin® Cosmetic 50 U vial	
1 ml	5/0.1
2 ml	2.5/0.1

As a higher dilution results in a wider denervation due to the broader spreading of the toxin, the risk of unwanted effects seems to increase. Furthermore, using small volumes can help to reduce the pain at the injection site.

Syringes and Needle for Injection

Depending on the volume of the reconstituted drug, different types of syringes can be used to inject. The most commonly used syringes are 1-mL insulin-type syringes with removable 30-gauge needles. Frequent changes of the needle may help to reduce the patients discomfort caused by dull needle tips.

Storage

According to the package insert, all botulinum toxin products should be protected from light. They should be stored in

the refrigerator at a temperature of 2°C to 8°C (36-46°F) no longer than 4h respectively 8h after reconstitution. However, this recommendation is for sterility purposes only and not because of a loss of efficacy. According to a study done by Hexsel et al., no statistical differences were observed in terms of toxin efficacy and duration in vials reconstituted at the time of injection, or at 2, 4, and 6 weeks before use [17]. Absence of contamination in vials diluted with a 0.9% saline solution without preservatives up to 7 weeks has been demonstrated [18]. However, because the product does not contain any antimicrobial agent, from a microbiologic point of view the storage of reconstituted product remains controversial and beyond FDA guidelines.

Dosing Recommendations

Dosing guidelines have not been standardized for individuals of varying racial and ethnic backgrounds. The final dosage for each individual treatment has to be adjusted in relation to the muscle bulk. Bigger muscles require a higher dose to achieve a similar effect. Besides that, wrinkle severity, variations in anatomy and patient's preference of a more natural or a more static look should be considered.

Literature

OnabotulinumtoxinA (Botox®)

The recommended total dose of onabotulinumtoxinA (Botox®) for treatments of glabellar rhytides is 20 U [19]. This dose has been proven to be efficient and safe in diverse clinical trials [20–23].

Carruthers A et al. demonstrated that in females 20–40 U onabotulinumtoxinA (Botox®) doses were significantly more effective at reducing glabellar lines than 10 U and resulted in a longer duration of benefit [22]. In the dose-finding study for men, the 40, 60, and 80 U doses of onabotulinumtoxinA (Botox®) were consistently more effective in reducing glabellar lines than the 20 U dose regarding the duration and clinical

Table 10.3 Dosing recommendations for BoNTA-ABO (Dysport®), BoNTA-ONA (Botox®), and BoNTA-INCO (Xeomin®).

Location/Sites	Muscle	Dose BoNTA-ABO	Dose BoNTA-ONA, BoNTA-INCO	Injection site/technique
Glabella	Corrugator supercilii	50–80 total	8–17 per side	Total U divided into five
	– medial		5–12 per side	areas 1 cm apart, keeping
	– lateral		3–5 per side	1cm above the supraorbital
	Procerus		5–10	ridge; adjusted for sex and
			20–50 total	muscle mass

response without any increase in the risk of drug-related adverse events [23]. According to these findings, the treatment of glabellar lines in men requires higher treatment doses of onabotulinumtoxinA (Botox®) than in women. The required doses for men start at approximately the double of the dose used in women.

AbobotulinumtoxinA (Dysport®)

The recommended total dose of abobotulinumtoxinA (Botox®) for treatments of glabellar rhytides is 50 U [24]. Two dose-finding studies considered 50 U abobotulinumtoxinA (Dysport®) being the optimal total dose for the glabellar line treatment [25, 26]. The 50 U should be equally distributed among the five injection points, with 10 U per point. Women injected with 50 U of abobotulinumtoxinA (Dysport®) were more likely to respond (investigator and subject assessments 93% and 83% respectively) than men (67% and 33%, respectively). This might be expected because men generally have a greater muscle mass that may require a dose higher than 50 U. Subjects aged 50 years and more had a lower degree of response than those younger than 50 [26]. This is not surprising, because there is a general loss of dermal elasticity with increasing age, which can affect the smoothness of the skin.

A study by Kane *et al.* demonstrated, that if the dose of abobotulinumtoxinA is being increased, the percentage of responders decreased at almost all times, as scored by blinded evaluator and patient self-evaluation. At day 30, 96% of patients receiving 50 U, 90%

of patients receiving 60 U, 81% of patients receiving 70 U, and 61% of patients receiving 80 U were considered responders by a blinded evaluator [27]. According to these findings, increasing the dose of abobotulinumtoxinA beyond a given amount does not significantly change efficacy when treating glabellar rhytides.

IncobotulinumtoxinA (Xeomin®)

The recommended total dose of incobotulinumtoxinA (Xeomin®) for treatments of glabellar rhytides is 20 U [28]. This dose was well tolerated and demonstrated significant efficacy in the treatment of glabellar frown lines [29–31].

Kane *et al.* demonstrated clinical equivalence of incobotulinumtoxinA and onabotulinumtoxinA for the treatment of moderate-to-severe glabellar frown lines at 20 U for each product within a prespecified margin of equivalence of 15% at the primary endpoint [32].

Given the lack of comparative assessments of the three competing BoNTA formulations, future head-to-head comparison studies are warranted [33]. In general, there is insufficient evidence demonstrating an increased efficacy or duration of benefit of any one BoNTA formulation relative to its competitors.

Anatomy

Facial rhytides and folds in this area results from depressor muscles, consisting of the

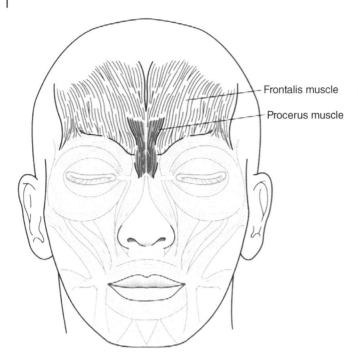

Frontalis muscle

Procerus muscle

Figure 10.1 Procerus and frontalis muscle. *Source:* Bassichis, Benjamin A., and J. Regan Thomas. The use of Botox to treat glabellar rhytids. Facial Plast Surg Clin N Am 13.1 2005;11–14.

procerus, the corrugator, the depressor supercilii and the orbicularis oculi.

The procerus is a thin pyramidal muscle that lies vertically between the eyebrows. It arises from the lower part of the nasal bone and upper part of the lateral nasal cartilage. It is inserted to the skin over the lower part of the forehead between the two eyebrows on either side of the midline. Its fibers merge with those of the frontalis muscle. Procerus contraction depresses the medial head of the eyebrows and induces horizontal lines (Figure 10.1).

The corrugator supercilii is a small, narrow, pyramidal muscle (Figure 10.2), arising from the medial end of the eyebrow beneath the frontalis and just above the orbicularis oculi. It inserts into the skin above the middle of the orbital arch. The corrugator draws the eyebrow downward, inward and medial ward and produces the vertical lines of the glabella. It is the 'frowning' muscle and may be regarded as the principal muscle in the expression of negative feelings. There is variability in the anatomy of the corrugator supercilii. Some patients have a short, narrow muscle located at the medial end of the supraorbital ridge, whereas other patients have a long, straight muscle, which extends along the supraorbital ridge to or beyond the mid-brow position [34]. The awareness of this anatomical variation is important, as in the presence of a long, narrow corrugator supercilii, the treating physician may extend the injections points more laterally to ensure that the whole muscle is treated. The best way to examine patient's individual anatomy is by watching the patient pull the eyebrows together or frown.

The depressor supercilii originates from the nasal process of the frontal bone and inserts into the skin at the medial aspect of the eyebrow, inferior to the corrugator supercilii.

The orbicularis oculi is a thin, broad muscle encircling the eye and adhering to the skin. The medial fibers of the orbicularis oculi originate from the medial orbital rim anterior to the origin of the corrugator. The medial fibers of the orbicularis oculi and the frontalis are intertwined with the corrugator and may contribute to wrinkle formation in this region.

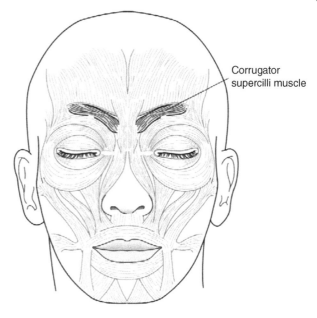

Corrugator supercilli muscle

Practical Part

Pretreatment Preparation

The first step during consultation should always be to analyze the patient's request, to discuss his expectations of the treatment outcome, and to inform about realistic results. It is sometimes helpful to give the patient a mirror to point out the area to be treated. Examine the patient's facial anatomy closely, at rest as as well as in movement. Each target area should be discussed separately.

The treatment plan should be based on the patient's request, facial anatomy, status of skin aging, and wrinkle type. Dynamic facial lines respond better to BoNTA injections than static rhytids. A patient may have more than one type of wrinkle and will therefore need combination treatment with other modalities such as fillers, peels, laser resurfacing, and thread lift.

In particular, the level of paralysis must be clarified. As frown lines often express negative feelings such as worry and anger, this area can be totally paralyzed. Other treatment sites, such as the forehead should keep some mobility, especially when a more natural look is intended. Pay attention to the difference between the patients' expectations and the realistic feasibility. The discrepancy between the patients' expectations and the actual outcome of treatment will determine the level of satisfaction.

It is recommended that beginners focus on the basic indications in the upper third of the face. They should only move on to dealing with the middle and lower parts of the face and other indications, after garnering adequate experience [35]. Injection in the mid and lower face and neck is reserved for experienced injectors and patients, who have had successful injections in the upper face [36]. An imprecise injection technique in the lower face may result in facial asymmetry and speech impediment.

Patients should be informed about the product, its mode of action, and its long history of safe use. Brochures elucidating further information, such as onset of action (approximately 3 days), maximal effect (after 1–2 weeks), duration of effect (3–4 months) and potential adverse events (headache, bruising, infection, eyelid drooping, facial asymmetry, speech changes, and dysphagia) should be provided. Patients should be informed that cosmetic injection in any site other than the glabella constitutes an off-label indication in the United States.

A consent form including the type of botulinum toxin, longevity expected, need for repeated treatments, and possible postoperative complications should be read, signed, and placed into the chart.

Photographs: It is strongly recommended to document any preexisting asymmetries by pretreatment photographs. For the glabella, pretreatment pictures may include:

- Neutral relaxed pose to document static rhytids.
- Frowning to document dynamic glabellar rhytids from procerus and corrugator muscle.

A follow-up appointment should be scheduled about 2 weeks after the initial injection to evaluate treatment outcome and level of satisfaction. If needed, patients can receive a touch-up treatment with small doses during this appointment.

Patient Preparation

The patient should be positioned in a sitting or semi-reclined/half-seated position with the chin down. All make-up has to be removed. The targeted areas should be examined closely, at rest and during movement. We suggest that particularly new injectors should mark the intended injection points. For disinfection, use nonalcoholic antiseptics because alcohol could be responsible for toxin inactivation. Since the injection is not very painful, topical anesthetics are usually not required. However, ice could be used as a numbing agent and could help to prevent bruising.

Note down treatment data: date of treatment, dilution of the drug, batch number of the drug, number of total units, units per point, and pattern of injection.

Injection Points and Technique

For complete improvement of glabellar lines, all muscles, which produce the glabellar complex (i.e., procerus, corrugator supercilii, and depressor supercilii and orbicularis oculi) must be treated. By asking the patient to frown and scowl, muscles of concern can be identified. Usually, a five-point injection is recommended. The middle injection point is used to inject the procerus and is located between the level of eyebrows and the root of the nose. The other four injection points are symmetrical. One site on each side is used to inject the corrugator (lateral), one site on each side is used to inject the orbicularis oculi and depressor supercilii (medial). The lateral injection point can be located at the midpupillary line or more medial, targeting the belly of the corrugator muscle. Some authors suggest that less experienced clinicians should inject at least 2 cm above the brow. The risk of eyelid ptosis can be reduced by targeting the medial part of the corrugator and by placing the injection points at least 1 cm above the bony supraorbital ridge, thus avoiding an injection near the levator palpebrae superioris.

To prevent a suboptimal aliquot of product, any air bubbles are expelled from the syringe and needle before injection. Then, the target muscles are palpated and stabilized or grasped with the clinician's nondominant hand. For cosmetic purposes, botulinum toxin is usually injected intramuscularly. If the toxin is injected subcutaneously or intradermally, more injection sites are needed to obtain the same effect. Intramuscular placement stings less and produces less local erythema but carries a higher risk of bruising. The injection should be perpendicular (90° angle) into the bulk of the noncontracted muscle, down to the last third of a 30G needle. The appropriate units of botulinum toxin are then injected as the needle is withdrawn.

A study performed by Rzany *et al.* showed that, injections in three essential sites, targeting the procerus and the corrugator muscle (three injections of 10 U) were essential for the treatment of glabellar wrinkles, while another injection site pattern, with two additional injections in the forehead region, did not significantly improve efficacy [37] (Figure 10.3 and Figure 10.4).

in the injected area. Advise the patient not to massage or manipulate the treatment area after injection. No heavy exercise should be done for 3–4 hours after the treatment. Patients should be instructed to remain in an upright position for the following 6 hours after injection to avoid ptosis caused by migration of toxin though the orbital septum.

Onset of Response

The median time for reaction to onset was determined to be 2–4 days [38–41]. In each study, responses as early as 24 hours after treatment were reported.

Duration

In the literature, the median duration of effect ranged from 3 to 5 months. In a repeated-treatment study, a small proportion of patients (2–7%) had a response that persisted up to 336 days (based on investigator assessment) [39]. In subgroup analysis, African American patients had a slightly longer duration of response, with a median time of 117 days and 129 days (based on assessment by investigators and patients respectively) compared to 109 days and 107 days for the entire population [27].

Efficacy with Repeated Treatments

Treatment efficacy with BoNTA has shown to be highly consistent among multiple

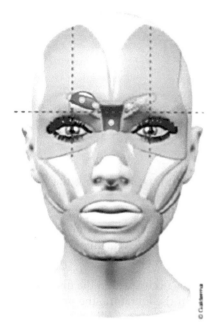

Figure 10.3 The injection points for glabellar line treatment with botulinum neurotoxin type A used in the European studies. *Source:* Rzany, B., B. Ascher, and G.D. Monheit, Treatment of glabellar lines with botulinum toxin type A (Speywood Unit): a clinical overview. J Eur Acad Dermatol Venereol 2010; 24(Suppl 1):1–14.

Posttreatment Care

Gentle pressure with gauze after injection can help to reduce oozing from the skin puncture sites and minimizing swelling and bruising. Ice packs applied for 5–10 minutes may help to reduce swelling and discomfort

Figure 10.4 Injection points. *Source:* Salti, G. and I. Ghersetich, Advanced botulinum toxin techniques against wrinkles in the upper face. Clin Dermatol 2008;26(2):182–191.

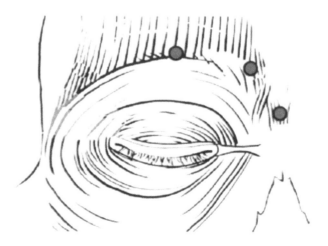

treatment cycles. No obvious loss of efficacy regarding median time to onset and median duration of effect was observed. When maintaining an interval between doses of at least 10 weeks, a cumulative effect after repeated injections is not expected [42]. To avoid short-term booster injections, it is generally recommended to use the lowest effective dose of the drug.

Treatment Interval

In a retrospective study including up to five treatments cycles, the median interval between two cycles was determined to be 5.9–6.5 months [42]. The between-treatment interval was longer than the duration of response reported in randomized and controlled studies [26, 27, 30, 40, 43]. This suggests that economic aspects may also play a role in treatment frequency because patients had to cover their own treatment expense during the retrospective study. In clinical practice, a treatment interval of about 6 months might be expected.

Safety Concerns and Adverse Events

Adverse events of botulinum toxin injection for cosmetic purpose are generally mild and transient. Adverse effects such as fatigue, malaise, nausea, muscle weakness and musculoskeletal pain, flulike symptoms, rash, dysphagia and dry mouth, headache, infection, and dysphonia have been described in patients receiving up to 1000 U of BoNTA-ABO for medical indications.

Clinically, the most common adverse events in cosmetic procedures are due to injection site reaction and include pain, hemorrhage, discomfort, anesthesia, swelling, bruising, irritation, stinging, erythema, or pruritus. The frequency of patients experiencing injection site reactions was the same for the placebo group as for the patients injected with BoNTA. This suggests, that

adverse events occurred because of the treatment procedure (insertion of a needle) rather than the injected toxin.

Brow/eyelid ptosis: The most common significant and least desired adverse effect is eyebrow or eyelid ptosis. Eyelid ptosis occurs from diffusion of the toxin through the orbital septum into the levator palpebrae superioris muscle. This complication can theoretically be minimized by

- injecting the toxin at least 1 cm above the bony superior orbital rim,
- not crossing the midpupillary line,
- using lower doses and injection volumes
- instructing the patient to remain in an upright position for 6 hours.

Eyelid ptosis generally occurs within the first 14–17 days (94%). In the literature, the percentage of patients reporting eyelid ptosis was between 1 and 4%. If ptosis occurs, patients should be informed that the symptom is temporary and usually subsides within a few weeks (39–85 days) and that no additional treatment is required [26].

Therapeutic Failure

Patients who do not respond at all to botulinum toxin treatments are designated as primary nonresponders. In contrast, secondary non-responders lose the response on subsequent injections after an initial successful use. Theoretically, these patients may have developed neutralizing antibodies from prior clinical exposure. When a loss of response occurs, the patients' physiologic response (weakness) to the toxin can be evaluated with a single test dose injection of 15 U BoNTA-ONA (Botox®) into the frontalis muscle.

Lack of response can be caused by many other conditions. Patients with nondynamic rhytides in origin (e.g., photodamage, age-related changes) do not respond. Treatment failure may also result from inadequate injection technique and therefore misplaced toxin, suboptimal dosing or inactivation respectively denaturation of the toxin by improper storage.

References

1 American Society of Plastic Surgeons. Plastic surgery statistics report [cited 2016 March 11]. www.surgery.org/sites/default/files/ASAPS-Stats2016.pdf.

2 Carruthers JD, Carruthers JA. Treatment of glabellar frown lines with C. botulinum-A exotoxin. J Dermatol Surg Oncol 1992;18:17–21.

3 Jankovic J, Hallet M (eds). *Therapy with Botulinum Toxin*. New York: Marcel Dekker, 1994.

4 Vita G. Cardiovascular reflex testing and single fiber electromyography in botulism, A longitudinal study. Arch Neurol 1987;44(2):202–206.

5 Jost WH, Kohl A, Brinkmann S, Comes G. Efficacy and tolerability of a botulinum toxin type A free of complexing proteins (NT 201) compared with commercially available botulinum toxin type A (BOTOX) in healthy volunteers. J Neural Transm 2005;112:905–13.

6 Claus D. Botulinum toxin: influence on respiratory heart rate variation. Mov Disord 1995;10(5):574–579.

7 Guyer BM. Some unresolved issues with botulinum toxin J. Neurol 2001;248(Suppl.1):11–13.

8 Dressler D, Wohlfahrt K, Meyer-Rogge E, *et al*. Antibody-induced failure of botulinum toxin A therapy in cosmetic indications. Dermatol Surg 2010; 36(Suppl 4):2182–2187.

9 Stengel G, Bee EK. Antibody-induced secondary treatment failure in a patient treated with botulinum toxin type A for glabellar frown lines. Clin Interv Aging 2011;6:281–284.

10 Stephan F, Habre M, Tomb R. Clinical resistance to three types of botulinum toxin type A in aesthetic medicine. J Cosmet Dermatol 2014;13(4): 346–348.

11 Borodic G. Immunologic resistance after repeated botulinumtoxin type A injections for facial rhytides. Ophthal Plast Reconstr Surg 2006;22(3):239–240.

12 Naumann M, Carruthers A, Carruthers J, *et al*. Meta-analysis of neutralizing antibody conversion with onabotulinumtoxinA (BOTOX®) across multiple indications. Mov Disord 2010;25(13):2211–2218.

13 Rzany B, Flynn TC, Schlöbe A, *et al*. Long-term results for incobotulinumtoxinA in the treatment of glabellar frown lines. Dermatol Surg 2013;39(1 pt 1):95–103.

14 Klein AW. Dilution and storage of botulinum toxin. Dermatol Surg 1998;24(11):1179–1180.

15 Trindade De Almeida AR, Di Chiacchio N, Neto DR. Foam during reconstitution does not affect the potency of botulinum toxin type A. Dermatol Surg 2003;29(5):530–531; discussion 532.

16 Redaelli A, Forte R. Botulinum toxin dilution: our technique. J Cosmet Laser Ther 2003;5(3–4):218–219.

17 Hexsel DM, De Almeida AT, Rutowitsch M, *et al*., Multicenter, double-blind study of the efficacy of injections with botulinum toxin type A reconstituted up to six consecutive weeks before application. Dermatol Surg 2003;29(5):523–529; discussion 529.

18 Alam M, Yoo SS, Wrone DA, *et al*. Sterility assessment of multiple use botulinum A exotoxin vials: a prospective simulation. Dermatol Surg 2006;55:272–275.

19 Allergan, Inc. Botox US prescribing information. http://www.allergan.com/assets/pdf/botox_cosmetic_pi.pdf. Accessed January 21, 2016.

20 Carruthers JA, Lowe NJ, Menter MA, *et al*. A multicenter, double-blind, randomized, placebo-controlled study of the efficacy and safety of botulinum toxin type A in the treatment of glabellar lines. J Am Acad Dermatol 2002;46(6):840–849.

21 Guo Y, Lu Y, Liu T, *et al*. Efficacy and safety of botulinum toxin type A in the treatment of glabellar lines: a meta-analysis of randomized, placebo-controlled,

double-blind trials. Plast Reconstr Surg 2015;136(3):310e–318e.

22 Carruthers A, Carruthers J, Said S. Dose-ranging study of botulinum toxin type A in the treatment of glabellar rhytids in females. Dermatol Surg 2005;31(4): 414–422.

23 Carruthers A, Carruthers J. Prospective, double-blind, randomized, parallel-group, dose-ranging study of botulinum toxin type A in men with glabellar rhytids. Dermatol Surg. 2005;31(10):1297–1303.

24 Ipsen Biopharmaceuticals, Inc. Dysport US prescribing information. https://www .dysport.com/pdfs/Dysport_Full_ Prescribing_Information.pdf. Accessed May 21, 2016.

25 Monheit G, Carruthers A, Brandt F, Rand R. A randomized, double-blind, placebo-controlled study of botulinum toxin type A for the treatment of glabellar lines: determination of optimal dose. Dermatol Surg 2007;33(1 Spec No.): S51–S59.

26 Brandt F, Swanson N, Baumann L, Huber B. Randomized, placebo-controlled study of a new botulinum toxin type a for treatment of glabellar lines: efficacy and safety. Dermatol Surg 2009;35(12):1893–1901.

27 Kane MA, Brandt F, Rohrich RJ, *et al.*, Evaluation of variable-dose treatment with a new U.S. botulinum toxin type A (Dysport) for correction of moderate to severe glabellar lines: results from a phase III, randomized, double-blind, placebo-controlled study. Plast Reconstr Surg 2009;124(5): 1619–1629.

28 Merz Pharmaceuticals, Inc. Xeomin US prescribing information. www.xeomin aesthetic.com/wp-content/uploads/2016/ 12/EM00451-02-Electronic-PI.pdf Accessed May 21, 2016.

29 Carruthers A, Carruthers J, Coleman WP III, *et al.* Multicenter, randomized, phase III study of a single dose of incobotulinumtoxinA, free from complexing proteins, in the treatment of glabellar frown lines. Dermatol Surg 2013;39:551–558.

30 Hanke CW, Narins RS, Brandt F, *et al.* A randomized, placebo-controlled, double-blind phase III trial investigating the efficacy and safety of incobotulinumtoxinA in the treatment of glabellar frown lines using a stringent composite endpoint. Dermatol Surg 2013;39:891–899.

31 Jones D, Carruthers J, Narins RS, *et al.* Efficacy of incobotulinumtoxinA for treatment of glabellar frown lines: a post hoc pooled analysis of 2 randomized, placebo-controlled, phase 3 trials. Dermatol Surg 2014;40(7):776–785.

32 Kane M, Gold MH, Coleman WP 3rd, *et al.* A randomized, double-blind trial to investigate the equivalence of incobotulinumtoxinA and onabotulinumtoxinA for glabellar frown lines. Dermatol Surg 2015;41(11): 1310–1319.

33 Bonaparte JP, Ellis D, Quinn JG, *et al.* A comparative assessment of three formulations of botulinum toxin type A for facial rhytides: a systematic review with meta-analyses. Plast Reconstr Surg 2016:137(4):1125–1140.

34 Janis JE, Gavami A, Lemmon JA, *et al.*, Anatomy of the corrugator supercilii muscle: part I. Corrugator topography. Plast Reconstr Surg 2007;120(6): 1647–1653.

35 Shetty MK. Guidelines on the use of botulinum toxin Type A. Indian JDermatol Venereol Leprol 2008 Jan;74(7 Suppl 1): 13–22.

36 Beer K, Cohen JL, Carruthers, A. Cosmetic uses of botulinum toxin A. In Ward AB, Barnes MP, eds, *Clinical Uses of Botulinum Toxins.* Cambridge University Press, 2007:328.

37 Rzany B, Ascher B, Fratila A, *et al.*, Efficacy and safety of 3- and 5-injection patterns (30 and 50 U) of botulinum toxin A (Dysport) for the treatment of wrinkles in the glabella and the central forehead region. Arch Dermatol 2006;142(3):320–326.

38 Beer KR, Boyd C, Patel RK, *et al.* Rapid onset of response and patient-reported

outcomes after onabotulinumtoxinA treatment of moderate-to-severe glabellar lines. J Drugs Dermatol 2011;10(1):39–44.

39 Moy R, Maas C, Monheit G, *et al.* Long-term safety and efficacy of a new botulinum toxin type A in treating glabellar lines. Arch Facial Plast Surg 2009;11(2): 77–83.

40 Rubin MG, Dovwer J, Glogau RC, *et al.* The efficacy and safety of a new U.S. Botulinum toxin type A in the retreatment of glabellar lines following open-label treatment. J Drugs Dermatol 2009;8(5):439–444.

41 Rappl T, Parvizi D, Friedl H, *et al.* Onset and duration of effect of incobotulinumtoxinA, onabotulinumtoxinA, and abobotulinumtoxinA in the treatment of glabellar frown lines: a randomized, double-blind study. Clin Cosmet Investig Dermatol 2013;6:211–219.

42 Rzany B, Dill-Müller D, Grablowitz D, *et al.* Repeated botulinum toxin A injections for the treatment of lines in the upper face: a retrospective study of 4,103 treatments in 945 patients. Dermatol Surg 2007;33(1 Spec No.):S18–S25.

43 Ascher B, Zakine B, Kestemont P, *et al.*, Botulinum toxin A in the treatment of glabellar lines: scheduling the next injection. Aesthet Surg J 2005;25(4): 365–375.

11

Treatment of the Forehead

Joel L. Cohen, MD (FAAD, FACMS)[1,2,3] and Ramin Fathi, MD[4]

[1] Director, AboutSkin Dermatology and DermSurgery, Greenwood Village and Lone Tree, Colorado, USA
[2] Associate Clinical Professor, University of Colorado Department of Dermatology, Denver, USA
[3] Assistant Clinical Professor, University of California Irvine Department of Dermatology, Irvine, USA
[4] Resident Physician, Department of Dermatology, University of Colorado, Aurora, USA

Introduction

The forehead, comprising over a third of the face, is a prominent and very expressive region of our emotional lexicon. Considering that forehead wrinkling is also one of the earliest indicators of aging, it is not surprising that transverse forehead rhytides or "worry lines" are a presenting concern of many patients seeking facial rejuvenation with botulinum toxin. The highly active musculature of the forehead contributes to repeated wrinkling of the overlying skin from a very young age, making this region extremely prone to the formation of transverse horizontal rhytides long before the cumulative effects of aging set in. Even in relatively young populations of patients, when the rest of the face still retains its youthful contour and skin texture, deep dynamic wrinkles can be easily observed on elevation of the brow (Figure 11.1).

The use of botulinum toxin type A (BoNTA) for the treatment of hyperfunctional facial rhytides has been successfully documented since the early 1990s [1]. It has become the most popular cosmetic procedure, primarily due to its temporary and minimally invasive nature, and because it avoids surgery-related risks [2]. Upper facial lines, including glabellar frown lines, lateral canthal lines and horizontal forehead lines were the first documented areas for aesthetic application of BoNTA and have the longest safety and efficacy record for aesthetic usage. When injected into muscles, BoNTA blocks the release of acetylcholine from the motor nerve end plate, thereby reducing muscle activity, which leads to smoother skin and improved patient quality of life measures [3]. There are three BoNTA formulations available in the United States at present, but several more in the FDA process of clinical trials. OnabotulinumtoxinA (Botox®, Allergan, Irvine, CA) was approved in April 2002, AbobotulinumtoxinA (Dysport®, Galderma, Switzerland) was approved in April 2009, and IncobotulinumtoxinA (Xeomin®, Merz, Germany) was approved in September 2011.

Treatment of the glabellar muscle complex (Onabotulinum, Abobotulinum, Incobotulinum) and lateral canthal rhytids (Onabotulinum) are the only FDA-labeled aesthetic indications of BoNTA. Nevertheless, physicians routinely inject BoNTA into the forehead region to soften horizontal forehead lines, and many clinical studies along with expert consensus recommendations are available to guide the approach to this region [4].

This chapter will serve to familiarize the injector with a thoughtful approach to the

Botulinum Toxins: Cosmetic and Clinical Applications, First Edition. Edited by Joel L. Cohen and David M. Ozog.
© 2017 John Wiley & Sons Ltd. Published 2017 by John Wiley & Sons Ltd.
Companion Website: www.wiley.com/go/cohen/botulinum

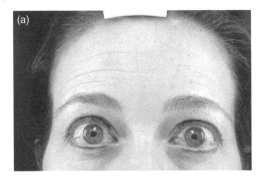 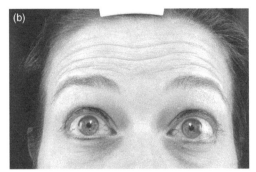

Figure 11.1 A 46-year-old woman (a) at rest showing some imprinting of forehead lines, (b) at animation lifting her eyebrows and contracting her frontalis muscle, demonstrating how lines at rest form over time.

aesthetic treatment of horizontal forehead rhytides using BoNTA. This approach requires careful consideration of eyebrow positioning to the extent that it is affected by musculature in the forehead area. This chapter will focus on the functional anatomy of the forehead and anatomic basis for various aesthetic changes that occur in this region that are amenable to rejuvenation with BoNTA. When injections with BoNTA are appropriately performed, desirable and reproducible results with high patient satisfaction can be achieved.

Anatomy

The anatomic boundaries of the forehead region are the supraorbital ridge and the root of the nose (inferiorly), the zygomatic arch (inferolaterally) and the hairline (superiorly) (Figure 11.2) [5]. The eyebrows are located at the inferior boundary of the forehead and their positioning is strongly influenced by muscle groups in this area. In cases with a receding hairline, the superior border of the forehead is determined by the superior extent of the frontalis muscle (Figure 11.3). The forehead may be further subdivided into a single central region that overlies the frontalis muscle and two lateral portions that extend into the temporal zones.

The skin of the forehead is the thickest skin of the face and is involved in many facial expressions. The skin is densely adherent to the underlying connective tissue layer and muscle layer via numerous transverse fibrous septa that are partially responsible for

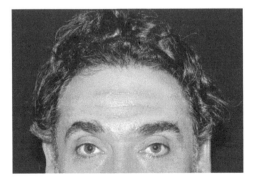

Figure 11.2 A 47-year-old at rest, showing imprinted lines in the forehead that demonstrate the anatomic boundaries of the forehead region.

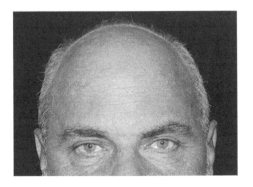

Figure 11.3 A 54-year-old man with a receding hairline.

the deep transverse forehead rhytides that develop over time [6].

The muscular layer of the forehead is below the subcutaneous tissue. This layer is composed of the elevator muscle (frontalis) at the superior aspect of the forehead and the depressor muscles (procerus, corrugator supercilii, and orbital portion of the orbicularis oculi) inferiorly (Figure 11.4). The frontalis is enclosed by a layer of fascia known as the galea aponeurosis, a thin sheet of connective tissue that encircles the entire skull [5, 7]. The galea is a fibromuscular extension of the superficial musculoaponeurotic system (SMAS) of the lower face, which invests and connects the muscles of facial expression. Contraction of the occipitofrontalis muscle-group tightens the scalp and allows for movement of the galea aponeurosis over underlying loose areolar tissue and periosteum.

The frontalis is comprised of two muscle bellies that originate superiorly from the galea with vertically oriented muscle fibers beginning approximately at the coronal suture. The frontalis bellies are sometimes discontinuous across the forehead, which creates a midline dehiscence or split. Cadaveric studies established average midline dehiscence locations at 3.5 cm in men and 3.7 cm in women above the superior orbital rim [7, 8]. Interestingly, a smaller interpupillary distance is predictive of a continuous or more midline frontalis muscles, indicating that those with a smaller head circumference are more likely to have active frontalis fibers across the entire forehead [8]. Clinically this means that women may have muscle fibers

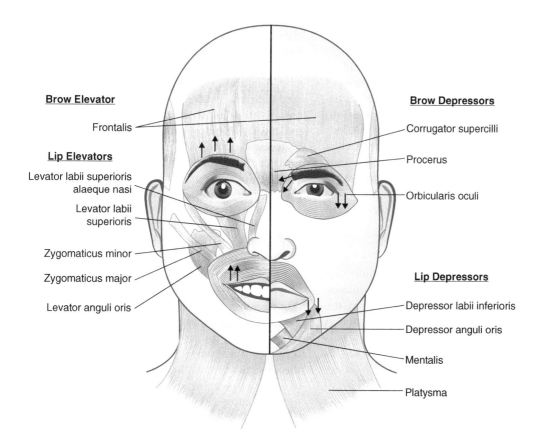

Figure 11.4 Protagonist/antagonist muscles of facial expression. Redrawn based on an original drawing by Margaret Ditré.

in the midline higher up on their forehead than men. In planning BoNTA intervention for transverse forehead rhytides, it is important to approximate the location of the dehiscence point, as injections above this area will not be focused at significantly active muscle fibers. From a practical clinical standpoint, however, many injectors simply examine the wrinkle pattern with animation, and inject in specific areas of movement.

The inferior insertion of the frontalis is at the level of the brow where it interdigitates with the three depressor muscles – the lateral fibers are blended with the pars orbitalis of the orbicularis oculi muscle, the medial fibers are continuous with the procerus and the intermediate fibers mixed with those of the corrugator supercilii. Contraction of the frontalis raises the eyebrows and creases the forehead skin transversely, antagonistic to the depressor actions of the orbicularis oculi, procerus, and corrugator supercilii muscles [9].

Sensory innervation of the forehead is via branches of the ophthalmic division of the trigeminal nerve (first branch of cranial nerve V). The ophthalmic nerve divides into the supraorbital and supratrochlear branches near the orbital rim. The nerves are part of neurovascular bundles with a corresponding artery and vein that supply the same region as the nerve. The facial nerve (cranial nerve VII) provides motor innervation to all the facial muscles. It innervates the muscles in the forehead region via its temporal branch [9].

It is important to keep in mind that the frontalis is the only elevator muscle of the forehead, thus any treatment of the frontalis may result in the unopposed action of the depressor muscles and vice versa. This becomes especially important when considering the effect of forehead BoNTA injections on the position and shape of the eyebrows, which is determined by the combined activity of the elevator and depressor muscles. Therefore, optimal outcomes are sometimes accomplished only through a calculated compromise of elevator and depressor

activity with well-planned BoNTA injection patterns.

Aging and the Forehead

Facial characteristics undergo several changes as a result of the cumulative effects of aging. Sebaceous activity declines, skin loses elasticity, subcutaneous tissue bulk decreases, attachments to underlying structures weaken allowing sagging due to gravitational forces, and bone resorption occurs [10, 11]. The combined effect of these factors is the formation of sagging redundancies in tissues evident as folds and wrinkles.

In the forehead, the effects of aging are compounded by repeated contraction of frontalis muscle that causes development of dynamic horizontal wrinkling during a variety of facial expressions as young as the 20s. Repetitive facial expression over many years eventually leads to the formation of static, etched-in lines present at rest – also, associated with and exacerbated by the decreased collagen content of the dermis and connective tissue with increasing age. For individuals with predominantly static wrinkles, inactivation of the frontalis with BoNTA will not yield as dramatic of an effect since BoNTA primarily addresses dynamic lines [12]. For this reason, we feel that BoNTA injections in the forehead are best suited for the younger to early mid-age patient who has not yet developed significant static wrinkles but would like to prevent them (Figure 11.5). The typical age range for this subset of patients is between 20 and 50 years depending on their intrinsic frontalis use for facial expression. With aging, the brow loses soft tissue support, which can result in a descent or loss of projection of the eyebrow causing brow-ptosis that tends to be more prominent laterally. The descent of the eyebrows below the supraorbital rim results in dermatochalasis or "hooding" of the upper lid with excess skin, which can often be exacerbated from significant sun-exposure and smoking.

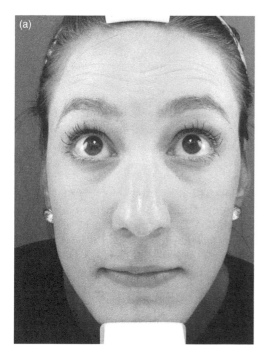
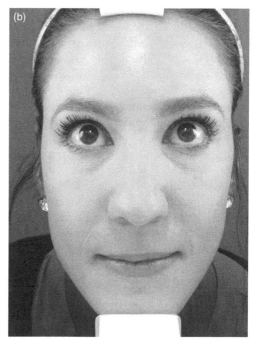

Figure 11.5 Forehead animation pretreatment (a) in a 29-year-old woman treated with 6 U Botox Cosmetic reconstituted 1 U/0.1 cm³ (b) and posttreatment.

The notion of aging prophylaxis with BoNTA is a concept that is being explored [13–15]. Many experts advocate initiating regular treatment with a neuromodulator in an individual's 20s or 30s with the argument that this will have a dramatic effect on the appearance of the face as seen in the person's 40s or 50s. There will be few, if any, lines of facial expression present [16]. Although no prospective, controlled clinical study has yet to examine aging prophylaxis with BoNTA, several case reports have suggested the potential of BoNTA for this purpose [13, 14]. A case-report examined prophylactic efficacy of BoNTA in identical 38-year-old twin sisters. One twin was regularly treated with BoNTA in the forehead and the glabella regions two to three times per year for 13 years. The second twin received only two total treatments with BoNTA in the forehead and the glabella within the previous 3 years [13]. In the twin undergoing regular treatment, photographic documentation showed no transverse forehead lines at rest, while the

minimally treated twin demonstrated static transverse rhytides in the forehead [13]. At 6-year follow-up (age 44), the treated twin continued to show diminished signs of facial aging and delayed appearance of hyperfunctional facial lines when compared to the sporadically treated twin [17]. Another case report examined two unrelated subjects in their 50s who were treated by the same clinician for over 7 years for non-reducible, hyperfunctional forehead lines [14]. Photographic documentation demonstrated effacement of static transverse lines at rest in both subjects, no evidence of the development of new wrinkles, and subjective improvement in skin quality over the 7-year treatment period [14]. Improvement in resting lines over repeat BoNTA injection has also been described by Carruthers through the reanalysis of previous clinical trial data [18].

While anecdotal and clinical data reveal the positive effect of BoNTA on resting lines, there are limited studies examining the biomechanical and anatomical factors involved. Current histological models of skin aging suggest that the development of static or nonreducible wrinkles could be secondary to actinic elastosis and the disappearance of microfibrils and collagen fibers from the dermal–epidermal junction [19]. It may be possible that BoNTA injections, by reducing the mechanical stress on the skin, enable the skin repair systems to work more efficiently, laying down connective tissue and improving skin quality. Of note, BoNTA has been shown to function in this capacity when used at the time of surgical repair of skin cancer defects and lacerations [20,21]. More studies are necessary to evaluate the cellular response secondary to muscle relaxation and the mechanisms behind long-term and prophylactic reduction of forehead lines.

Approaching the Patient (Evaluation and Selection)

When approaching a cosmetic patient, the physician should be aware that a "good result" always depends on the physician meeting the patient's expectations and pleasing the patient. A Treat-to-Goal (TTG) approach was recently described to objectively define start points and treatment goals for BoNTA treatment, utilizing the Merz Aesthetics Scale [22]. The Merz Aesthetics Scale is a visual tool that facilitates assessment of wrinkle severity via a dynamic 5-point photonumeric scale. This was developed as an effort to standardize means of establishing patient expectations and measuring treatment success as an integral part of the consent process. The rationale of the TTG approach is that with a standard consent, patients are not provided with an objective assessment of the likely cosmetic effect of their treatment. The study by Jandyhala demonstrated that the TTG approach represented a significant improvement over the standard consent approach because it enabled patients to gain a fuller understanding of what they should expect from their treatment [22].

The evaluation should begin with a discussion of what the patient perceives as undesirable in their appearance and the specific goals that the patient has for the treatment. The notion that BoNTA produces an unnatural "frozen" look is a common misconception and is an adverse outcome that has been frequently depicted in the media as overzealous cosmetic intervention. From surveys that examined parameters of patient satisfaction, it is clear that the trend in BoNTA rejuvenation is towards a "natural and relaxed look" [15]. Subjective patient satisfaction with BoNTA treatment is achieved when patients feel they look as good as possible for their age, look rested and relaxed without looking like they had any treatments performed, and convey less negative emotions while maintaining some degree of expression [15]. It is important the patient and physician discuss the degree of muscle softening versus overall paralysis they want to achieve – which will then determine the optimal treatment dosage. Although patients may welcome more extensive paralysis in the glabellar area (which is associated with conveying mostly negative emotions), highly expressive patients may desire only partial effect in the forehead to retain some animation activity (Figure 11.6). Two important consensus papers only 4 years apart document the trend of patients and physicians toward more forehead movement and less overall dosing of BoNTA in the frontalis (Table 11.1) [4, 23]. Recommended forehead dosages were reduced by about 50% in the subsequent paper in favor of less muscle immobilization and an overall more "natural" appearance.

Active and resting tranverse forehead rhytides will be assessed at the initial consultation. The patient should be asked to elevate the brows to determine the strength of the frontalis muscle as well as the location of the lines that are generated by forceful contraction. As described earlier, dynamic wrinkles generated by muscle contraction will benefit the most from treatment with BoNTA. If static wrinkles are the primary

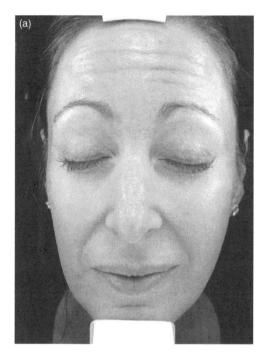 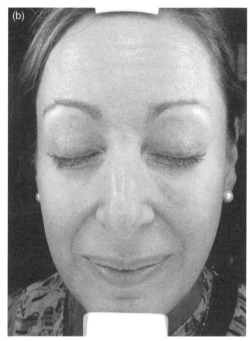

Figure 11.6 Forehead animation pretreatment (a) and posttreatment (b) in a 42-year-old woman treated with 3 U Botox Cosmetic.

concern of the patient, the treatment plan should encompass skin-resurfacing and sometimes volume replacement strategies in combination with BoNTA [24–28]. During forceful contraction, the clinician should evaluate the degree of muscle contraction in the midline to assess the level of dehiscence or continuity of the frontalis. Muscles should be palpated at rest and with contraction to assess muscle mass, tonicity, and the contribution of underlying subcutaneous tissue and facial skeleton to overall contour.

Resting transverse forehead lines are often most prominent if the frontalis is used as a compensatory mechanism to clear the superior visual field when it is compromised by brow ptosis, dermatochalasis, upper lid ptosis alone or in combination. In contrast to treating other areas of the upper face with BoNTA where there may be few functional consequences to relaxing the musculature, treatment of the frontalis requires careful additional consideration. Any current brow ptosis, extra eyelid hooding or reduction

Table 11.1 Treatment guidelines for horizontal forehead lines.

Target indication	Muscles involved	Recommended No. injection points	Total starting dose	
			Botox/Xeomin	Dysport
Horizontal forehead lines	Frontalis, possible interactions with procerus, corrugators, and orbicularis oculi	4–9, spaced at least 1 cm apart and dictated by overall forehead shape	Women: 6–15 U; Men: 6–15 U	20–60 U

Adapted and updated from Carruthers 2008 [23] and Ascher 2010 [51].

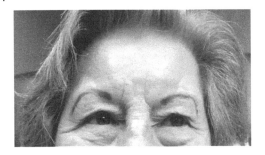

Figure 11.7 A 78-year old woman demonstrating profound dermatochalasis. Her eyelids are literally hanging over her eyelashes, and she is using her frontalis muscle even at rest to try to hoist up her eyebrows.

of the visual field must be noted because BoNTA in these patients may exacerbate the descent of the brow resulting in a tired look or compromised visual field. Patients that rely on the frontalis to constantly elevate the brow can be identified by multiple fine low-lying wrinkles immediately above the eyebrow (Figure 11.7). These patients should be made aware of these low-lying lines and advised on other options rather than botulinum toxin – such as ablative laser resurfacing, deeper chemical peel or even dermal fillers [29].

Any clinical assessment of the forehead requires close attention to brow position, which is of primary importance in conveying a range of emotions and moods. The physician should note the brow's shape and position, and also the relationship to the superior orbital rim as well as any potential redundancies of the eyelid itself. The eyebrow usually extends in a smooth arch laterally but often shows variation between ethnic groups and genders. In men, the eyebrows are generally straighter with less lateral arching than in women, and they are located more inferiorly, level with the superior orbital rim. In women, the eyebrows are usually located above the orbital rim and have a natural lateral arch that peaks superior to the lateral limbus at the lateral third of the brow [30, 31].

All patients should be evaluated for pre-existing asymmetry. Almost all faces will have a natural degree of asymmetry that is often overlooked by the patient. Pre-treatment asymmetry and scars should always be pointed out to the patient and documented in the patient's chart. Pre- and post-procedure photographs are of critical importance in managing patient expectations and assessing outcomes. Patients who do not consent to having their pictures taken should be approached with extra caution. The physician should explain the mode of action of BoNTA, the estimated onset and duration of effect (shorter durations are expected with lower dosing used for "more natural look"), the potential for adverse events, and the treatment options for undesired outcomes should they occur. Patients should be clearly informed that they are about to receive injections at an off-label site. Consent is typically in the form of an oral discussion as well as the standard signed written document that is completed before treatment is performed.

To assess treatment outcome, especially for new patients or more challenging patients, a follow-up appointment is often recommended 2 to 3 weeks after initial injection – when there is expected to be more maximal BoNTA effect. This will provide an opportunity to compare before and after treatment photographs, and assess the patient's level of satisfaction. At this optional follow-up appointment, patients can receive any necessary touch-up treatment with small doses to correct residual frontalis activity or asymmetry if present. Accurate documentation is key to successful utilization of BoNTA. In addition to taking photographs, recording the specific sites of injection and the total units injected during each procedure will allow the clinician to duplicate successful treatment in the future or modify treatment where outcomes could be improved.

Toxin and Dosage Selection

Several commercial preparations of BoNTA products are available for clinical usage. Though these are covered comprehensively in individual chapters, it is helpful to review here as a preface to some of the important toxin comparison studies that are relevant to the forehead region. Among these botulinum toxin agents, Botox (onabotulinumtoxinA) (Allergan Inc., Irvine, CA, USA) and Dysport (abobotulinumtoxinA) (Galderma, Switzerland) are the two most widely used from an aesthetic standpoint. They are produced from different strains of bacteria, purified and stabilized via different methods and therefore have distinct biological properties. As such, the units of these BoNTA preparations are not interchangeable. Bioassays that determine the potency of a neurotoxin quantify 1 unit (U) of purified BoNTA-Botox as the amount that is lethal to 50% of female Swiss Webster mice, known as the mean lethal dose (LD_{50}). To distinguish between the different preparations and potencies, BoNTA-Dysport is quantified in Speywood Units (s.U.). Both preparations contain the 150 kDa neurotoxin, but they differ in the size of their complexing proteins. The Botox product consists of uniformly sized complexes of 900 kDa, while Dysport is composed of a heterogeneous mixture of 500–900 kDa complexes [32, 33]. Additionally, in the United States a third preparation of BoNTA, Xeomin (incobotulinumtoxinA) (Merz Pharmaceuticals, Frankfurt, Germany) has been FDA approved for the treatment of cervical dystonia and blepharospasm, and obtained FDA approval for aesthetic use in the glabella in 2011. Xeomin is free from complexing proteins and contains only the 150 kDa neurotoxin component, which the manufacturer claims may result in a lower immune response, but this has not yet been validated clinically [34, 35]. The current clinical conversion rate of Botox to Xeomin is reported as 1:1 in the treatment of focal dystonias, with Xeomin demonstrating comparable efficacy, duration of effect, and tolerability as compared to Botox [36–38]. A recent randomized, double-blinded trial of 250 females aged 18–50 years old investigated the dose equivalence of Xeomin and Botox for glabellar frown lines. The investigators found 20 U of both products had equivalent primary efficacy at 1 month and 4 months after treatment with similar tolerability by the patient [39].

Several studies have looked at comparative dosages of Botox and Dysport preparations, with a wide range of 2–4 s.U. of Dysport required to achieve the same therapeutic effect as 1 U Botox [40–44]. However, many experienced physicians seem to agree that the most suitable dose equivalence is between 2.5 s.U. of Dysport and 1 U of Botox based on several studies. Additionally, the FDA approved dosages in the glabella are 20 U Botox and 50 s.U. Dysport. One double-blind, randomized study that examined the conversion ratio of 1:2.5 (Botox:Dysport) for the treatment of mild-to-moderate moderate facial lines found that both products produced similar improvements from baseline at 8 and 12 weeks. However, differences emerged at the 16-week follow-up – showing a greater duration of effect for Botox, indicating that a larger dose of Dysport may be necessary to achieve duration equality [42]. A dosing study evaluating the Botox:Dysport conversion ratio of 1:4 for the cosmetic treatment of hyperfunctional facial lines, including transverse forehead rhytides, investigator assessment found Dysport statistically superior in reducing horizontal forehead lines at maximum contraction [45]. The adverse event profile showed no differences between the different formulations, leading the investigators to conclude that a larger dose ratio of Botox:Dysport can be safely utilized in the upper face.

Various lines of research suggest that the two commonly employed formulations of BoNTA (Botox and Dysport) exhibit different diffusion tendencies from the site of injection. Diffusion rates, or the "spread" of the toxin from the site of injection, result in different "fields of effect" or surface area that is affected by the toxin. The diffusion potential of BoNTA is dependent on various factors including most importantly the dose injected as well as likely the volume of injection, but potentially also the molecular size, structure, and subtype of the toxin, and site of injection. The possibility of diffusion is of great clinical relevance in certain areas with small, thin, and closely positioned muscles of the upper face (but also the lower face as well). When planning the choice of BoNTA (including dilution ratios and injection sites), it is imperative to understand the anticipated migration of the toxin in the thin frontalis muscle and the effect this will have on the treatment outcome. The impact of neurotoxin complex size on diffusion potential is, at least theoretically, based on the principle that larger proteins diffuse more slowly through an identical aqueous medium compared with smaller proteins, predicting that BoNTA formulations of greater molecular weight will have lower diffusion potential [46]. However, it has been shown that the complexing proteins immediately disassociate from the naked neurotoxin literally right after dilution of each of the BoNTA formulations. Therefore, other factors may play a greater role in the diffusion properties – such as the total injection volume. When diffusion was evaluated in relation to the injected volume and BoNTA concentration, Hsu *et al.* [47] found that higher dilutions (lower concentration in a higher volume) were associated with a wider area of effect in the forehead. They saw a 50% increase in the treatment zone by diluting the same concentration of BoNTA in a five-fold larger volume leading to the conclusion that a higher dilution and a larger volume can be utilized for broad, flat muscles with fewer injection points [47]. However, this was a small study involving 10 patients that investigated only the Botox preparation and did not correlate higher injected volume to any indication of duration of toxin action.

Building on these findings, several groups attempted to contrast the diffusion potential between Botox and Dysport. In a double-blinded study of 20 patients, diffusion of Botox and Dysport were compared by assessing forehead hyperhidrosis [44]. Patients were randomly injected with 3 U of Botox or Dysport at a conversion ratio of 1 : 2.5, 1 : 3, and 1 : 4 in four areas of the forehead. Identical volumes (0.06 ml) were used for all injections. Patients were assessed by using the starch–iodine test after 24 hours, 1 week, 2 weeks, and monthly up to 6 months to evaluate anhidrotic halos. Dysport produced a larger area of anhidrosis in 93% of comparisons at all dose ratios [44]. Another study compared 12 healthy volunteers who were randomly assigned to receive three 0.1 ml intradermal injections in their forehead: 4 U Botox on one side, 12 s.U. Dysport (conversion ratio of 1 : 3) on the contralateral side, and saline in the center [48]. Anhidrosis was assessed by the starch-iodine test at the 14-day follow-up visit. A higher mean area of anhidrosis was observed on the Dysport side in 11 of the 12 subjects. The authors concluded that Dysport has a higher migration potential than Botox [48]. However, another study failed to duplicate these diffusion results when a lower volume of injection was used [49]. This latter smaller volume study was an open-label, randomized study treating 18 subjects for dynamic rhytides in the frontal region. Investigators examined the diffusion potential of Dysport and Botox by assessing the action halo, or degree of muscle paralysis, and the zone of anhidrosis. Only one conversion ratio of 1 : 2.5 (Botox : Dysport) was utilized in an equal volume of 0.02 ml, delivering 2 U and 5 s.U. respectively on opposite sides of the frontalis at the midpupillary line. Evaluations were performed at 28-day follow-up. Results showed no statistical difference between the average area of action halos for muscular weakness or anhidrosis between Botox and Dysport. However, the action halo for muscular relaxation was bigger than the anhidrotic halo for both preparations, albeit this was not statistically validated [49]. A higher diffusion potential will likely result in fewer required injections in the treated area. This can be beneficial in patients who bruise easily or are very injection-phobic, but it could be detrimental in patients with a redundant brow-lid complex where tight control of diffusion is necessary to prevent brow ptosis. More studies are needed to determine if an increased field of effect provides an advantage in clinical outcomes and patient satisfaction, and how to best utilize the migration potential of BoNTA when planning patient care.

While it may not be ideal to compare dilution ratios, it is important to know the relative dosages of the different toxins, since patients sometimes switch to a different preparation of BoNTA for various reasons including personal preference or even recommendation from someone for aesthetic or even logistical reasons. For most forehead patients, it is recommended to start with a small initial dose to avoid the "frozen" look. The dosage recommendations from the 2008 Facial Aesthetics Consensus group reflect the Botox experience of a multidisciplinary group of aesthetic experts [23]. The current set of guidelines updates the previous Botox specific recommendations, decreasing the initial starting dose by about 50% in the forehead [4, 23]. The current recommended total starting dose for injecting the forehead in women is approximately 6–15 5 BoNTA for the Botox formulation with 3–5 t per injection point. The consensus recommendation in men is to also start with 6–15 5; however, greater dosages are frequently employed due to the greater muscle mass in men (Figure 11.8). On average, treatment of the forehead in men will require an additional 25–50% of toxin (especially for those who want the muscle pretty much immobile) when compared to women with a similar degree of wrinkling. The only BoNTA study that was specifically undertaken to examine BoNTA dosing in men examined the dose-response relationship in the glabella [50]. In this glabellar study, the authors' conclusions supported starting men at a dose approximately twice the standard dose used in women – but again, this

was a glabella specific study where the muscles are typically fully-treated, rather than "minimized" as is more "natural" of a look in the forehead. In current clinical practice when treating the forehead, the authors commonly use 4–6 Botox/Xeomin in women (10–15 5 Dysport) and 8–12 2 Botox/Xeomin in men (20–30 0 Dysport).

There is currently no dose-optimization study with Dysport performed for transverse forehead rhytides. The 2010 international consensus recommendation for this preparation is a total dose of 20–60 s.U. with 5–10 s.U. per injection point (Ascher 2010). The consensus recommendation for the Dysport formulation did not include specific recommendations based on gender [51]. Previous guidelines on Dysport for different aesthetic regions, published by Matarasso and Shafer in 2009, also recommended 30–60 over three to six injection sites into the frontalis, but also did not make specific gender-based dosing recommendations [52].

One of the authors of this chapter (JLC) uses Botox in the forehead with a 4 ne^3 dilution and in the glabella and crow's feet with 1 it^3 dilution. For Dysport, JLC uses a 3 di^3 dilution in forehead and 1 di^3 in glabella. Tighter control of dilution in the glabella is usually much more important, whereas facilitating some spread in the forehead helps limit injection sites but also may help to achieve a more natural overall smoothness to the forehead as more areas of the large frontalis may be softened.

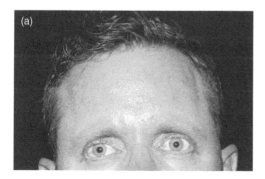 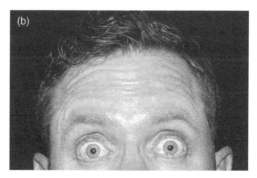

Figure 11.8 A 40-year-old male patient demonstrating significant muscle mass of the frontalis from eyebrow all the way up into the hairline.

Toxin Administration

Given the natural individual variation of the frontalis muscle, there is no single technique or landmark that is followed when choosing injection points. Each patient's distinctive musculature, wrinkle pattern, and eyebrow position must be considered. Individualization of the treatment is key to a successful outcome and patient satisfaction.

The dimensions of the forehead, and thus the frontalis muscle, differ from one patient to another [8, 53, 54]. Forehead injections of BoNTA are generally placed over four to nine injection sites. A vertical length of over 70 mm between the glabella and the frontal midline hairline characterizes a wide forehead, which may benefit from two rows of injection sites. A vertical length of less than 60 mm characterizes a narrow forehead which can often be treated with a single row of injection sites [53]. As illustrated by the anhidrosis diffusion studies, the effect of BoNTA is not confined to the area where it is injected. Diffusion of the toxin into surrounding tissue leads to spread of the effect in an area roughly 3 cm in diameter. In patients with particularly narrow foreheads, there is a larger potential for brow asymmetry and brow ptosis due to diffusion of toxin. To minimize diffusion-related complications, injections should generally not be placed any closer than 1.5 cm above the bony orbital rim with Botox and about 1.5–2 cm above the bony orbital rim for Dysport. Another potentially useful guideline is to avoid treatment of the first row of horizontal rhytides above the brow, or consider just a very low-dose in this area to simply "soften" the musculature slightly without fully knocking it out to avoid significant repositioning of the brow downward.

In female patients, injection sites should often follow the curve of the brow to preserve the natural arch (Figure 11.9). In men, it is more common for rhytides to extend up to the superior portion of the frontalis near the hairline. Failure to treat these superior rhytides can result in patient

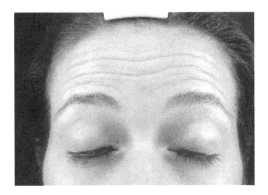

Figure 11.9 Animating forehead demonstrating the relationship of the frontalis musculature on shape and positioning of the eyebrows.

dissatisfaction and an unnatural appearance. In men with a receding hairline, recruitment of more superior frontalis fibers can occur after mid-forehead injection – leading to the appearance of new rhytides superiorly at the attachments of the frontalis to the galea. It is important to identify the potential for this compensatory mechanism and treat balding patients with at least two rows of injections (Figure 11.10).

The authors most commonly use the BD 0.3 ml or 0.5 ml insulin syringes with a 31 gauge, short incorporated needle (BD. Franklin Lakes, NJ, USA). This syringe type allows for precise treatment and accurate dosing due to the small volume of solution

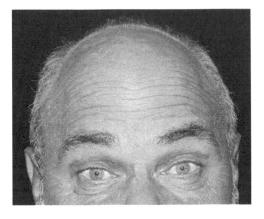

Figure 11.10 Receding hairline with high recruitment of muscle fibers, particularly laterally.

that is loaded. Multiple syringes are often used for a single treatment providing a sharp, less painful needle that is discarded after a few injections. The patient is treated in a seated or semireclined position to allow for better visualization of the anatomy of the muscles. It is important, especially for newer injectors, to mark the planned injection points (we use a dry-erase marker that wipes off easily with water) to ensure accurate injection. Injections are placed adjacent to but not through the marker ink to avoid a potential ink tattoo. With the patient's forehead at rest, botulinum toxin injections are injected intramuscularly or often superficially raising blebs on the skin surface. Care should be taken to avoid injecting below the muscular layer of the frontalis or into the periosteum, where injections are more painful for the patient and can potentially have a reduced clinical effect. If the bony skull is felt while injecting, withdraw the needle about 3–4 mm before infiltrating BoNTA. Postinjection, the area is often iced to try to prevent possible significant swelling or ecchymosis, and the patient is advised not to manipulate the treated area for a couple of hours after the injection [55, 56].

BoNTA rejuvenation is very often requested in more than one facial area. A placebo-controlled, double blind study examined the efficacy and safety of treating the forehead, glabellar area, and crow's feet in a single session with the Botox formulation. No significant adverse events were reported, and the study validated the common clinical experience that Botox can be used safely and effectively to treat multiple areas of the upper face [57]. However, for novice injectors, it is recommended to split up the treatment areas – treating the glabella before the forehead. Otherwise, if the forehead is treated first, the depressor function of the glabellar muscles may predispose to brow ptosis. When BoNTA rejuvenation is planned in combination with fillers, it is recommended to stage the treatments – treating first with BoNTA and then with filler [25]. This allows for the assessment of residual static

lines after the onset of BoNTA action, and has been shown to increase the durability of the filler correction as well [25]. In all combination treatments, the most important consideration is careful documentation of the injection sites and units placed.

Key Points of Technique

Avoid treating the most inferiorly positioned horizontal forehead line in patients who demonstrate excessive eyelid skin, or dermatochalasis [58]. While sagging eyelids are usually a cosmetic concern, they can lead to visual field loss, ocular or eyelid irritation, and headaches due to forced brow elevations to increase the visual field. Significant and independent risk factors for sagging eyelids included age, male sex, lighter skin color, and higher body mass index according to a large study of 5578 patients with sagging eyelids [58]. Prior to injection, evaluation of the eyelids should occur, especially in higher risk patient populations to ensure dermatochalasis is not induced or worsened.

Contraindications and Complications

BoNTA is contraindicated in the presence of infection at the proposed injection site and in patients with a known hypersensitivity to any ingredient in the formulation. Caution should be exercised in treating patients with peripheral neuropathic disease or neuromuscular junction disorders such as myasthenia gravis, Lambert–Eaton syndrome, or amyotrophic lateral sclerosis. Concomitant aminoglycoside antibiotics may interfere with neuromuscular transmission and potentiate the effects of BoNTA [56]. Use in pregnant and breastfeeding women has not been clinically evaluated and there is no reliable human data available to define the degree of risk in these situations. Therefore, treatment of pregnant or breastfeeding women is not recommended. In cases where there is a previous history of surgery to the area, caution should be exercised as the underlying anatomy may be altered. For example, one study of patients with cervical dystonia treated with BoNTA found an odds ratio of 9.8 ($p = 0.013$) for secondary nonresponse if they had a prior surgical treatment for cervical dystonia [59].

As with other regions of BoNTA treatment, injection-site reactions such as erythema, edema, and ecchymosis are the most common adverse events of treatment in the forehead. Patients are cautioned to consider avoiding any agents that may inhibit clotting such as nontherapeutic aspirin (as long as patients are not on aspirin for a specific medical purpose such as a history of a heart attack, stroke, blood clot or atrial fibrillation) as well as nonsteroidal anti-inflammatory drugs and alcohol for at least several days prior to treatment, but this is certainly not mandatory. Focal firm pressure and ice are always recommended postinjection if an injection site displays immediate bleeding or significant swelling. Removal of makeup and gentle cleansing of the treatment area with alcohol are recommended prior to all BoNTA treatments in our office.

The primary complication of concern with forehead BoNTA injections is brow ptosis, which is cosmetically unacceptable and sometimes visually significant. If encountered, this complication is not completely treatable, but the patient can be reassured that it is temporary and will fully reverse in 3–4 months, although clinically significant improvement is often noted as soon as 4–6 weeks. Some patients with a lateral brow ptosis, however, may benefit from injection of the superior aspect of the lateral orbicularis oculi area to lead to a functional brow lift by decreasing the baseline downward pull of this portion of the orbicularis oculi. Similarly, some patients with a medial brow ptosis may benefit from injecting the brow depressors of the glabella to try to lift this area of the brow. Due to the lack of complete treatment of this complication, the best strategy

is a judicious and fastidious technique in the first place. For these reasons performing inferior injections at least 1.5 cm above the eyebrows, or at least significantly lower doses in this area, for the entire width of the frontalis muscle is recommended as well as avoidance of treating patients with significant frontalis compensation at baseline for brow ptosis – as is common in older patients. As with most cosmetic procedures, it is always possible to add more product to touch-up some residual activity rather than overdo it in the first place. It is suggested that the initial starting dose of any preparation of BoNTA be reduced in older patients who are more reliant on the frontalis to elevate the brow. This subset of patients should be carefully counseled about the risks of brow ptosis and the possibility that the aesthetic result they seek will be more amenable to surgery.

One of the most common forehead complications from BoNTA is caused from glabella injections either treated too broadly or too high, resulting in a partially treated forehead and an unnatural appearance (Figure 11.11). This usually happens with novice injectors

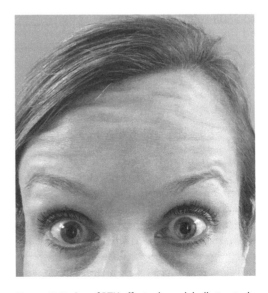

Figure 11.11 Arc of BTX effect when glabella treated too broadly, and adjacent spread makes the cut-off of treated versus untreated forehead too distinct. *Source:* Courtesy of David M. Ozog.

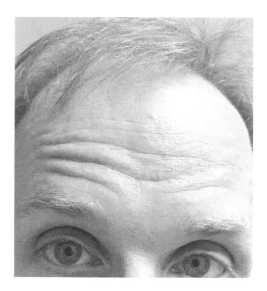

Figure 11.12 Missed area on right forehead after forehead BTX treatment by a novice injector. *Source: Courtesy of David M. Ozog.*

and inappropriately high dosing and is best resolved by treating the remainder of the forehead with neuromodulator. Novice injectors are also more likely to miss areas as they get accustomed to injecting small aliquots in the forehead (Figure 11.12).

A quizzical or cock-eyed appearance of the eyebrow (Mephisto or "Mr. Spock" brow) can be seen when the medial forehead is paralyzed and the lateral frontalis fibers remain functional. Injecting 1–3 t BoNTA Botox formulation into untreated lateral fibers that are causing the upward pull can correct this. Some asymmetry may result despite consistent technique due to intrinsic patient variability. It is best to evaluate any reports of asymmetry at least 10 days posttreatment to allow the full onset of effect of the BoNTA in case one side responds quicker than the other side.

Utilization of greater doses than those recommended for the forehead may lead to the suboptimal outcome of the "frozen" look or a state of inexpressivity [15]. Although some patients may express the desire for a high degree of immobility, it is up to the practitioner to adjust the patient's expectations

to a more realistic and aesthetically pleasing outcome. Patient education during every visit and by all members of the treatment team is the best approach for correcting misinformation regarding BoNTA practice and to foster a long-term and trusting relationship with the patient. We generally counsel patients that ideal outcomes in forehead treatment often require relatively low dosing that may necessitate more frequent injections every 2–3 months for maintenance (versus other areas that typically receive higher doses and are usually treated every 3–4 months or even longer).

Although there is more than one preparation of BoNTA available, caution must be utilized in using different varieties of BoNTA concurrently in the same patient – particularly if they are new to botulinum toxin treatment in your office. It is advised by some experts to start treating the patient with a single type of toxin. Otherwise, should an adverse event occur, or should a patient have an extremely rare reaction precipitated by treatment, it will be difficult to tell which toxin is causing it. This can result in the patient discontinuing all further interventions with BoNTA and abandoning the treatment plan.

Conclusions

- Patient education and counseling are integral parts of BoNTA treatment. It is essential for patients to have a realistic expectation of the treatment outcome to achieve satisfaction with the treatment and the provider.
- In general, beginning practitioners need to understand precise regional anatomy and the muscle vectors that contribute to the aesthetic concern.
- Common considerations include toxin agent, dose, dilution, and patient selection.
- Keep in mind the greater muscle mass in men when planning total forehead dose. But overall, the forehead musculature is commonly "softened" or "minimized"

rather than fully knocked-out like in other areas of treatment.

- BoNTA use for cosmetic applications in the forehead rarely produces serious

adverse events; however, caution should be utilized when treating low-lying rhytides that may cause toxin diffusion below the orbital rim.

References

1 Carruthers JD, Carruthers JA. Treatment of glabellar frown lines with C. botulinum-A exotoxin. The Journal of dermatologic surgery and oncology. 1992;18(1):17–21.

2 The American Society for Aesthetic Plastic Surgery (2016) Top 5 surgical and non-surgical cosmetic procedures. Highlights of the ASAPS 2016 statistics on cosmetic surgery. 2016 10 April 2016. Available from: http://www.surgery.org/sites/default/files/ASAPS-Stats2016.pdf

3 Cox SE, Finn JC. Social implications of hyperdynamic facial lines and patient satisfaction outcomes. International ophthalmology clinics. 2005; 45(3):13–24.

4 Carruthers J, Fagien S, Matarasso SL. Consensus recommendations on the use of botulinum toxin type a in facial aesthetics. Plast Reconstr Surg 2004; 114(6 Suppl): 1s–22s.

5 Sherris DA, Larrabee WF, editors. *Principles of Facial Reconstruction*. New York: Raven Press; 1995.

6 Tarbet KJ, Lemke BN. Clinical anatomy of the upper face. Int Ophthalmol Clinic 1997; 37(3):11–28.

7 Abramo AC. Anatomy of the forehead muscles: the basis for the videoendoscopic approach in forehead rhytidoplasty. Plast Reconstr Surg 1995; 95(7):1170–1177.

8 Spiegel JH, Goerig RC, Lufler RS, Hoagland TM. Frontalis midline dehiscence: an anatomical study and discussion of clinical relevance. J Plast Reconstr Aesthet Surg 2009; 62(7):950–954.

9 Zimbler MS, Kokoska MS, Thomas JR. Anatomy and pathophysiology of facial aging. Facial Plast Surg Clinics North Am 2001; 9(2):179–187, vii.

10 Coleman SR, Grover R. The anatomy of the aging face: volume loss and changes in

3-dimensional topography. Aesthet Surg J/Am Soc Aesthet Plast Surg 2006; 26(1s): S4–S9.

11 Imayama S, Braverman IM. A hypothetical explanation for the aging of skin. Chronologic alteration of the three-dimensional arrangement of collagen and elastic fibers in connective tissue. Am J Pathol 1989; 134(5):1019–1025.

12 Branford OA, Dann SC, Grobbelaar AO. The quantitative assessment of wrinkle depth: turning the microscope on botulinum toxin type A. Ann Plast Surg 2010; 65(3):285–293.

13 Binder WJ. Long-term effects of botulinum toxin type A (Botox) on facial lines: a comparison in identical twins. Arch Facial Plast Surg 2006; 8(6):426–431.

14 Bowler PJ. Dermal and epidermal remodeling using botulinum toxin type A for facial, non reducible, hyperkinetic lines: two case studies. J Cosmet Dermatol 2008; 7(3):241–244.

15 Carruthers A, Cohen JL, Cox SE, *et al.* Facial aesthetics: achieving the natural, relaxed look. Journal of cosmetic and laser therapy : official publication of the Eur Soc Laser Dermatol 2007; 9(Suppl 1):6–10.

16 Hamilton HK, Arndt KA. When is "too early" too early to start cosmetic procedures? JAMA Dermatol 2013; 149(11):1271.

17 Rivkin A, Binder WJ. Long-term effects of onabotulinumtoxinA on facial lines: a 19-year experience of identical twins. Dermatol Surg 2015; 41(Suppl 1): S64–S66.

18 Carruthers A, Carruthers J, Lei X, *et al.* OnabotulinumtoxinA treatment of mild glabellar lines in repose. Dermatol Surg 2010; 36(Suppl 4):2168–2171.

19 Bosset S, Barre P, Chalon A, *et al.* Skin ageing: clinical and histopathologic study of permanent and reducible wrinkles. Eur J Dermatol 2002; 12(3):247–252.

20 Flynn TC. Use of intraoperative botulinum toxin in facial reconstruction. Dermatol Surg 2009; 35(2):182–188.

21 Gassner HG, Brissett AE, Otley CC, *et al.* Botulinum toxin to improve facial wound healing: A prospective, blinded, placebo-controlled study. Mayo Clinic Proc 2006; 81(8):1023–1028.

22 Jandhyala R. Improving consent procedures and evaluation of treatment success in cosmetic use of incobotulinumtoxinA: an assessment of the treat-to-goal approach. J Drugs Dermatol 2013; 12(1):72–78.

23 Carruthers JD, Glogau RG, Blitzer A. Advances in facial rejuvenation: botulinum toxin type a, hyaluronic acid dermal fillers, and combination therapies – consensus recommendations. Plast Reconstr Surg 2008; 121(5 Suppl):5S–30S; quiz 1S–6S.

24 Carruthers J, Carruthers A, Zelichowska A. The Power of Combined Therapies: BOTOX and Ablative Facial Laser Resurfacing. Am J Cosmet Surg 2000; 17(3). http://journals.sagepub.com/doi/abs/10.1177/074880680001700302

25 Carruthers J, Carruthers A. A prospective, randomized, parallel group study analyzing the effect of BTX-A (Botox) and nonanimal sourced hyaluronic acid (NASHA, Restylane) in combination compared with NASHA (Restylane) alone in severe glabellar rhytides in adult female subjects: treatment of severe glabellar rhytides with a hyaluronic acid derivative compared with the derivative and BTX-A. Dermatol Surg 2003; 29(8):802–809.

26 Carruthers J, Carruthers A, Maberley D. Deep resting glabellar rhytides respond to BTX-A and Hylan B. Dermatol Surg 2003; 29(5):539–544.

27 Kadunc BV, Trindade De Almeida AR, Vanti AA, Di Chiacchio N. Botulinum toxin A adjunctive use in manual chemabrasion: controlled long-term study for treatment of upper perioral vertical wrinkles. Dermatol Surg 2007; 33(9):1066–1072; discussion 72.

28 Kenner JR. Hyaluronic acid filler and botulinum neurotoxin delivered simultaneously in the same syringe for effective and convenient combination aesthetic rejuvenation therapy. J Drugs Dermatol 2010; 9(9):1135–1138.

29 Alam M, Dover JS, Klein AW, Arndt KA. Botulinum a exotoxin for hyperfunctional facial lines: where not to inject. Arch Dermatol 2002; 138(9):1180–1185.

30 Gunter JP, Antrobus SD. Aesthetic analysis of the eyebrows. Plast Reconstr Surg 1997; 99(7):1808–1816.

31 Pham S, Wilhelmi B, Mowlavi A. Eyebrow peak position redefined. Aesthet Surg J 2010; 30(3):297–300.

32 Lietzow MA, Gielow ET, Le D, *et al.* Subunit stoichiometry of the *Clostridium* botulinum type A neurotoxin complex determined using denaturing capillary electrophoresis. Protein J 2008; 27(7–8): 420–425.

33 Schantz EJ, Johnson EA. Properties and use of botulinum toxin and other microbial neurotoxins in medicine. Microbiol Rev 1992; 56(1):80–99.

34 Naumann M, Carruthers A, Carruthers J, *et al.* Meta-analysis of neutralizing antibody conversion with onabotulinumtoxinA (BOTOX®) across multiple indications. Mov Disord 2010; 25(13):2211–2218.

35 Xeomin [package insert]. Frankfurt, Germany: Merz Pharmaceuticals; 2011.

36 Dressler D. Comparing Botox and Xeomin for axillar hyperhidrosis. J Neural Transm (Vienna) 2010; 117(3):317–319.

37 Jost WH, Blumel J, Grafe S. Botulinum neurotoxin type A free of complexing proteins (XEOMIN) in focal dystonia. Drugs 2007; 67(5):669–683.

38 Roggenkamper P, Jost WH, Bihari K, *et al.* Efficacy and safety of a new botulinum toxin type A free of complexing proteins in the treatment of blepharospasm. J Neural Transm (Vienna) 2006; 113(3):303–312.

39 Kane MA, Gold MH, Coleman WP 3rd, *et al.* A Randomized, double-blind trial to investigate the equivalence of incobotulinumtoxinA and

onabotulinumtoxinA for glabellar frown lines. Dermatol Surg 2015; 41(11): 1310–1319.

40 Durif F. Clinical bioequivalence of the current commercial preparations of botulinum toxin. Eur J Neurol 1996; 2: 17–18.

41 Karsai S, Raulin C. Current evidence on the unit equivalence of different botulinum neurotoxin A formulations and recommendations for clinical practice in dermatology. Dermatol Surg 2009; 35(1): 1–8.

42 Lowe P, Patnaik R, Lowe N. Comparison of two formulations of botulinum toxin type A for the treatment of glabellar lines: a double-blind, randomized study. J Am Acad Dermatol 2006; 55(6):975–980.

43 Sampaio C, Costa J, Ferreira JJ. Clinical comparability of marketed formulations of botulinum toxin. Mov Disord 2004; 19(Suppl 8):S129–S136.

44 Trindade de Almeida AR, Marques E, de Almeida J, et al. Pilot study comparing the diffusion of two formulations of botulinum toxin type A in patients with forehead hyperhidrosis. Dermatol Surg 2007; 33(1 Spec No.):S37–S43.

45 Lowe NJ, Shah A, Lowe PL, Patnaik R. Dosing, efficacy and safety plus the use of computerized photography for botulinum toxins type A for upper facial lines. J Cosmet Laser Ther 2010; 12(2):106–111.

46 de Almeida AT, De Boulle K. Diffusion characteristics of botulinum neurotoxin products and their clinical significance in cosmetic applications. J Cosmet Laser Ther 2007; 9 Suppl 1:17–22.

47 Hsu TS, Dover JS, Arndt KA. Effect of volume and concentration on the diffusion of botulinum exotoxin A. Arch Dermatol 2004; 140(11):1351–1354.

48 Cliff SH, Judodihardjo H, Eltringham E. Different formulations of botulinum toxin type A have different migration characteristics: a double-blind, randomized study. J Cosmet Dermatol 2008; 7(1):50–54.

49 Hexsel D, Dal'Forno T, Hexsel C, et al. A randomized pilot study comparing the action halos of two commercial preparations of botulinum toxin type A. Dermatol Surg 2008; 34(1):52–59.

50 Carruthers A, Carruthers J. Prospective, double-blind, randomized, parallel-group, dose-ranging study of botulinum toxin type A in men with glabellar rhytids. Dermatol Surg 2005; 31(10):1297–1303.

51 Ascher B, Talarico S, Cassuto D, E et al. International consensus recommendations on the aesthetic usage of botulinum toxin type A (Speywood Unit) – Part I: Upper facial wrinkles. J Eur Acad Dermatold Venereol 2010; 24(11):1278–1284.

52 Matarasso A, Shafer D. Botulinum neurotoxin type A-ABO (Dysport): clinical indications and practice guide. Aesthet Surg J 2009; 29(6 Suppl):S72–S79.

53 Ozsoy Z, Genc B, Gozu A. A new technique applying botulinum toxin in narrow and wide foreheads. Aesthet Plast Surg 2005; 29(5):368–372.

54 Ozsoy Z, Genc B, Gozu A. A new technique for the application of botulinum toxin in short and tall foreheads. Plast Reconstr Surg 2005; 115(5):1439–1441.

55 Hsu TS, Dover JS, Kaminer MS, et al. Why make patients exercise facial muscles for 4 hours after botulinum toxin treatment? Arch Dermatol 2003; 139(7): 948.

56 Huang W, Foster JA, Rogachefsky AS. Pharmacology of botulinum toxin. J Am Acad Dermatol 2000; 43(2 Pt 1):249–259.

57 Carruthers J, Carruthers A. Botulinum toxin type A treatment of multiple upper facial sites: patient-reported outcomes. Dermatol Surg 2007; 33(1 Spec No.): S10–S17.

58 Jacobs LC, Liu F, Bleyen I, et al. Intrinsic and extrinsic risk factors for sagging eyelids. JAMA Dermatol 2014; 150(8): 836–843.

59 Ferreira JJ, Colosimo C, Bhidayasiri R, et al. Factors influencing secondary non-response to botulinum toxin type A injections in cervical dystonia. Parkinsonism Relat Disord 2015; 21(2): 111–1115.

12

Treatment of the Periocular Area – Crow's Feet, Brow, and Bunny Lines

Girish S. Munavalli, MD (MHS, FACMS),[1] Anthony V. Benedetto, DO (FACP, FCPP),[2,3]
Brian S. Biesman, MD (FACS),[4] and Carolee M. Cutler Peck, MD[5]

[1] *Medical Director, Dermatology, Laser, and Vein Specialists of the Carolinas, PLLC, Charlotte, USA*
[2] *Clinical Professor of Dermatology, Perelman School of Medicine, University of Pennsylvania, PA, USA*
[3] *Medical Director, Dermatologic SurgiCenter, Philadelphia and Drexel Hill, PA, USA*
[4] *Assistant Clinical Professor Ophthalmology, Dermatology, Otolaryngology, Vanderbilt University Medical Center, Nashville, TN, USA*
[5] *Ophthalmic and Plastic and Reconstructive Surgeon, SouthEast Eye Specialists, Knoxville, USA*

Introduction

The eyes have long been appreciated as centrally important to the cosmetic appearance of the face. Indeed, long before Cicero noted "The eyes are the window to the soul", in the book of Matthews in the Old Testament, it is quoted, "The light of the body is the eye: if therefore thine eye be single, thy whole body shall be full of light." (Matthew 6:22–23). A single or complex interplay of factors can cause one's eyes to look less than desirable. It is critically important to understand exactly what feature of the periocular region is of most concern to the patient before making therapeutic recommendations. Some patients blame a chronic lack of sleep on "looking tired" when in fact they are concerned about extrinsic aging factors such as loss of skin tone, excessive eyelid skin (dermatochalasis), eyebrow ptosis, or dark circles under the eyes, hollowness in the tear trough area (medial lower eyelid below the orbital rim). Some patients will be concerned about lower eyelid bags, festooning or bulging orbital fat pads. Certain other less structurally severe conditions, such as "hypertrophic" pretarsal orbicularis oculi muscle, and/or deep lateral canthal rhytids can also be concerning. These rhytids can be effectively addressed with readily available neuromodulators such as botulinum toxin.

Considered to be an off-label treatment, botulinum toxin types A and B have both been employed for the reduction of periocular rhytides with excellent clinical results [1–4]. The best candidates for periocular botulinum toxin injections are those with mild to moderately deep lateral canthal rhytids and/or those who develop a "roll or mound" of pretarsal orbicularis muscle, just inferior to the lid margin, as they smile. There are very few absolute contraindications to periocular botulinum toxin injection. Caution should be employed in patients with true dry eye syndrome or systemic diseases that may produce dry eyes such as Sjogren's syndrome and severe rheumatoid arthritis, and lastly, patients with ocular myasthenia gravis or other conditions that may affect extraocular muscle function. It should be used with great caution in patients with lagophthalmos (inability to completely close the eyes) due to previous 7th nerve palsy, thyroid eye disease, or previous blepharoplasty [5]. More recently, Goldman described a case report of new-onset festooning of the lower lids after botulinum injection in a male patient who had a history of transcutaneous lower lid blepharoplasty [6].

Anatomic Considerations

Effective botulinum toxin treatment of the periocular area involves a though understanding of facial anatomy, with special attention to periorbital anatomic structures and their functional correlation to ocular and facial aesthetics. Eyelid skin is among the thinnest in the body with little underlying subcutaneous tissue. By its very nature, it is dynamic and moves frequently with gaze and blinking. It is also located in an anatomic region that receives extensive exposure to sunlight. All these factors predispose eyelid and periocular skin to actinic injury with thinning, loss of elasticity, dyspigmentation, and the development of fine wrinkling [7].

Downward movement of the eyebrows is another common occurrence with aging. Eyebrow ptosis may present as "hooding" of the upper eyelids, horizontal forehead rhytids from chronic brow elevation, horizontal rhytids at the nasion, and even headache and fatigue. Brow ptosis develops insidiously and many affected patients fail to recognize this change themselves. A history of "looking better" when a towel has been wrapped around the head after showering is highly suggestive of brow ptosis. Significant brow ptosis can also accentuate superiorly located lateral canthal "crow's feet" lines. Failure to recognize brow ptosis can have disastrous consequences if Botulinum toxin injections are administered in an effort to treat horizontal forehead rhytids. In this scenario, relaxation of the frontalis muscle will prevent elevation of the brows leaving an uncompensated ptosis. This is referred to as latent brow ptosis and can be identified by manually holding the brows in a fixed position as the patient gazes straight ahead. This simple, but important maneuver is performed by asking the patient to hold their head parallel to the floor while they fixate their gaze on an object across the room (not too close) at eye level. The forehead is then observed for the presence of horizontal rhytids and frontalis muscle activation. Gentle palpation of the skin overlying the forehead rhytids will allow the examiner to detect underlying frontalis muscle activity.

Brow configuration varies widely from patient to patient. In many cases it is impossible to determine whether the brows have actually fallen or whether they were always low. When asked, most patients provide an unreliable history of this. The good way evaluate if brow position has changed is to examine old photographs of the patient, preferably looking at multiple photos over a period of time per decade starting back with high school pictures. Repositioning of brows via surgical or chemical techniques can be highly rewarding but can also change a patient's fundamental appearance. This must be carefully discussed prior to treatment.

Eyelid position relative to the eye itself must also be carefully assessed. The eyelids should be studied both at rest and while animating. Normally the upper eyelid margin covers the superior 1–2 mm of the cornea while the lower eyelid margin rests at the corneoscleral limbus. The white colored sclera should not be visible at either the 6:00 or 12:00 positions. The distance between the edge of the upper and lower eyelids while the patient gazes straight ahead in primary position is referred to as the palpebral fissure or palpebral aperture. Barring normal variations in the population, the normal palpebral fissure is 8–11 mm [7]. The palpebral fissure normally narrows with smiling. Failure of this subtle change to occur with facial animation may be interpreted by others as unnatural or insincere. Upper eyelid position is usually judged relative to the pupil or superior limbus. There is a wide range of "normal" with some patients having naturally low upper lids while others have a wide palpebral fissure. Blepharoptosis is the term used to describe a lid that is in a lower than desirable position. Ptosis is thus a relative as opposed to an absolute condition. A ptotic upper eyelid may occlude some, none, or even the entire pupil [8]. Many patients are highly sensitive to changes in their upper eyelid position although most do not become aware of their eyelid position until after undergoing a periorbital procedure such as botulinum toxin injection or blepharoplasty surgery. The value of preoperative photographs and identification of pretreatment asymmetry cannot be overstated.

Lower eyelid position is also somewhat dependent on the position of the eye relative to the orbital rim. With increasing laxity, the lid will sag visibly exposing the sclera below the inferior corneoscleral limbus. This condition is best known as ectropion. Many patients have enough residual canthal tendon tone that the lower eyelid position remains acceptable from functional and aesthetic standpoints; however, there isn't enough structural integrity to avoid ectropion formation when additional stresses such as botulinum toxin injections or surgery are introduced. Lower eyelid integrity may be assessed with the "snap" or "pinch" tests. The snap test is performed by pulling the lid downward and letting the lid return to its resting position. A brisk return is considered normal. A slow, gradual response is abnormal and suggestive of excessive laxity and thereby, increased risk for ectropion formation or tearing following botulinum toxin injections. The pinch test, somewhat less popular than the snap test, is performed by pinching the lower eyelid between the thumb and forefinger and distracting it from the globe. Less than 6 mm is considered normal. If the lid stretches further than 6 mm, caution should be undertaken when performing lower eyelid procedures. While upper eyelid position is highly variable, lower eyelid position is less so. Rounding of the lateral canthus or temporal ectropion can be interpreted as a sad or artificial look and should be avoided. Potential changes in lower eyelid position must be discussed prior to botulinum toxin injection.

Beneath the eyelid skin is found the orbicularis oculi muscle, which forcibly closes the eyelids when contracted. The orbicularis oculi muscle is divided into three components: pretarsal, preseptal, and orbital. The pretarsal component overlies the tarsal plates, the collagenous "backbone" of the eyelid while the preseptal portion overlies the

orbital septum, a fibrous membrane separating the orbital contents from more superficial structures. If the pretarsal orbicularis muscle is rendered inactive while the preseptal portion of the muscle is allowed to contract, the preseptal portion of the muscle can move upward in an "overriding" fashion, turning the eyelashes and lid margin in against the globe, a condition known as entropion. Relative hypertrophy of the pretarsal orbicularis muscle produces "bunching" of the lower eyelids that occurs with smiling. If this condition is treated with botulinum toxin, the injections should be administered into the pretarsal and superior preseptal muscle. The orbital portion of the orbicularis oculi muscle overlies the orbital rim and blends with the frontalis, procerus, depressor supercilii and corrugator supraciliaris muscles of the eyebrow superiorly and the temporalis and zygomaticus major and minor muscles laterally and inferiorly. The temporal portion of the orbital orbicularis oculi muscle is the primary eyebrow depressor [9].

The orbital portion of the orbicularis muscle is highly variable in size and shape, especially laterally and inferiorly. Temporally the orbicularis oculi muscle fans out from the lateral canthus toward the ear. In some patients, the muscle extends only as far as the outer aspect of the orbital rim while in others it extends almost to the tragus [7]. The muscle also extends to a variable degree superiorly and inferiorly. The distribution of the orbicularis oculi muscle is assessed by asking the patient to forcibly close their eyes. Digital palpation is then used to determine the muscle's size and shape. Asymmetry of the orbicularis oculi muscle is common so the muscle should be assessed on each side prior to botulinum toxin injection. The dose and distribution pattern of the toxin is entirely dependent on the orbicularis oculi muscle size and shape. Although general guidelines can be created, the concept of a "standard" dose and distribution pattern of botulinum toxin does not apply in the periorbital region.

Lines emanating from the lateral canthal region in a fan shaped distribution are commonly referred to as "crow's feet" lines. These lines can be one of the first signs of aging. Depending on a person's skin type, history of sun exposure, and muscle strength, crow's feet can appear in someone as young as 20 years of age [10]. The natural thinness and abundance of the skin in the lateral periorbital area make this site prone to wrinkling. These lateral canthal lines initially appear only during animation, they soon accentuate while smiling, laughing, or squinting and become increasingly noticeable with time. Their presence causes a perpetually tired and fatigued appearance, which can make the person look even older than their actual current age. Presence of these lines may have a slightly different societal perception depending on gender, in the sense that lines in women are considered undesirable, especially when make-up accumulates in the depths of the creases. For men, crow's feet may be perceived as a masculine, rugged feature [10].

These lines may be caused by contraction of the orbicularis oculi muscle alone but skin laxity and contraction of zygomaticus major may contribute to varying degrees as well. Some patients have deep rhytids in repose while others only demonstrate deep lines with animation. These types of wrinkles are always present whether or not a person is actively animating and therefore are referred to as static wrinkles. When the bulk of crow's feet are the result of long-term static wrinkles, injections of botulinum toxin A will be less effective but will improve the static appearance over time (Figure 12.1a, b). In this case, a resurfacing procedure or a soft tissue filler may help minimize static wrinkling of the lateral canthus. When the bulk of crow's feet are produced by the hyperactivity of the lateral orbital orbicularis oculi, then injections of botulinum toxin A can play a significant role in diminishing the wrinkling. Lastly, it is extremely important to distinguish between lines caused by orbicularis contraction versus those produced by a wrinkling effect as contraction of the zygomaticus muscles "pushes" skin into the periorbital region

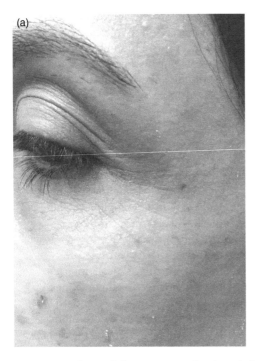 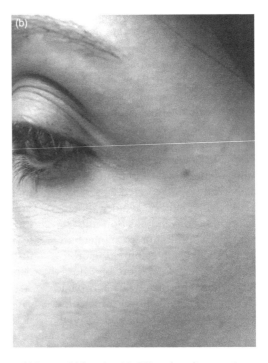

Figure 12.1 Before and after treatment of early static lines of 36 year old female with 8 U onabotulinumtoxin.

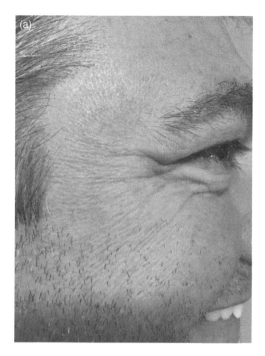 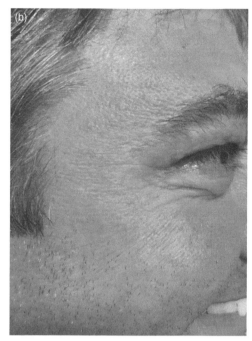

Figure 12.2 Before and after treatment of moderate crows feet of 50 year old male with 12 U of incobotulinumtoxin. Note the zygomaticus muscles "pushes" skin into the periorbital region in both the before and after photo and is not improved with toxin injection.

(Figure 12.2a, b). The latter phenomenon is difficult to treat without risking facial droop or an unnatural appearance as overtreatment of the zygomaticus muscle will decrease the natural cheek elevation and fullness that occurs with smiling. Again, a resurfacing procedure or a soft tissue filler may help in this instance.

Patient Selection/Pretreatment Evaluation

It is critically important to understand exactly what feature of the periocular region is of most concern to the patient before making therapeutic recommendations. Some patients complain of "looking tired" when in fact they are concerned about loss of skin tone, excessive eyelid skin (dermatochalasis), eyebrow ptosis, dark circles under the eyes, hollowness in the tear trough area (medial lower eyelid below the orbital rim), bulging orbital fat pads, "hypertrophic" pretarsal orbicularis oculi muscle, and/or deep lateral canthal rhytids. Periocular rejuvenation is a complex topic and addressing only one of many needs may or may not provide a satisfactory result.

Evaluation of the patient begins from the time the person first walks into the examination room. The patient's facial features are assessed for typical facial stigmata of aging including lentigenes, erythema, fine wrinkling, loss of skin laxity, eyebrow and/or eyelid ptosis (or chronic eyebrow elevation to correct latent brow or lid ptosis), midfacial ptosis, jowling, loss of facial volume, and deep dynamic rhytids in the glabellar, perioral, and periocular regions. It is particularly important to view the patient as a whole before concentrating on the periocular (or any other individual) region as the goal of any treatment is to create a harmonious facial appearance. Any pre-existing asymmetry should be noted and documented prior to treatment.

The patient is then evaluated from a frontal perspective. Particular attention is paid to the presence of rhytids at rest, eyebrow contour and position, horizontal forehead rhytids that may be indicative of chronic brow elevation, extent of photoaging, presence of dermatochalasis (excess skin laxity) in the upper eyelid, position of the upper eyelid margin relative to the pupil, and lower eyelid position. If white sclera is visible above the superior limbus or below the inferior corneoscleral limbus, additional ophthalmic evaluation is warranted. The presence of horizontal forehead rhytids may either indicate overactive use of the muscles or facial expression or a compensatory response to eyebrow ptosis. One must make this distinction as weakening the frontalis muscle in the latter setting will uncover a previously latent eyebrow ptosis. Patients who have been unknowingly compensating by elevating their eyebrows continuously to prevent impairment of their superior visual field will no longer be able to do so if their frontalis muscle is weakened.

The examiner can identify the patient with latent brow ptosis by studying the patient when the frontalis muscle is completely relaxed (instruct the patient to relax their forehead). If the eyebrows assume a lower position when the frontalis muscle relaxes, botulinum toxin should not be injected into the forehead. These patients need eyebrow and/or eyelid surgery to correct their underlying problem. Next, the patient is asked to gently (not forcibly) close the eyes to ensure complete apposition of the upper and lower lids. Some patients who have had prior surgery, trauma, or thyroid disease may be able to forcibly close their eyes but have an incomplete blink that leaves them highly vulnerable to symptomatic dry eyes if the orbicularis oculi muscle is weakened. The patient is then instructed to forcibly close the eyes. This permits evaluation of the pretarsal orbicularis oculi muscle in its dynamic state. The appearance of a prominent "bulge" in the pretarsal region is suggestive of "hypertrophic" orbicularis oculi muscle. Importantly, this condition must be differentiated from a "bunched" lower eyelid occurring as a result of cheek tissue recruitment with contraction of the zygomaticus major and minor muscles.

Horizontal rhytids in the lateral canthal region should be evaluated in both frontal and lateral views. The patient is viewed from each side first at rest, then with gentle eyelid closure and finally during forced closure. This series of maneuvers permits the examiner to differentiate between fine skin wrinkles due to loss of elasticity and rhytids caused by action of the orbicularis oculi muscle. Next, a "map" of the orbicularis oculi muscle should be constructed by asking the patient to repeatedly squeeze their eyes tightly while the examiner palpates the lateral canthal region with the tip of the index finger. The orbicularis oculi muscle may be relatively small and confined to the region overlying the lateral orbital rim or may extend nearly to the tragus laterally, into the lateral extent of the temporal region superiorly, and into the upper region of the midface inferiorly. It is important to map the orbicularis oculi muscle on both sides as its distribution may be asymmetric.

Finally, the position of the eye is assessed relative to the orbital rim. Patients with prominent eyes due to high myopia (a condition in which the globe is actually longer than normal), thyroid eye disease, or shallow orbits should be treated with greater care as they are more prone to lagophthalmos and change in lower eyelid position after botulinum toxin injection.

Botulinum toxin may be used in the periorbital region to diminish dynamic rhytids in the lateral canthal region, to weaken eyebrow depressors and thereby elevate or contour the brows, and to treat "hypertrophic" orbicularis oculi muscle in the lower eyelid. In any given patient, it may be desirable to accomplish one or more of these goals. They are not mutually exclusive and should be considered independently.

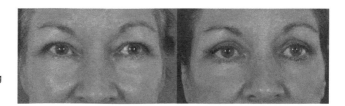

Figure 12.3 Complete treatment of hypertrophic orbicularis oculi muscle will reduce the muscle bulk upon smiling but will also make the eyes appear to be open wider. Patient also had upper blepharoplasty contributing to outstanding aesthetic outcome.

When treating lateral canthal rhytids, the injector must distinguish between those lines due to the action of the orbicularis oculi muscle, those caused by contraction of zygomaticus major and minor muscles (causing upward movement of the cheek with smiling) and those due to photoaging of the skin. Only those lines clearly caused by contraction of the orbicularis oculi muscle should be treated with botulinum toxin [11–13]. Treatment at the most inferior-medial orbicularis may produce an unnatural appearance when smiling, facial asymmetry or, in the most extreme circumstance, facial drooping. The safest approach is to use the least amount of toxin necessary to produce the desired clinical effect while still providing adequate efficacy. One can start conservative and add more in subsequent weeks as needed. Use of too much toxin will minimize the action of the orbicularis oculi muscle to the point where the lateral canthus does not wrinkle at all with smiling and other facial expression. This can signal the appearance of insincerity in some patients, and thus over aggressive injection in the crow's feet region should be avoided.

Careful documentation should be kept and first-time patients are usually followed up 2 weeks after their injection. At the follow up visit, the treatment goals should be reviewed and compared to the clinical results. If additional injections are needed, this is a good timepoint to intervene, as all the neuromodulatory effect should be present. If the patient isn't satisfied with the results, careful notes should be made about adjustments that need to be made in dosage, placement, or both.

As another subtle, yet effective periocular treatment, botulinum toxin can also be used to weaken the pretarsal orbicularis oculi muscle. This can reduce the prominent "roll" that appears with smiling in patients with "hypertrophic" orbicularis muscle and can also increase the size of the palpebral fissure (the distance between the upper and lower eyelids). While these goals are separate, they are indistinct as it is difficult to accomplish one objective without the other; that is, treatment of hypertrophic orbicularis oculi muscle will not only reduce the muscle bulk upon smiling but will also make the eyes appear to be open wider. (Figure 12.3).

Further, some patients who complain of "bunching" of their lower eyelid with smiling or animation have either excess eyelid skin or a normal amount of eyelid skin that is compressed into a small area by the upward movement of the cheek associated with strong contraction of the zygomaticus muscles. These patients will not benefit significantly from botulinum toxin injection into the lower eyelid. Thus, a careful examination and discussion about realistic goals is needed prior to treatment.

The dosage of botulinum toxin A injected into the periorbital region should be determined by the treatment goal, the size and strength of the orbicularis oculi muscle, and the position of the globe relative to the orbit. With regards to dosage amounts, it should be noted that one size definitely does not fit all. The size and distribution of the orbicularis oculi muscle may vary dramatically from patient to patient and even within individuals from one side of the face to the other.[12] Additionally, distinct crow's feet patterns were further identified and quantified by Kane *et al.* in a recent retrospective photographic review [13]. The looked retrospectively at 2,699 photographs from 1,392 subjects who had previously participated in neuromodulator

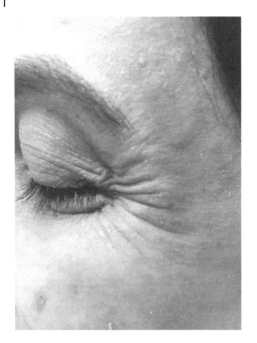

Figure 12.4 Full-fan pattern as described by Kane *et al.* [14] (crinkling of lateral canthal skin from lower lateral brow across the upper eyelid, through the lateral canthus, and across the lower eyelid/upper cheek junction).

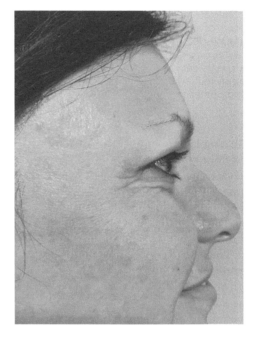

Figure 12.5 Central-fan pattern as described by Kane *et al.* [14] (severe wrinkles only in the skin immediately surrounding the lateral canthus).

studies. Full-fan pattern (crinkling of lateral canthal skin from lower lateral brow across the upper eyelid, through the lateral canthus, and across the lower eyelid/upper cheek junction) (Figure 12.4), lower-fan pattern (wrinkling in both the lower lid and upper cheek area), central-fan pattern (severe wrinkles only in the skin immediately surrounding the lateral canthus) (Figure 12.5), and upper-fan pattern (wrinkles only in the upper eyelid skin down to the lateral canthus were quantified at rest and animation. The incidence of full fan, lower fan, and central fan patterns at rest and animation was approximately one third for each, while upper fan was quite uncommon, seen in only 4.2% of patients at maximum smile and 6.4% of patients at rest. Individuals with muscle distributed over a large area or with relatively hypertrophic muscle will require larger doses of toxin than may be considered "standard". Similarly, patients with smaller muscles that do not contract as forcefully should receive relatively lower doses

of toxin. The dosage should also be reduced when injecting the lower eyelid and inferior lateral canthal region of patients with prominent globes due to shallow orbits, thyroid eye disease or myopia (extreme near-sightedness due to a longer than normal eye) as these patients are at higher risk for ectropion or incomplete eyelid closure [12].

The authors recommend that when dosing this area, it may be helpful to think in terms of number of units per injection site than the total dose required to treat the entire region. As a general rule, 2.5–5.0 U of onabotulinum or incobotulinum toxin per site is adequate in the lateral canthal area. When treating the inferior pretarsal orbicularis oculi muscle only 1–2 U should be used per site.

Injection Technique

It is impossible to construct an injection site map or scheme that can be applied to patients in a generic manner. While some general

Figure 12.6 Relaxation of the temporal brow depressor (orbicularis oculi) leading to brow elevation. The patient also had her glabellar complex treated.

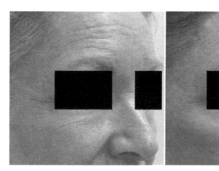

guidelines can be applied, it is not feasible or appropriate to recommend a fixed number of injection sites, total dose of toxin, or the exact location of injection sites; treatments must be individualized to each patient. Asymmetry in orbicularis oculi muscle distribution does occur [13]. This often necessitates varying the dose of toxin between the 2 sides of the face. When injecting in the lateral canthal region, the risk of toxin diffusion into the orbit increases with proximity to the canthal angle as well as depth. While there has yet to be a study to address this issue directly, it seems that injecting 1–1.5 cm from the lateral canthal angle minimizes the risk of clinical effects of toxin on the extraocular muscles.[12]

Because this can be a sensitive area for treatment, pain management techniques for periorbital botulinum toxin injections are often employed. Topical anesthetic agents, such as 4–6% topical lidocaine can be used with appropriate incubation times. Additionally, some have used of ice packs immediately prior and after injection for pain control, vasoconstriction of periocular vessels, and containment of new-onset purpura. Extremely anxious patients may very rarely request oral sedation prior to injection. Of course, transportation arrangements must be made as driving while sedated cannot be permitted. If a topical anesthetic agent such as 4% lidocaine cream, is applied, it should be thoroughly removed before injection. Residual cream can occlude the small caliber 30–32 G needles and result in lost time and wasted product.

Regarding brow contouring/shaping with botulinum toxin, some of the finer points

of treatment should be discussed. The rationale for using botulinum toxin A to change eyebrow position is based on the selective relaxation of brow depressors [16]. Centrally the corrugator, depressor supercilii, and procerus muscles are all important brow depressors. Temporal to the papillary midline, the orbicularis oculi muscle is the sole brow depressor. The orbicularis oculi is opposed by the frontalis muscle medial to the temporal line of fusion (conjoined tendon) and is unopposed temporal to this landmark (in the region overlying the temporalis muscle). Therefore, relaxation of the temporal brow depressor leads to brow elevation (Figure 12.6).

For placement of these injections, anecdotal reports suggest a variety of options including directly into the tail of the brow, above the tail, and below the lateral brow. Providing the orbital orbicularis oculi muscle is affected by the toxin, the exact placement of the injection is probably not critical. Avoiding unintended diffusion into the inferior aspect of the frontalis muscle is to be strictly avoided. Those injectors using a higher dilution (e.g. 4 cm^3 of saline) and thus a greater volume may be well advised to inject relatively more superiorly to avoid unexpected diffusion of toxin into the levator muscle. Another option is to utilize a more potent/less diluted injection solution. The authors have found that a 1 cm^3 dilution gives very precise control over the treatment area. Injections given along the superior orbital rim should be performed with care. In this manner, injections can be safely performed in this area. As an example, the authors routinely treat patients with intractable blepharospasm, injecting 5 U of onabotulinumtoxinA each of three positions along the superior orbital rim (a total of 15 U) along with an additional 2.5–5.0 U in the medial and lateral portions of the upper eyelid itself (a total of 5–10 U), without adverse sequelae (Dr. Biesman, personal communication). Always direct the needle away from the orbit as directing the toxin toward the eye may result in diffusion of toxin into extraocular muscles or even serious injury if the patient were to move suddenly during the injection.

The novice injector may wish to either stabilize their injecting hand against the patient or "smart" hand as it rests on the patient. This will prevent inadvertent perforation of veins or the eye in the event of an unexpected movement. When injecting into the periorbital region, always point the needle away from the eye itself. To minimize the risk of ecchymosis in the lateral canthal region, it is helpful to identify the vessels when possible. Visualization with good overhead room lighting, a dermatoscope, transillumination, or use of a cross-polarized light source can help with this. This is easier with type I–III patients and atrophic skin. The authors recommend very superficial intradermal injections, akin to a superficial bleb (Figure 12.7). When possible, injecting immediately overlying an obvious vessel should be avoided.

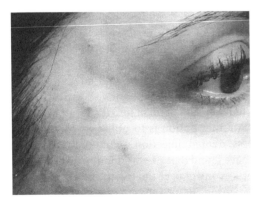

Figure 12.7 Superficial blebs demonstrating placement depth of neuromodulator in periocular area will minimize all potential complications.

Finally, injections should be administered from the side and never from in front of the patient to avoid having the needle directed towards the orbit. If immediate bleeding or bruising does occur, holding point pressure with a fingertip or cotton-tipped applicator for 1–2 minutes will help minimize spread. Additionally, use of the pulsed dye laser can hasten the clearance of new-onset purpura.

Although it is generally true that absolute rules about dosage and number of injection sites should not be made, great care should be taken when injecting the pretarsal orbicularis oculi muscle. This muscle can be injected in its central portion (immediately below the pupil) or alternately, may be injected in two sites, roughly corresponding to the medial and lateral corneoscleral limbus. If a single central injection is planned, a dose of no more than 2 U of onabotulinumtoxinA should be injected initially. Additional injections can be administered as needed at the 2-week follow up visit. If two separate sites are used, no more than 1.0–1.5 U should be delivered at each site. Excessive delivery of toxin in this region can impair eyelid closure and may lead to tearing, ectropion, and even inward turning of the eyelid against the eye (entropion). Entropion can occur when the preseptal orbicularis oculi muscle contracts forcefully in the setting of an immobile pretarsal muscle. In this situation, the preseptal muscle moves upward overriding the pretarsal muscle and pushing the pretarsal muscle and eyelid margin inward toward the eye. This usually produces severe ocular pain and irritation. When administering lower eyelid injections, it is advisable to deliver the toxin subcutaneously to avoid diffusion into the inferior oblique muscle which occupies a relatively anterior position in the orbit. If the inferior oblique muscle is affected, vertical and/or torsional diplopia can result.

The final area of treatment to be discussed in this chapter is treatment of the oblique lines overlying the nasal root and dorsum, the so-called "bunny lines." This pattern of dynamic rhytides can be elicited by scrunching the nose, or with expressions of displeasure or a forced smile. Additionally, this pattern can often be seen in concert with the appearance of crow's feet, because both are elicited by chronic squinting. These lines should be differentiated from transverse lines resulting from procerus activity.

Bunny lines can result from contracting the transverse portion of the nasalis. This portion arises from the maxilla and runs diagonally across the bridge of the nose. It expands into a thin aponeurosis and is continuous with that of the muscle of the opposite side and with the aponeurosis of the procerus [14]. The nasalis muscle has two main parts, the transverse or compressor part (also known as compressor naris), which constricts the nostril, and the alar or dilator part (also known as dilator naris), which flares the nostril [15]. An alternate etiology of these lines is due to contraction of the levator labii superioris alequae nasi in some patients, analogous to zygomaticus causing lateral canthal lines.

Injection technique

When treating this area, it is imperative that injections avoid the levator labii superioris alaeque nasi and the levator labii superioris to prevent drooping of the upper lip. A series of one to three injection points along the midline nasal dorsum and along the upper nasal sidewall, superficially in the nasalis muscle, should be sufficient to soften or eliminate these lines. Performing the injections superficially is critical to avoid bruising in this highly vascular area [16, 17]. Typically, 1–3 U of onabotulinumtoxinA per injection point is sufficient to achieve the desired effect. The injector can also consider including an injection of 1–2 U per side of the upper nasalis when treating the glabellar area, to prevent recruitment. As previously noted, the authors recommend a 1 cm^3 dilution to avoid diffusion in this area, which could result in lip ptosis.

In summary, enhancement of the periocular area of the face with botulinum toxin can be challenging and technique-dependent. Careful evaluation of the area, with attention to any pre-existing asymmetry, underlying compensatory muscle action, and natural brow positioning is critical to achieving good treatment outcomes. Using the approach and techniques described in this chapter can facilitate reproducibly good results for rejuvenation of this cosmetically sensitive region.

References

1 Frankel AS. Botox for rejuvenation of the periorbital region. Facial Plast Surg 1999; 15(3):255–262.

2 Flynn TC. Periocular botulinum toxin. Clin Dermatol 2003 Nov–Dec;21(6):498–504.

3 Matarasso A, Glassman M. Effective use of botox for lateral canthal rhytids. Aesthet Surg J 2001 Jan;21(1):61–63.

4 Matarasso SL, Matarasso A. Treatment guidelines for botulinum toxin type A for the periocular region and a report on partial upper lip ptosis following injections to the lateral canthal rhytids. Plast Reconstr Surg 2001 Jul;108(1):208–214.

5 Biesman, B. Periorbital rejuvenation. In Hirsch R., Sadick N., and Cohen JL (eds), *Aesthetic Rejuvenation – A Regional Approach*. New York, McGraw Hill, 2008: 100–115.

6 Goldman MP. Festoon formation after infraorbital botulinum A toxin: a case report. Dermatol Surg 2003 May;29(5): 560–561.

7 Schwartz RJ, Burns AJ, Rohrich RJ, *et al.* Long-term assessment of CO_2 facial laser resurfacing: aesthetic results and complications. Plast Reconstr Surg 1999; 103(2):592–601.

8 Biesman BS. Anatomy of the eyelid, forehead, and temporal region. In Biesman BS (ed), *Lasers in Facial Aesthetic and Reconstructive Surgery*. Baltimore. Williams and Wilkins 1999:15–27.

9 Aguilar GL, Nelson C. Eyelid and anterior orbital anatomy. In Hornblass AH (ed.) *Oculoplastic, Orbital and Reconstructive Surgery*. Baltimore, Williams and Wilkins 1988;4–22.

10 Benedetto AV. *Botulinum Toxins in Clinical Aesthetic Practice*, 2nd ed. New York: Informa Healthcare, 2011:64.

11 Fagien S. Botox for the treatment of dynamic and hyperkinetic facial lines and furrows: adjunctive use in facial aesthetic surgery. Plast Reconstr Surg 1999;103: 701–708.

12 Biesman BS, Arndt KA. Periocular treatment. In Carruthers A and Carruthers J (eds). *Botulinum Toxin. Procedures in Cosmetic Dermatology*. 2005 Elsevier, Inc.:45–57.

13 Kane MAC. Classification of crow's feet patterns among caucasian women: the key to individualizing treatment. Plast Reconstr Surg:2003 Oct 112(5);33S–39S.

14 Kane AC, Cox SE, Jones D, *et al.* Heterogeneity of crow's feet line patterns in clinical trial subjects. Dermatol Surg 2015 Apr;41(4):447–456.

15 Carruthers J, Fagien S, Matarasso SL. Consensus recommendations on the use of botulinum toxin type a in facial aesthetics. Plast Reconstr Surg 2004 Nov;114(6 Suppl): 1S–22S.

16 http://www.med.umich.edu/lrc/ coursepages/m1/anatomy2010/html/ anatomytables/muscles_head_neck.html

17 Maas CS, Kim EJ. Temporal brow lift using botulinum toxin A: an update. Plast Reconstr Surg 2003 Oct;112(5 Suppl): 109S–112S.

13

Contouring of the Lower Face and of the Lower Leg and Calf

Mee young Park, MD (PhD),¹ Dennis A. Porto, MD,² and Ki Young Ahn, MD (PhD)³

¹*Department of Neurology, Yeungnam University, College of Medicine, Daegu, South Korea*
²*Department of Dermatology, Henry Ford Hospital, Detroit, USA*
³*Director, Dr. Ahn's Aesthetic & Plastic Surgical Clinic, Daegu, South Korea*

Contouring of the Lower Face

Introduction

In 1994, Smyth [1] first reported the medical utility of botulinum toxin type A (BoNTA) in benign masseter hypertrophy (BMH). BoNTA injection was suggested as a potential aesthetic procedure for lower face contouring by von Lindern *et al.* in 2001 [2] and was simultaneously being employed by early physician adopters in Korea and elsewhere in Asia [3, 4].

The mechanism of lower facial contouring by BoNTA differs from that of treatment of dynamic rhytides and various facial neuromuscular disorders [3, 5] such as blepharospasm and hemifacial spasm. Facial contouring, instead, relies on the temporary but significant effects of muscle atrophy and partial muscle paralysis due to acetylcholine blockade at the neuromuscular junction.

The facial muscles (which are traditional targets of BoNTA injection for treating rhytides) are relatively thin and if atrophy occurs after repeated injections, it may not be clinically apparent. In contrast, the masseter muscle is thicker, making it an ideal target for facial contouring and amenable to treatment for BMH.

Body contouring with neurotoxins continues to be refined, and investigators have made forays into calf, shoulder, and neck sculpting as well. More research is necessary to fully define the role of neurotoxins in this blossoming discipline.

Contouring

Some women tend to prefer oval and almond-shaped faces and dislike a square jaw, which they believe is more masculine. Differences in facial preferences between Caucasians and Asians derive in part from ethnic differences in the craniofacial shape, with those of European origin often having a long, narrow face compared to shorter, wider faces among some Asian women [6]. Many Asian women tend to dislike a square shaped jaw as it can accentuate a wider face. Men tend to prefer a defined jaw and therefore masseter injections are rare in this group; however, we are happy to accommodate men who are seeking a slenderer appearance or those interested in gender confirmation procedures.

Contouring of the mandible is a relatively common aesthetic procedure in Asia, although it is rare among Caucasians. At present, operative treatment is limited to resection of the angle or body of the mandible, masseter resection, and liposuction. These surgical procedures have many disadvantages, including risks of persistent swelling, hematoma, and postoperative pain.

Botulinum Toxins: Cosmetic and Clinical Applications, First Edition. Edited by Joel L. Cohen and David M. Ozog.
© 2017 John Wiley & Sons Ltd. Published 2017 by John Wiley & Sons Ltd.
Companion Website: www.wiley.com/go/cohen/botulinum

In addition to these immediate complications, prominent scars may occur on the neck with the extraoral approach, and partial palsy of the facial nerve has been reported [2, 7].

Patients who desire neurotoxin facial contouring are generally 20–40 years old and often have social responsibilities that make surgical procedures difficult. Therefore, the use of botulinum toxin type A (BoNTA) for contouring of the lower face could offer a simple alternative to the risks of surgery.

BoNTA injections are gaining acceptance for lower facial contouring in Korea. This procedure is beginning to be used as frequently as surgical mandiblectomy and sometimes the two are used in combination.

The goal has been to establish a procedure that avoids the risks of surgery while offering a predictable and clinically significant improvement. Since 2001, we have worked to achieve this goal and the remainder of this chapter delineates our findings.

The Anatomy of the Masseter Muscle

The masseter is the most superficial and one of the strongest muscles of mastication. The masseter is a thick, somewhat quadrilateral muscle, consisting of two heads: superficial and deep. The fibers of the two heads are continuous at their insertion. The superficial head is larger and originates with thick and tendinous aponeuroses from the zygomatic process of the maxilla and from the anterior two-thirds of the inferior border of the zygomatic arch. Its fibers pass inferior and posterior and insert into the angle of the mandible and inferior half of the lateral surface of the ramus of the mandible. The deep head is much smaller, yet more muscular. It originates from the posterior third of the lower border of the zygomatic arch and from the whole of the medial surface of the zygomatic arch. Its fibers pass ventral and inferior, to be inserted into the upper half of the ramus as high as the coronoid process of the mandible. The deep head of the muscle is partly concealed, anteriorly, by the superficial portion. Posteriorly, it is covered by the parotid gland.

Along with the other three muscles of mastication (temporalis, medial pterygoid, and lateral pterygoid), the masseter is innervated by the mandibular division (V3) of the trigeminal nerve.

The action of the muscle during bilateral contraction of the entire muscle is to elevate the mandible, raising the lower jaw. Elevation of the mandible occurs during the closing of the mouth. The action of the masseter parallels the medial pterygoid muscle, but it is stronger.

We performed a cadaveric dissection to better characterize landmarks and other properties of the masseter to refine our technique. The masseter is approximately 8 cm and its thickness varies along its length with a maximum of about 1 cm (Figure 13.1) The majority of the masseter volume is below the line from the subnasale to the tragus (Figure 13.2).

We recruited 12 women between the ages of 20 and 40 without masseter hypertrophy in order to study the masseter with ultrasound and CT scans. The mean (SD) thicknesses of masseter muscles in these normal control subjects by ultrasound were 12.1 ($\pm$1.0) mm on the left side and 12.1 ($\pm$1.1) mm on the right side. By CT scans, these figures were 12.1 ($\pm$1.2) and 12.5 ($\pm$1.8) mm, respectively. These data are also similar to the results of Qingfeng Li *et al.* in China, published in the 2014 [8].

These are the only published measurements of masseter thickness, and therefore are the reference when establishing whether a patient has BMH.

Preinjection Considerations

It is important to review with patients the possible causes of masseter hypertrophy. These include chewing gum or cuttlefish, bruxism, various dental treatments, and temporomandibular joint pain. If bony protuberance of the mandibular angle is instead suspected, this can be confirmed with xray. If TMJ is suspected, this should be confirmed with TMJ X-rays, CT and/or MRI. BoNTA

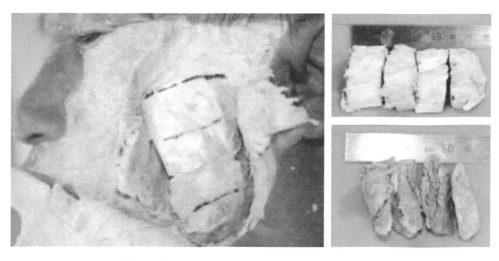

Figure 13.1 A cross-sectional view of the masseter muscle along its length.

injection may lead to adverse effects among these patients.

Injection Technique

As with other neuromodulator use, there is considerable variability among authors on neuromodulator type, dose, volume, injection points, and intervals for repeat injections.

We reconstitute 100 U vials of onabotulinumtoxin (Botox®) with 2 ml of normal saline to yield 5 U per 0.1 ml. We then ask the patient to clench their jaw so that the borders and volume of the masseter muscle can be palpated. We define a safe area of injection by drawing a line from the subnasale to the tragus and connecting this to the palpated anterior, inferior, and posterior margins of the masseter. Percutaneous intramuscular injections of the masseter are performed without electromyographic guidance. Between 25 and 30 U are injected into each masseter, divided between five to six points. In male patients, up to 40 U are sometimes used. We inject deep into the masseter itself with a 29 gauge, 12.7 mm BD insulin syringe. Most patients were injected with a total of 50 U to 60 U (Figure 13.3).

It is important to inject both masseter muscles, even in patients with asymmetric hypertrophy, because both muscles contract simultaneously; however, an additional 5–10 U can be injected into the hypertrophic side (Figure 13.4).

Figure 13.2 The topographic relationship between the masseter and nose, lips, ear. The majority of the masseter volume is below the line from the columella to the tragus in Frankfort horizontal position. (a) Subnasale; (b) the highest point of the upper vermillion border; (c) the lateral oral commissure.

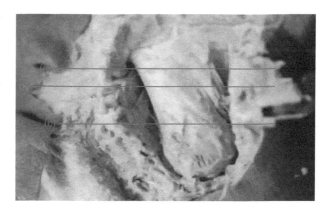

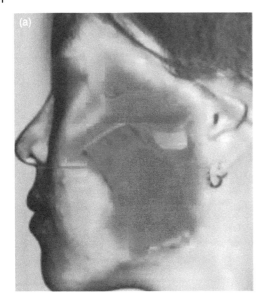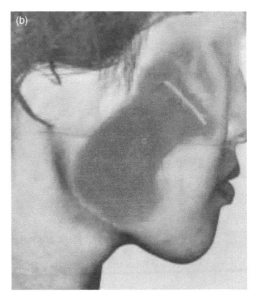

Figure 13.3 Injection points. A checkerboard pattern is used to create five or six injection points for each masseter.

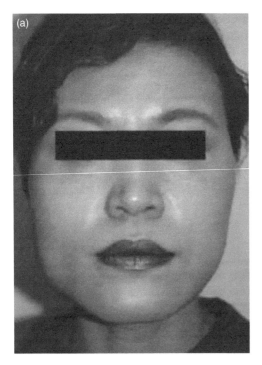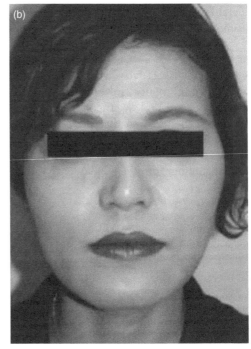

Figure 13.4 A 34 year old female patient, treated with 25 U of Botox® on the left masseter and 30 U on the right masseter. (a) Preinjection; (b) 3 months after injection.

Reduction in Hypertrophy Measured by Ultrasound and CT

To better evaluate the reduction in masseter volume after BoNTA injections, CT and ultrasound imagining were performed at follow-up. Due to the variable thickness of the masseter along its length, it was necessary to use well-defined landmarks and patient positioning to make meaningful measurements.

Serial measurements of the thickness of the masseter were made by ultrasound and CT scans before the injections and at 1 and 3 months thereafter. Two males and 43 females participated in the study. Ages ranged between 24 and 48 years, with a mean of 35. Among the total of 45 patients, 15 underwent all three ultrasound scans, whereas 14 received all three CT scans. The mean masseteric thickness before injection was 14.0 (1.9) mm on the left side and 14.4 (2.2) mm on the right side, as measured by ultrasound. Using CT, these measurements were 14.9 (2.2) and 15.5 (3.3) mm, respectively. Mean masseteric thicknesses at 1 and 3 months after injection by ultrasound were 11.2 (1.6) and 11.5 (1.4) mm on the left side and 11.5 (1.6) and 11.9 (1.4) mm on the right side, respectively. By CT scan, these respective figures were 13.3 (2.1) and 12.0 (1.7) mm and 14.2 (2.6) and 12.7 (2.2) mm (Table 13.1).

In this study, the average amount of thickness change of masseter in ultrasound and CT measurement studies was approximately 2.8–2.9 mm, and these changes were equivalent to approximately 18–20% of the muscle thickness of the masseter at preinjection. This change was statistically significant. In an extreme case, one patient who was excluded from the quantitative analysis of the thickness change showed an approximate 30% masseter thickness change.

In 2001, several studies attempted to quantify the change in masseter thickness after BoNTA. A report by von Lindern et al. [2] found that seven patients with unilateral or bilateral hypertrophy of the masseter and temporalis muscles that were treated with an average of 100 U of Dysport® showed a 50% reduction in masseter thickness. That result was considered to be aesthetically satisfactory after a single injection in four of the seven patients. To et al. [7] described five patients with unilateral and bilateral hypertrophy of the masseter who were treated with 200–300 U of Dysport® per side, and demonstrated improvement confirmed by ultrasound. Three of five patients needed a secondary injection within 1 year. Mandel and Tanakan [9] reported that one patient with unilateral hypertrophy of the masseter was treated with 5 U of Botox, and the effect lasted approximately 4 months, although no long-term results were reported.

Table 13.2 is a summary of other recent reports that attempt to quantify masseter improvement with neuromodulator use.

Outcomes Measured by Serial Photography

The outcome most important to our patients is the improvement in their clinical appearance. This can be easily, inexpensively, and accurately measured by anterior-posterior (A-P) photography. We collected serial photographs of multiple patients and measured

Table 13.1 Descriptive analysis of observed data for the masseter thickness in both sides (mean [SD]).

Time methods	Preinjection		Postinjection 1 Month		Postinjection 3 Months		Controls (N = 12)	
	Lt	Rt	Lt	Rt	Lt	Rt	Lt	Rt
CT (N = 14)	14.9 (2.2)	15.5 (3.3)	13.3 (2.1)	14.2 (2.6)	12.0 (1.7)	12.7 (2.2)	12.1 (1.2)	12.5 (1.8)
SONO (N = 15)	14.0 (1.9)	14.4 (2.2)	11.2 (1.6)	11.5 (1.6)	11.5 (1.4)	11.9 (1.4)	12.1 (1.0)	12.1 (1.1)

Lt, Left; Rt, Right; Mo, Month; SONO, Ultrasound; CT, Computerized tomography.

Table 13.2 Comparison of several reports of botulinum toxin for masseter hypertophy.

Reference	Aesth Plast Surg (2011) 35:452–455	Plast Reconstr Surg 134:209e, 2014	Plast Reconstr Surg, March 2005 115:919	Dermatol Surg 2015;41: S101–S109	Dermatol Surg 2003;29: 484–489
Corresponding author	C. S. Chang et al. [10]	Qingfeng Li et al. [8]	Nam Ho Kim et al. [11]	Chuanchang Dai et al. [12]	Kyle Seo et al. [4]
Type of BoNTA	Dysport®	HengLi® (similar to Botox®)	Dysport®	BTX-A (unspecified type)	Botox®
Concentration and dilutent	200 U/cm³ in sterile distilled water	unknown	125 U/cm³ in sterile distilled water	unknown	100 U/cm³ in sterile saline
Injection points per masseter	6	unknown	3–4	4	6
Total injected dose per masseter	120 U	20–40 U based on masseter thickness	100–140 U based on masseter volume	35 U	30 U
Approximate measured improvement	30% decreased volume	32% decreased thickness	31% decreased thickness	31% decreased thickness	22% decreased volume

their improvement using a standardized technique. To quantify improvement, the width of the lower face at the level of the oral commissure (A) was measured and compared to the unchanging width between the left and right ala (B). With these values, the percent reduction in width of the lower face can be determined using this formula:

The reduction rate of the width of the lower face at oral commissure level (%) =

$$\frac{\text{A/B (preinjection)} - \text{A/B (postinjection)}}{\text{A/B (preinjection)}} \times 100$$

This ratio is also demonstrated in Figure 13.5.

We used this method of measurement for a patient and found a 3.7% reduction in facial width 1 month after injection. Maximum efficacy was at 3 months with a 6.9% improvement before eventuating in a 4% improvement at 1 year postinjection (Figure 13.6). This is in keeping with our clinical experience, in that maximal efficacy is noted

at month 3 or 4 with a gradual return to baseline over many months. In this way, improvement from BoNTA injection is more dynamic and reversible when compared to a procedure like mandibulectomy or liposuction.

Our patients were very satisfied after treatment with a single injection. At 10 months' postinjection, 37 of 45 patients were either very satisfied or satisfied. These numbers are similar to other published reports.

Repeat injections

Improvements in masseter hypertrophy after BoNTA injection tend to subside over the proceeding months and years, so repeat injections are often necessary. Some authors allow patients to decide when they require reinjection while others have a structured reinjection schedule. Further, some authors adjust the dose of the BoNTA injection based on masseter size while others use the original dose for all subsequent injections.

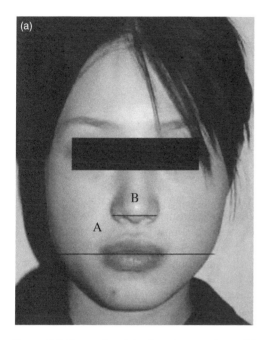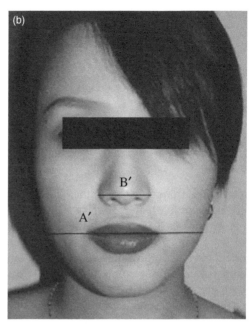

Figure 13.5 Pre- and post-treatment comparison of the static distance between the left and right nasal ala, and the improved width of the lower face at the level of the oral commissure.

We studied a group of patients that were reinjected every 6–12 months at the same dose as their initial injection (typically 25–30 U per masseter, as described above). We then used serial photographic measurements to track facial width. We followed 13 patients over several years during which they received at least three injections. On average, patients completed 5.5 sessions and returned about every 11.5 months. We analyzed patients in two groups: those with irregular reinjection intervals between 7 and 12 months, and those

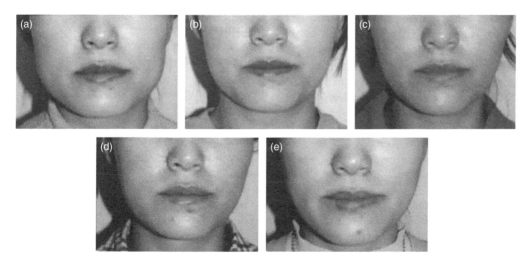

Figure 13.6 Serial photography over the course of one year post-injection with maximum efficacy at three months.

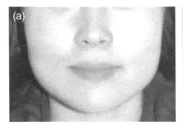 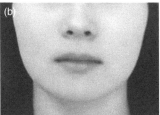 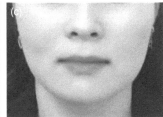

Figure 13.7 Significant improvement of masseter hypertrophy in a patient treated every six months with botulinum toxin.

with regular reinjections every 6 months. The mean reduced width of the lower face in the former group was 8.15% and in the latter group was 12.42%. Further, duration of improvement after cessation of injections was longer in the 6 month group compared to the 7–12 month group (Figure 13.7).

There are few reports that examine the durability of improvement after repeat injection.

Kim *et al.* [13] studied 121 patients treated for more than 1 year with BoNTA, receiving anywhere from two to eight injections. At each visit, masseter thickness was measured with ultrasound. Patients were injected with 100–140 U of Dysport in each masseter, based on thickness. Average masseter muscle thickness was reduced from 13.32 mm at the baseline visit to 9.94 mm at the last visit on average (a 25.4% improvement). The dose of Dysport was adjusted downward at return visits as the masseter's thickness decreased.

In a randomized control trial of 98 patients, Jiao Wei *et al.* [14] found that patients instructed to exercise their masseter early after BoNTA injection had the effect of delaying the return of masseter hypertrophy.

Effect on the mandible and other muscles of mastication

Chang *et al.* [10] examined the mandible with three dimensional CT before and three months after BoNTA injection of bilateral masseter muscles. They evaluated ten female patients and measured mandibular cortex thickness, bone thickness, and mandibular volume and found that there were no

significant changes during this time interval preinjection and postinjection. They believed that these results supported the continued practice of BoNTA masseter injection combined with mandibular surgery in selected patients. Further, Chung-Chih Yu *et al.* [15] used CT to confirm no significant changes in other mastication muscle volume of after masseter injection.

Side effects

Patients may notice an ache at the site of injection, difficulty with hard food, and speech disturbances 1–4 weeks after injection; these complaints are transient. There are also reports of visible masseter fasciculation, dry mouth, and asymmetry including a prominent zygoma or sunken cheek. Kim *et al.* [13] have suggested that sunken cheeks may be attributed to injections that are too high or too anterior on the masseter and may be more common in those with poor skin elasticity.

The most common side effect is a transient and mild masticatory weakness with easy fatigue while chewing, or weakened bite with tough food. Such changes are mild and tolerable and should be anticipated with BoNTA injection into the masseter.

Using a bite-force transducer, we quantified this reduction in masseter strength [15]. We measured bite force prior to injection of BTX-A 25 U bilaterally, and at 2, 4, 8, and 12 weeks' postinjection. While the maximum bite force was significantly reduced after injection, it slowly recovered by 12 weeks. Chung-Chih Yu [16] completed a similar study that found that bite force was decreased 1 week postinjection and that it reached its lowest point in week 3. But by month 3, bite force completely recovered despite improvements in masseter hypertrophy. This discrepancy is thought to be due to compensation by the other muscles of mastication.

Other side effects are similar to BoNTA injections elsewhere on the body and include headache, body ache, and rare allergy. Further, there are rare reports [17] of antibody-induced therapy failure with multiple injections.

Ideal facial contouring with BoNTA maximizes reduction in masseter hypertrophy while minimizing masseter weakness. Reports of temporomandibular joint disturbances or antibody formation are thought to be related to high doses of administered BoNTA. As in Sloop's dose–response curve [18], beyond a certain point, additional units of BoNTA do not lead to additional efficacy. Therefore, it is preferable to use the lowest necessary dose while scheduling appropriate reinjections to prevent complications.

Contouring of the Lower Leg

Introduction

More and more women are interested in contouring and slimming of the lower leg, in part due to popular clothing styles that highlight this area (e.g., high-heeled shoes, shorts, skirts, capris). Often, women requesting this are former professional or amateur athletes or those with jobs that require a lot of standing (including professional models), leading to calf hypertrophy. Men rarely request calf contouring. In fact, the authors have not treated a male patient with this procedure, although it could feasibly be part of a gender confirmation procedure.

Over the past 15 years, many surgical approaches to calf slimming have been attempted, but most require invasive procedures with inherent risks. These include liposuction, endoscopic partial resection of the hypertrophic calf, and severing branches of the tibial nerve that innervate the medial head of the gastrocnemius. In addition to the usual surgical risks of ecchymosis, swelling, hematoma, scarring, and infection, there are also reports of long postoperative recoveries and gait disturbances [19].

The surface appearance of the calf is influenced not only by the underlying muscle, but also the abundance or paucity of subcutaneous fat, the exposed Achilles' tendon, and the shape of the tibia and fibula. Large calves can be divided into three etiologic groups: lipodystrophic (often with a slim ankle), hypertrophic (often with visible fasciculation when walking), and combined lipodystrophic and hypertrophic (often with a larger ankle circumference and "radish-like" appearance).

Patients in the lipodystrophic group benefit most from liposuction. In the past, patients in the hypertrophic group have been treated with endoscopic resection of the hypertrophic parts of the calf and severing of branches of the tibial nerve that innervate the medial head of the gastrocnemius. Patients in the mixed lipodystrophic/hypertrophic group have been treated with a combination of these modalities.

Calf contouring with BoNTA began in the past 15 years in Korea among physicians who had positive experiences using these injections for lower face contouring. BoNTA injection was thought to be potentially a safer, temporary but effective alternative to the invasive surgical procedures used previously. As expected, patients with large calves due primarily to muscular hypertrophy stand to benefit most from BoNTA injection.

Anatomy

The target muscles of calf reduction and contouring procedures with BoNTA are the gastrocnemius and soleus muscles located on the posterior surface of the low leg. The primary action of these muscles is plantar flexion (i.e., "tip-toeing") [21]. Among these, the soleus is the more important postural muscle, and is persistently active during ordinary standing to prevent the person falling forward; thus,

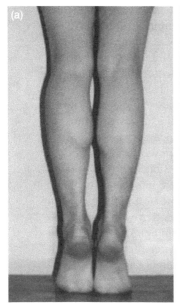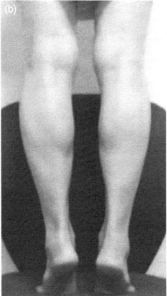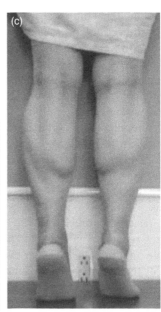

Figure 13.8 The various types of muscular hypertrophy calf. the prominent medial head (a), the prominent medial and lateral heads (b), and the diffusely prominent calf (c).

soleus paralysis is likely to disturb gait and stability.

The gastrocnemius muscle is more superficial and thus contributes more to the superficial contour of the calf. The lateral head of the gastrocnemius originates from the lateral condyle of the femur and the medial head originates from the medial condyle of the femur. Together with the soleus muscle, the gastrocnemius forms the Achilles' tendon which inserts onto the posterior surface of the calcaneus. While the gastrocnemius also contributes to plantar flexion, it plays a lesser role and therefore is unlikely to disturb gait if weakened. Therefore, the target muscle for BoNTA (at least initially) is the gastrocnemius.

Injection Technique

Prior to injection, the most hypertrophic portions of the calf are identified and marked with the patient in plantar flexion. Patients are injected with 100 U of Botox® reconstituted in 10 cm³ of normal saline, yielding 10 U/cm³. The gastrocnemius is a relatively thick and dense muscle, so we use a 23G, 1.25 inch, 10 cm³ Profi syringe® for injection.

Among patients with muscular calf hypertrophy, we find that their anatomy most often falls into one of three categories: the prominent medial head, the prominent medial *and* lateral heads, and the diffusely prominent calf (Figure 13.8a–c).

We inject 50–100 U per each calf, divided between 5 and 10 injection points with 5–10 U of BoNTA per point. The injections should be deep within the substance of the muscle, thus requiring a 1.25 inch syringe. Most patients are injected with a total of 100–200 U each session. To limit the risk of gait abnormality, it is sometimes advisable during the patient's first session to limit injections only to the medial gastrocnemius.

Clinical effect

Calf contouring with BoNTA remains a relatively rare procedure due to expense and comparatively short duration of effect. Furthermore, objectively measuring improvement with CT or ultrasound have proven

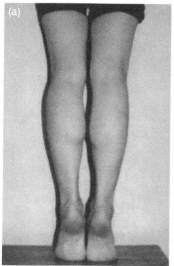
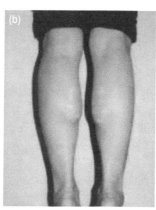
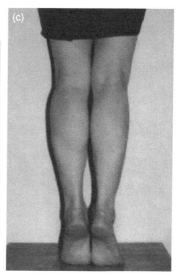

Figure 13.9 (a) Pre-injection; (b) injection points; (c) attenuation of the medial head of the gastrocnemius.

difficult and cost prohibitive. For these reasons, there is very little published on this technique. We will review several demonstrative cases below.

Case 1

A 28-year-old patient with hypertrophy of the medial head of the gastrocnemius was injected with 50 U of Botox® in each calf, divided among the medial head as shown in Figure 13.9. Eight weeks after injection, the border of the medial head of the gastrocnemius was softened.

Case 2

A 41-year-old patient with prominent medial and lateral heads of the gastroctemius received yearly injections of 50 U Botox® per side for a total of four sessions. She returned 3 years after her fourth injection with persistent slimming of the lower legs (Figure 13.10).

Case 3

A 56-year-old patient with diffusely prominent calves was injected with Xeomin® 100 U per calf every 6 months. Both the gastrocnemius and soleus were injected. Six months after the second injection, the lower legs are slimmer with attenuated surface contouring (Figure 13.11).

In the authors' experience, clinical improvement in calf hypertrophy tends to be evident at 3–4 weeks' postinjection and from month 6 to 12 begins to return to baseline. This course is similar to our experience in lower face contouring. Park et al. [19] have found that 50–150 U of BoNTA per calf led on average to a decrease in calf circumference of 0.7–1.58 cm (12.5–24.8% improvement) 6 months' postinjection. According to Park et al. [19], 50–150 U of BoNTA on each calf region and followed up for 6 month. This percent improvement is also similar to what can be expected with masseter injection. Apart from changes in calf circumference, many patients also are pleased with improvement in calf contour.

Side effects

The most common side effects were minor ecchymosis or dull and transient discomfort at the sites of injection. Uncommonly, standing instability or fatigue (especially with high heels) were noted. This instability also tends to subside within a month and is related to higher administered doses and injections

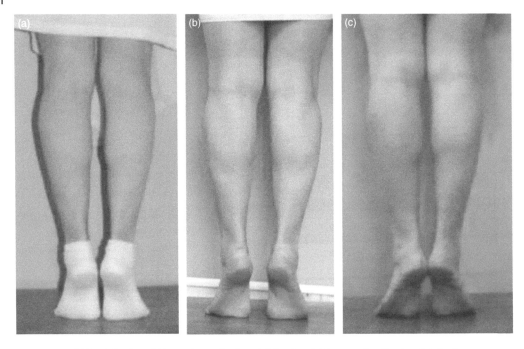

Figure 13.10 (a) Pre-injection; (b) just prior to the fourth injection; (c) 3 years after the fourth injection.

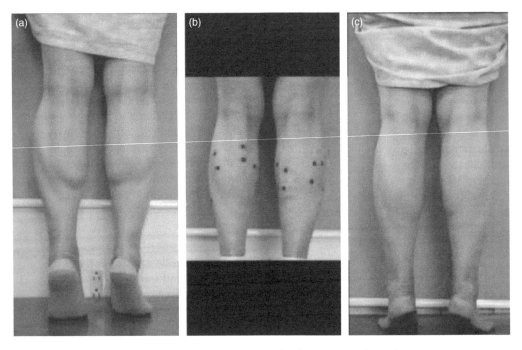

Figure 13.11 (a) Pre-injection; (b) injection points; (c) 6 months after the second injection.

outside the gastrocnemius. The authors have not observed gait disturbance or antibody formation leading to BoNTA inefficacy, although these are theoretical risks. To reduce the likelihood of antibody formation (especially considering the high doses of BoNTA required), injection intervals of 6 months or longer are recommended. To limit side effects and cost, efforts should be made to use the minimal dose of BoNTA necessary to achieve the desired clinical endpoint.

Concluding Remarks: Masseter and Calf Contouring

Basic principles of BoNTA injection apply to both masseter and calf injection, and principles in one muscle group can help inform the other. Calf muscles, for example, are much larger than the masseter and therefore 100 U of Botox® are diluted in 10 cm³ of normal saline for the calf and we only dilute with 2 cm³ for the masseter. For both muscle groups, injections should be distributed evenly over the body of the muscle, including origins and insertions. Failure to ensure even distribution can result in compensatory hypertrophy or fasciculation.

In the authors' experience, clinical response to BoNTA varies considerably among individuals based on a myriad of factors including gender, age, anatomy, and ethnicity. Further, reduction in hypertrophy tends not to be as idealized as Sloop's curve. Instead, from our experience and from the available literature, the reduction of both masseter and calf hypertrophy seems to approximate 20–30% regardless of the maximal dose injected. Thus, every effort should be made to use as little BoNTA as necessary to achieve an excellent clinical outcome. Both muscle groups require regular repeat injections for sustained improvement. The high doses of BoNTA required in these procedures put the patient at increased risk for antibody development leading to treatment failure, so repeat injections are not recommended more frequently than every 6 months. As BoNTA treatment of larger muscle groups (trapezius, deltoids, thighs) gain popularity, this concern is even greater.

Critically, the most desirable clinical endpoint is typically not the greatest reduction in muscle mass; instead, the goal should be beauty. Beauty is in part related to principles like symmetry and the golden ratio, but in part is beyond objective definition and relies on the artistic acumen of the physician.

References

1 Smyth AG. Botulinum toxin treatment of bilateral masseteric hypertrophy. Br J Oral Maxillofac Surg 1994;32:29–33.
2 von Lindern JJ, Niederhagen B, Appel T, Berge S, Reich RH. Type A botulinum toxin for the treatment of hypertrophy of the masseter and temporal muscle: an alternative treatment. Plast Reconstr Surg 2001;107:327–332.
3 Park MY, Ahn KY, Jung DS (2003) Botulinum toxin type A treatment for contouring of the lower face. Dermatol Surg 29:477–483; discussion 483.
4 Kim HJ, Yum KW, Lee SS, Heo MS, Seo Kyle Effects of botulinum toxin type A on bilateral masseteric hypertrophy evaluated with computed tomographic measurement. Dermatol Surg 2003;29:484–489.
5 Park, MY, Ahn KY. Follow-up; Botulinum toxin A for the treatment of facial hyperkinetic wrinkle lines in Koreans. Plast Reconstr Surg 2003;105:148(s).
6 Satoh K. Mandibular contouring surgery by angular contouring combined with genioplasty in Orientals. Plast Reconstr Surg 1998;101:461–472.
7 To EW, Ahuja AT, Ho WS, et al. A prospective study of the effect of botulinum toxin A on masseteric muscle hypertrophy with ultrasonographic and

electromyographic measurement. Br J Plast Surg 2001;54:197–200.

8 Yun Xie, Jia Zhou, Haizhou Li, Cheng Cheng, Tanja Herrler, Qingfeng Li. Qingfeng Li Classification of masseter hypertrophy for tailored botulinum toxin type A treatment. Plast Reconstr Surg 2014; 134:209e–217e.

9 Mandel L, Tanakan M. Treatment of unilateral masseteric hypertrophy with botulinum toxin: case report. J Oral Maxillofac Surg 1999;57:1017–9.

10 Chang. CS, Bergeron L, Yu CC, Chen PKT, Chen YR. Aesth Plast Surg 2011;35:452–455.

11 Kim NH, Chung JH, Park RH, Park JB. The use of botulinum toxin type A in aesthetic mandibular contouring. Plast Reconstr Surg 2005;115:919–929.

12 Yun Xie, Jia Zhou, Haizhou Li, Cheng Cheng, Tanja Herrler, Qingfeng Li. Classification of masseter hypertrophy for tailored botulinum toxin type A treatment. Plast Reconstr Surg 2014;134:209e–218e.

13 Kim NH, Park RH, Park JB. Botulinum toxin type A for the treatment of hypertrophy of the masseter muscle. Plast Reconstr Surg 2010;125:1693–1705.

14 Jiao Wei, Hua Xu, Jiasheng Dong, Qingfeng Li, Chuanchang Dai. Prolonging the duration of masseter muscle reduction by adjusting the masticatory movements after the treatment of masseter muscle hypertrophy with botulinum toxin type A injection. Dermatol Surg 2015;41: S101–S

15 Ahn KY, Kim ST. The change of maximum bite force after botulinum toxin type A injection for treating masseteric hypertrophy. Plast Reconstr Surg 2007; 120:1662–1666.

16 Chung-Chih Yu, Philip Kuo-Ting Chen, Yu-Ray Chen. Botulinum toxin A for lower facial contouring: A prospective study. Aesth Plast Surg 2007;31:445–451.

17 Lee HH, Kim ST, Lee KJ, Baik HS. Effect of a second injection of botulinum toxin on lower facial contouring, as evaluated using 3-dimensional laser scanning. Dermatol Surg 2015;41:439–444.

18 Sloop RR, Escutin RO, Matus JA, Cole BA, Peterson GW. Dose–response curve of human extensor digitorum brevis muscle function to intramuscularly injected botulinum toxin type A. Neurology 1996;46:1382–1386.

19 Park JM, Ha JS, Lee KC, Kim SK, Lee GN, Lee MJ, Lee KH. The effect of botulinum toxin A on calf reduction. J Korean Soc Plast Reconstr Surg 2005;32:85–92.

20 Suh IS. Neurectomy of nerve branch to medial gastrocnemius muscle for calf reduction. J Korean Soc Aesth Plast Surg 2007;13;95–104.

21 Lee HJ, Lee DW, Park YH, Cha MK, Kim HS, Ha SJ. Botulinum toxin A for aesthetic contouring of enlarged medial gastrocnemius muscle Dermatol Surg 2004;30:867–871.

22 Han KH, Joo YH, Moon SE, Kim KH. Botulinum toxin A for lower leg contouring. J Dermatol Treat 2006;17: 50–254.

14

Treatment of the Perioral Area

Shawn Allen, MD (FAAD, FACMS),[1,2] Roberta Sengelmann, MD,[3] and Rachel Simmons, MD (FAAD)[4]

[1] *Director and Founder, Dermatology Specialists, Boulder, USA*
[2] *Assistant Clinical Professor, University of Colorado, Department of Dermatology, Boulder, USA*
[3] *President and Owner, Santa Barbara Skin Institute, Associate Clinical Professor, UCI Dermatology, Santa Barbara, USA*
[4] *Dermatologist, Dermatology Specialists, Boulder, USA*

Introduction

Rejuvenation of the aging face can take on many different forms and methods ranging from laser and surgical approaches, injectable fillers and topical cosmeceuticals. Much of the aging of the central face may be attributed to the chronic use of the perioral muscles as well as loss of bony and structural support around the mouth. Minimally invasive procedures to address these concerns such as soft tissue filler and neurotoxin injections have grown in popularity due to the minimal downtime, good safety profile, increased efficacy, and reproducibility of results. Chemical denervation with botulinum toxins plays an important role in minimally invasive facial rejuvenation, particularly in the perioral area.

Although current FDA-approved cosmetic indications for botulinum toxins do not include treatment of the perioral area, this is a common location where experienced injectors can take advantage of the muscle relaxing effects of neurotoxins to reduce facial lines, wrinkles, and folds as well as to reshape the face. Some of the perioral uses of botulinum toxins include treating hyperfunctional vertical lip lines, reshaping the face by lowering the upper lip or elevating the corners of the mouth, smoothing the dimpled skin

of the chin, as well as restoring symmetry. Because the mouth is critical to many daily activities, care should be taken to have a thorough understanding of muscular anatomy and neurotoxin properties to avoid complications when attempting to rejuvenate this area.

In general, due to the important functional considerations around the mouth, injection doses in the lower face tend to be lower than those in the upper face. The need to maintain normal function of the mouth for eating, speaking, drinking, and daily activities makes overdosing in this area more than just a cosmetic concern. Therefore, special caution should be used when injecting patients, especially those who make a living from using their mouths professionally such as wind instrument musicians, singers, speech therapists, and public speakers. In contrast to treating the glabellar complex where the goal of treatment is to minimize or eliminate movement, the goal of treating the perioral region is to weaken the muscles while preserving function. Patients must therefore be educated that more subtle results (than those achieved in the glabella) are to be expected when treating this area.

In this chapter we review the common uses of neurotoxins in the perioral area. We will focus on improvement of hyperdynamic vertical lip lines, relaxing the upper lip to alleviate a "gummy smile", lifting the down-turned corners of the mouth and correcting the dimpling of the chin. When available, we will provide consensus recommendations as well as author preferences for dosing and injection location. Please note that recommended dosing will vary depending on the choice of neuromodulator used. For the purposes of this chapter, we will limit the dosage discussion to the botulinum toxins FDA-approved for cosmetic use on the face at the time of publication: abobotulinumtoxinA (Dysport®), onabotulinumtoxinA (hereafter referred to as Botox®), and incobotulinum-toxinA (Xeomin®). Other neurotoxins that become available for cosmetic use will need to be dosed according to product-specific published studies or guidelines. Please note that botulinum toxin units may not be interchangeable between different products as one must consider the different diffusion characteristics, units of measurement, onset of action, duration, potency, and side effects associated with each commercially available product; however, it is generally agreed that Botox and Xeomin may be compared at a 1 : 1 ratio. As the authors have more clinical experience with Botox/Dysport, the reader may comfortably substitute Xeomin doses when only Botox doses are stated.

Lip Area: Vertical Lip Lines

Upper and lower radiating vertical lip lines are primarily caused by the large sphincter muscle called the orbicularis oris. This muscle contracts to purse the lips and results in radial lip lines when fully contracted. Its function is critical in daily activities such as eating and drinking, the use of straws, the ability to enunciate letters such as "p" and "q" and the ability to whistle. The goal in treating the orbicular oris is to weaken (rather than immobilize) the muscle to decrease lip pursing and the formation of vertical lines. Overdosing this area can lead to difficulty in phonation, eating, drinking, and kissing [1].

Some predisposing factors to the early onset of static radiating vertical lip lines include daily practices that cause frequent pursing of the lips. For example, smokers, athletes who frequently drink from water bottles, and professional wind instrument musicians will have an increased risk of developing premature vertical lip lines due to their frequent pursing motion of their lips. The primary author has noted a significant trend for women, far greater than men, to have early or late signs of vertical lip lines.

Vertical lip lines may be dynamic or static in nature. The end result of a chronic untreated dynamic line, resulting from muscle contraction, is a static line. Once static lines are created, they may be softened by neurotoxin injections but usually not erased. This will usually require the addition of soft tissue fillers and/or chemical or laser resurfacing procedures. Therefore, early treatment with botulinum toxins may help to prevent and/or delay the creation of these static lines. In addition to relaxing vertical lip lines, it has been reported that injection into the vermilion border of the lip may also result in the appearance of slight lip pseudoaugmentation due to the decreased centripetal sphincter tone with subsequent eversion of the lip [1].

Treatment of the vertical lip lines in conjunction with other aesthetic procedures can have a synergistic beneficial effect. When toxin in the perioral area is combined with soft-tissue fillers, the presence of toxin in this highly dynamic area can increase the duration of the filler. Toxin can also improve the outcome of perioral laser resurfacing as the healing time is decreased with minimized muscular contraction theoretically [2].

Injection points for vertical lip lines will vary from individual to individual based upon the shape of the mouth, the strength of the orbicularis oris, and the location and severity of the vertical lines with animation. Injections of botulinum toxins for vertical lip lines can be administered to the upper or bottom lip alone or both simultaneously. Many patients will benefit from injections at the vermilion border only while others will need the

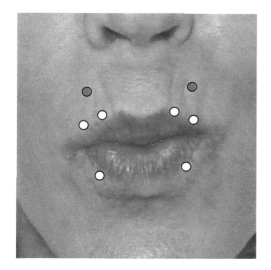

Figure 14.1 Pursing the lips will assist in determining the amount and location of the injections. Typical injection points along the vermilion border of 2.5–5 DU or 1–2BU/XU per site are identified by white circles. Additional injection points are located in red but may increase risk of oral incompetence.

vermilion and focal areas of the cutaneous lip injected to best address their concerns. Having the patient animate by pursing their lips will help to assess where, how much, and how many injections are needed (see Figure 14.1).

Several scales for classifying severity of aging in the perioral area are available. An aesthetic rating scale which classifies perioral lines at maximal contracture (POLM) is particularly relevant to the treatment of this area with neurotoxin. Patients can typically expect one grade of improvement in POLM score with successful treatment of botulinum toxin to the vertical lip lines. Reference to severity scales in clinical practice can be useful in patient consultation as education about anticipated improvement can help temper patient expectations and gauge patient satisfaction [3].

Published consensus recommendations and author preferences for vertical lip line injections include the following for Dysport® and Botox®/Xeomin®. Locations of injections of Dysport units (DU),Botox units (BU), and Xeomin units (XU) are essentially the same. Volume dilution should be modified to

patient needs and desired effects. For moderate dynamic lip rhytides, the vermilion border of the upper lip should be injected at 2–4 injection points within 2–5 mm of the vermilion border with 2–4 DU and 1–2 BU/XU per site. Two additional injection points with similar doses in the mid cutaneous lip can be performed for patients with long radiating lines; however, these injections may have a higher likelihood of impairing lip function and should be performed cautiously. Because of its less dynamic lines, the lower lip is usually injected at only two points located just below the vermilion border with 2–3 DU or 1–2 BU/XU per site. The dose range in the upper lip is 2.5–16 DU and 4–6 BU/XU and the range for the lower lip is 2.5–7.5 DU and 2–3 BU/XU [4, 5].

Cohen et al. compared the dose response of onabotulinumtoxinA (BU) 7.5 BU to 12 BU for injection in the upper and lower lips to minimize perioral lines. The authors found that the 7.5 BU dosing (two injection points per lip with 5 BU in the upper lip and 2.5 BU in the lower lip) was optimal for most patients as it was highly effective for up to 16 weeks with lower potential for AEs. Examples of treatment-related AEs in this study included lip weakness, lip numbness, difficulty eating, lip dryness, lip fullness, lip swelling, and inability to kiss [1]. Care should be taken to avoid overdosing in this area [2]. Options to minimize the risk of lip ptosis and functional compromise include treating at the lower range and having the patient return in 2 weeks for reassessment and additional units as needed. Some injectors may also choose to treat the upper lip only to maintain the integrity of the lower lip's pursing effect. Keeping injections superficial [6] and within 5 mm of the vermilion border will also help to avoid further excessive effect. Having the patient purse their lips prior to injecting will help to gauge the strength and integrity of the muscle and to adjust toxin doses accordingly (Figure 14.2). Some other key points to consider include avoiding injections too laterally as this can cause drooping of the mouth and drooling if the integrity of the oral

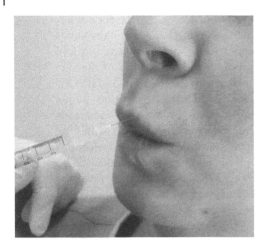

Figure 14.2 Having the patient pucker the lips will help to assess where along the vermilion border to place your injection of 2.5-5 DU or 1-2BU/XU per site. A 32 gauge needle with a 1cc no waste syringe is used.

the muscles but typically does not result in static changes.

The mentalis muscles are the main contributors not only for dimpling of the chin but also for the creation of the mental crease, along with the depressor labii inferioris muscles. Once a mental crease or groove has been formed, it may be softened by neurotoxin injections but usually not erased. This may require the addition of soft tissue fillers or other chin implant procedures for full correction. Therefore, early treatment with botulinum toxins for chin dimpling may also help prevent and/or delay the creation of the mental crease.

Injections of botulinum toxins for chin dimpling can be done as a single injection centrally or in 2 separate symmetrical sites. Palpating the mentalis muscles while having the patient animate by pushing the lower lip up toward the top lip or pulling the lower lip in towards the lower teeth will help assess where to place the injections. The mentalis muscles are the deepest muscles in the chin and should be targeted deeply just above the level of the periosteum. Injections should be placed in a caudal location within 10 mm of the bony rim of the chin (Figure 14.3). Alternatively, more superficial injections may target the more superficial fibers of the mentalis but may carry a higher risk for involving the depressor labii inferioris and may risk oral compromise. Care must also be taken to avoid injecting too laterally or superiorly as this can cause oral incompetence and drooling of the mouth due to involvement of the depressor labii inferioris.

Published consensus recommendations and author preferences for mentalis injections include the following. Locations of injections of both products are essentially the same. Depending all toxins on the volume dilution and desired effect they should be modified accordingly. For mild to moderate mentalis muscle volume and strength, a single injection point within 5 to 10 mm of the chin apex with 5–10 DU and 2.5–5 BU/XU is recommended. Alternatively, two separate injection points may be more effective for

commissure is compromised. Also, avoid injections too medially as this may cause softening or loss of the cupids bow shape.

Lastly, in the authors' experiences the low doses typically used as well as the constant activity of the large underlying sphincter muscle contributes to a shorter duration of action of botulinum toxins in this area. Therefore, realistic expectations and counseling regarding the possible need for frequent treatments as well as adjunctive modalities such as laser or chemical resurfacing procedures and or soft tissue fillers should be discussed prior to treatment in this area.

Chin Area: Chin Dimpling and Mental Crease

Chin dimpling, also referred to as "peach pit chin," "apple dumpling chin" or "golf ball chin" is caused mainly by the activity of the mentalis muscle. The muscles originate from the incisive fossa near the apex of the chin and the paired muscles ascend in opposite superolateral directions toward the lower lip to insert into the skin of the chin [7]. The chin dimpling occurs with the dynamic contraction of

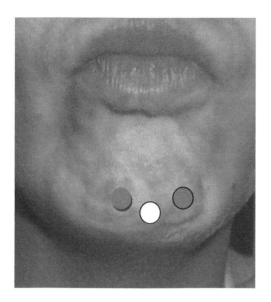

Figure 14.3 Patient animating to help identify the mentalis muscles. Single injection point of 10 DU or 5 BU/XU located in white. Alternatively, 2 separate injection points of 2.5-5 DU or 2.5-5 BU/XU each, identified by red circles.

wider stronger mentalis muscles. Each site receives 5- 10 DU or 2.5–5 BU/XU (See Figure 14.3). The dose range is 5–20 DU and 2.5–10 BU. It may be helpful to lower the dose and bring the patient back at 2 weeks and touch up the area as needed. Some experienced injectors may choose to try to treat the dimpled chin and mental crease with a more cephalad injection. This can be done, but again risks some degree of oral incompetence if the depressor labii inferiors is inadvertently injected.

Care should be taken to avoid overdosing and injecting too cephalad in this area as this may lead to oral functional compromise. Options to minimize this risk include treating at the lower range and having the patient return in 2 weeks for reassessment and additional units as needed. Keeping injections deep and caudal within 5 to 10 mm of the bony chin border will also help to avoid further unwanted side effects. Having the patient animate prior to injecting will help to gauge the strength and integrity of

the muscle and help in adjusting doses and location accordingly.

Downturned Commissures: Mouth Frown

Downturned corners of the mouth can create a frowning appearance at baseline. The sad or angry appearance is caused mainly by the activity of the depressor anguli oris (DAO) muscles. The lateral fibers of the depressor labii inferioris (DLI) muscles and platysmal bands also play a more minor role in this effect. The DAO muscles originate from the oblique line of the bony rim of the mandible and are intercalated with the platysma at their origin. The paired muscles ascend in an arcuate and superolateral then superomedial direction toward their respective corners of the mouth where they then intercalate with the orbicularis oris and the risorius muscles.[5] The down turning of the mouth corners occurs by unopposed or hyperactive downward pull of the muscles and typically does not result in static changes although there can be some accentuation of the oral commissure crease and marionette lines. Once an oral commissure crease or groove has been formed, it may be softened by neurotoxin injections but usually not erased. The addition of soft tissue fillers are often most helpful for full correction. Early treatment with botulinum toxins for downturned mouth corners may help prevent and/or delay the creation of the oral commissure crease.

Injections of botulinum toxins for downturned oral commissures are usually done as a single injection per side. Palpating the DAO muscles while having the patient animate by showing their lower teeth will help assess where to place the injections. The DAO muscles are superficial muscles in the lateral chin and should be targeted intramuscularly and in a caudal location within 5 mm of the bony rim of the chin. Alternatively, more superficial injections may target the more superficial fibers of the DAO, but may carry a higher risk for involving the depressor labii inferioris which would lead to oral incompetence. Injections located too high along the lateral chin will likely cause some functional compromise by either denervating more muscle mass than desired and or inadvertently involving the DLI muscles and ascending platysmal fibers.

Published consensus recommendations and author preferences for DAO injections include the following. Locations of injections are essentially the same. Depending on the volume dilution and desired effect, they should be modified accordingly. For mild to moderate DAO muscle volume and strength, a single injection point within 5 mm of the bony rim of the chin with 5–10 DU or 2.5–5 BU/XU is usually adequate (See Figure 14.4). The total dose range is 10–20 DU and 5–10 BU/XU. Advanced injectors may choose to try to treat the DAO with a more cephalad injection. This can be done as a second site with low doses with 2.5 DU and 1 BU/XU but may risk functional compromise with drooling.

Care should be taken to avoid overtreatment in this area which may lead to oral incompetence. It is also important to avoid injecting too cephalad as this can also lead

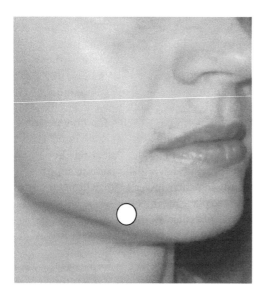

Figure 14.4 Injection of the DAO at the mandible border (white dot) with 5-10 DU or 2.5-5 BU/XU will allow for upturned corner of the mouth.

to oral incompetence and drooling due to inadvertent denervation of the DAO and DLI. Options to minimize this risk include treating at the lower range and having the patient return in 2 weeks for reassessment and additional units as needed. Keeping injections caudal and within 5 mm of the bony chin border will help to avoid unwanted side effects. Having the patient animate prior to injecting will help to gauge the strength and integrity of the muscle and aid in adjusting doses and location accordingly.

Gummy Smile

A gummy smile is defined as excessive gingival show (greater than 3 mm) [8] when smiling, and is caused mainly by the over activity of the levator labii superioris alaeque nasi (LLSAN) muscles. The other lip levators such as the levator labii superioris (LLS), levator anguli oris (LAO), risorius, zygomaticus minor (ZMi) and zygomaticus major (ZMa) may also play a role in creating a gummy smile. Mazzuco and Hexsel further classified the gummy smile into 4 categories based on the contraction of the specific above listed muscle(s) responsible for the gingival show [9].

In addition, genetic or acquired changes in gingival tissue and maxillary bone formation can play a role in accentuating the gummy smile [10]. Although botulinum toxins may be ideal for treating many patients [11], surgical lip repositioning, gingival laser treatments and other procedures performed by oral surgeons, orthodontists or periodontists may also be considered. The LLSAN muscles originate from the bony aspect of the nasal sidewall and frontal process of the maxilla and insert at the deep border of the orbicularis oris of the upper lip [7]. The muscles travel from the nasal sidewall, along the edge of the alar crease below the LLS, and then intercalate with the orbicularis oris. Early descending fibers assist in dilating the nares, while the longitudinal fibers assist in elevating the lip. The excess gummy show of the smiling mouth occurs by unopposed upward pull of the muscles, but does not result in static changes. There can also be some baseline elevation and asymmetry of the upper lip which may be corrected with botulinum toxins.

The LLSAN and the LLS muscles are the main contributors for the creation of the gummy smile and intersect near the junction of the nose, lip and cheek. As opposed to some perioral concerns, a gummy smile may be softened by neurotoxin injections and often fully corrected by neurotoxins alone. As mentioned, other procedures such as surgical revision of the lip and gums, laser gum treatments, dental appliances and maxillary surgery may be needed in the most extreme cases.

Injections of botulinum toxins for excessive gingival show are usually done as a single injection per side [12]. Palpating the LLSAN muscle while having the patient animate by smiling will help to assess where to place the injections. The LLSAN muscles should be targeted deeply at the level of the junction of the alar crease and the upper lip (see Figure 14.5). Injections in this area may be started at a lower dose with a touch up planned at 2 weeks. Injections at higher doses may cause some functional compromise or inability to smile symmetrically and effectively.

Published consensus recommendations and author preferences for LLSAN injections include the following. Locations of injections are essentially the same. Depending on the volume dilution and desired effect they should be modified accordingly. For mild to moderate gummy smile, use a single injection point within 5–10 mm of the junction of the upper lip, nose, and cheek (just lateral to the alar crease) with 5–10 DU or 2.5–5 BU/XU per side (See Figure 14.5). The total dose range is 10–20 DU and 5–10 BU/XU.

Care should be taken to avoid overtreatment and injecting too caudal and lateral in this area as this may lead to oral incompetence by immobilizing the distal fibers of the LLSAN, LLS and ZM. Options to minimize the risk of oral functional compromise include treating at the lower range and having the patient return in 2 weeks for

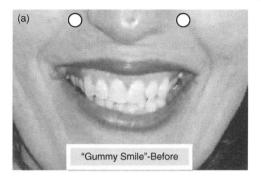

(a) "Gummy Smile"-Before

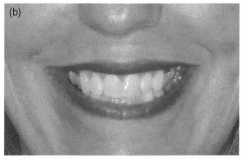

(b)

Smile 2 Months After 5U Dysport per side (total 10U)

Figure 14.5 Gummy smile at baseline (a) and 2 months post treatment with 5 DU to a single injection point per side (white dots) 1 cm lateral to the ala and at the level of the alar rim (b).

reassessment and additional units as needed. Keeping injections within 5–10 mm of the alar crease at the junction of the upper lip and cheek will also help to avoid further unwanted side effects. Having the patient animate prior to injecting will help to gauge the strength and integrity of the muscle and help in adjusting doses and location accordingly.

Summary

Treating the lower face requires a detailed understanding of facial anatomy. The perioral area is balanced by opposing muscles as well as muscles that intercalate with each in several key areas. Injectors should be aware of the effect of denervating muscles that have an opposing muscle so as to avoid asymmetry and overcorrection. Strategic injection placement at the periphery of the perioral area helps to minimize the risk of loss of function. It should be noted that all of the above recommended injection points are located either at the central border or the peripheral border of the perioral area (Figure 14.6). This location helps to ensure that only certain fibers of the targeted muscles are denervated. Because of the critical function of the perioral musculature, this area should be treated by experienced injectors. Careful informed consent and pretreatment photographs at rest, smiling, and while pursing the lips should take place prior to injection. Understanding the anatomy, starting with lower doses and having patients return for a touch up in 2 weeks will help to ensure adequate treatment while minimizing risks in this sensitive area.

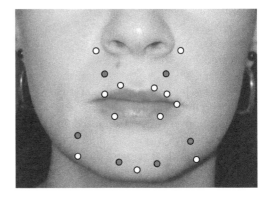

Figure 14.6 Summary of recommended injection points marked in white. Red circles indicate additional alternative injection points to consider with caution. Note that the white injection points are at the periphery of the muscles in the perioral area. Red injection points are more central and may carry a higher risk of functional compromise.

References

1 Semchyshyn N, Sengelmann RD. Botulinum toxin A treatment of perioral rhytides. Dermatol Surg 2003 May;29(5): 490–495.

2 Cohen J, Dayan Sn. OnabotulinumtoxinA dose-ranging study for hyperdynamic perioral lines. Dermatol Surg 2012;38: 1497–1505.

3 Cohen J, Thomas J, Paradkar D, *et al.* An interrater and intrarater reliability study of 2 photographic scales for the classification of perioral aesthetic features. Dermatol Surg 2014;40:663–670

4 Kane M, Donofrio L, Ascher B, *et al.* Expanding the use of neurotoxins in facial aesthetics: a consensus panel's assessment and recommendations. J Drugs Dermatol. 2010 Jan; 9;(1 Suppl);S7-S22, quiz S23–S25.

5 Carruthers J, Fagien S, Matarasso SL; Botox Consensus Group. Consensus recommendations on the use of botulinum toxin type A in facial aesthetics. Plast Reconstr Surg. 2004 Nov;114 (6 Suppl): 1S–22S.

6 Caruthers J, Carruthers A. Clinical indications and injection technique for the cosmetic use of botulinum A exotoxin. Dermatol Surg 1998; 24:1189–1194.

7 *Gray's Anatomy: The Anatomical Basis of Clinical Practice*. 40th edition (2008).

8 Garber DA, Salama MA. The aesthetic smile: diagnosis and treatment. Periodontol 2000 1996;11:18–28.

9 Mazzuco R. Hexsel D. Gummy smile and botulinum toxin: A new approach based on the gingival exposure area. J Am Acad Dermatol 2010 Dec;63(6):1042–1051.

10 Hwang WS, Hur MS, Hu KS, *et al.* Surface anatomy of the lip elevator muscles for the treatment of gummy smile using botulinum toxin. Angle Orthod 2009;79: 70–77.

11 Polo M. Botulinum toxin type A (Botox) for the neuromuscular correction of excessive gingival display on smiling (gummy smile). Am J Orthod Dentofacial Orthop. 2008; 133:195–203.

12 Carruthers A, Carruthers J. Cosmetic uses of botulinum A exotoxin. In: Klein AW, eds. *Tissue Augmentation in Clinical Practice: Procedures and Techniques*. New York: Marcel Dekker; 1998:207–236.

15

Neck Rejuvenation

Koenraad De Boulle, MD,[1] Lakhdar Belhaouari, MD,[2] and Julia D. Kreger, MD[3]

[1] Aalst Dermatology Clinic, Aalst, Belgium
[2] Director, Centre de Chirurgie Esthétique et Medecine Esthétique Jules Guesde, Toulouse, France
[3] University of Colorado Dermatology, Colorado, USA

Throughout the ages, men and women have wanted to make themselves attractive, preserve the freshness of their youth, and even to turn back time. 3500 years ago, an Egyptian papyrus was already extolling the virtues of an abrasive paste of milk and honey with particles of alabaster for smoothing the surface of the skin and removing imperfections. But humans, "late arrivals in an already old world", are subject to aging, defined as the action of time on the body. This physiological phenomenon is irreversible, slowly progressive, and inevitable in all living matter. From a morphological perspective, its signs are revealed in their most obvious and irreversible form in the face and neck.

The Anatomical and Functional Basis of Aging

The signs of aging in the face and neck are based on a trilogy: sagging, wrinkles and atrophy. Sagging in the neck occurs through loss of elasticity, and manifests as loss of tension and tone of the different components: skin, subcutaneous fat, aponeurosis and muscle [1, 2].

The Skin of the Neck and Its Subcutaneous Fatty Tissue

The skin loosens, thins, and becomes less elastic through the loss of its mechanical properties in the derma (fewer collagen fibers, fewer elastic fibers). This explains the loss of definition of the mandibular edge and the cervicomental angle, and also the shrivelled skin, more pronounced jowls, and "turkey neck" appearance [3]. In short, the laxity which explains why for ages men and women have looked at themselves in a mirror, or in a pool of water before mirrors existed, said to themselves "wouldn't it be good if …" and pulled the skin of the face and neck up and back, imitating the procedure of the facelift. In fact, it was they who first imagined the face lift, and not the brilliant and dedicated surgeons – such as Charles Conrad Miller in the United States, the dermatologist Suzanne Noël, Raymond Passot, and Julien Bourguet in France, and Eugen Hollander and Erich Lexer in Germany – who at the beginning of the twentieth century had the genius and daring to perform the first procedures. These pioneers were followed by many other outstanding surgeons throughout the twentieth century, culminating in today's techniques [1, 2].

Above all else, it is vital for a doctor to understand anatomy. Anatomy is essentially a fundamental science and its knowledge is indispensable to any doctor, regardless of specialty, for understanding a treatment physiologically, functionally, and clinically, before attempting its technical execution. This is equally true whether the treatment is surgical or nonsurgical, such as with the injection of botulinum toxin.

The Platysma Muscle

Platysma means "flat plate" in Greek. It is the cutaneous muscle of the neck: a thin, flattened, very broad, quadrilateral, paired, symmetric sheet. It covers the anterolateral region of the neck but also the inferior part of the face, passing above the horizontal branch of the lower jaw, and stretches from the thorax to the inferior maxilla and cheek (Figure 15.1).

Its caudal origin is in the deep part of the skin that covers the acromion and the deltoid and subclavian regions, and it proceeds somewhat obliquely upward, forward and medially in a splitting of the superficial fascia covering the anterolateral region of the neck [4–7].

The two parts of the platysma, which are separated at their base, proceed upward and come closer together on the upper cervical median line. Their median, anterior edges form the platysmal bands. These platysmal bands interlace below the chin in 75% of cases at a height of 1–2 cm; they remain separated without decussation in 10% of cases, or in 15% of cases, they interlace and reconnect further up and form a continuous muscular sheet with the thyroid cartilage [8].

The upper insertion points are both bony and cutaneous:

- After interlacing, the anterior fibers attach to the skin of the mental eminence and the mental protuberance.
- The middle fibers attach to the lower edge of the mandible on the anterior part of its external oblique line and the lateral part of the mental protuberance. Some of these fibers contract from adhesions by entwining, proceeding and interlacing with fibers of the depressor anguli oris and the depressor labii inferioris muscles.
- The posterior and lateral fibers cover the gonion and extend to the labial commissure and the skin of the cheek. At the cheek, the most lateral fibers entwine with the risorius muscle fibers (although according to some anatomists this muscle may only be an extension of the platysma) [5,6].

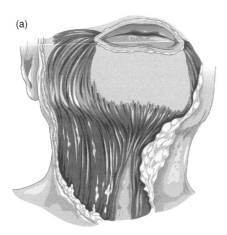
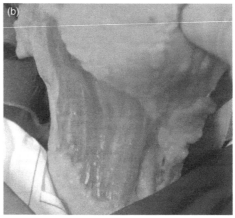

Figure 15.1 (a) *Source*: Reprinted courtesy L. Belhaouari from Ref. [3]; © 2013, L. Belhaouari. (b) Dissection by L. Belhaouari and F. Lauwers., Department of Anatomy Toulouse University, France. *Source*: Reproduced from Ref. [3] courtesy L. Belhaouari; © 2013.

Function: Its anterior fibers draw the skin of the chin downwards, its middle fibers pulls the angle of the mouth and lower lip down by unfolding it, and its posterior fibers draw the skin of the cheek downward and the labial commissure laterally and down. It also tenses and creases the skin of the neck and lifts the skin of the pectoral region. It contracts during exertion (forced inspiration) and in anger, and it forms the platysma bands. Its atrophy as a result of aging results in "turkey neck": unsightly vertical creases that affect elderly people.

How Does the Platysma Age?

As with the skin of the neck and its subcutaneous tissue, the platysma atrophies and loses its tone. It should logically become more flaccid and stretched out through the loss of its mechanical and viscoelastic properties, but unlike the skin, the muscle is a reactive tissue, and responds to this stretching out by muscular hypertonia. This contraction combats the theoretical stretching of aging, resulting in shortening of the muscle, giving a pseudo-muscular resting tone [9].

As a result, this originally flat muscle loses its homogeneity. Its fibers shrink up into bundles (the platysmal bands), leaving empty or loosely dense fiber spaces between these bands, and thus genuine open gaps in the flat surface of the platysma. This is an essential consideration, since if botulinum toxin is injected subcutaneously in the neck and the injected toxin encounters one of these open spaces, it will inevitably diffuse deeper into the neck, since there is no muscular barrier to absorb it. If the doses are large, adverse effects could result.

Consequently, the platysmal bands arise from these two factors: shortening of the resting muscle and union with bundles of fibers between them.

Muscles Associated with the Platysma

The Depressor Anguli Oris (DAO)

Triangular in shape (the origin of its "triangular muscle" name in French), its inferior base arises from the anterior third of the external oblique line of the mandible. Its fibers then proceed upward, by criss-crossing and entwining with the anterior fibers of the platysma, and continue upwards towards the labial commissure. Some of these fibers attach to the skin of the angle of the mouth to transform the labial commissure, resulting in the expression of sadness. Other fibers, after interlacing with the other muscles that form the muscular knot termed the modiolus, go back up into the upper lip and (with the upper fascias of the buccinator muscle) form the external orbicularis oris muscle of the lips before attaching beneath the skin of the lips at the philtral ridge. These superficial extrinsic fibers thus contribute to the relief of the philtrum (said in folklore to be the indent from God's finger on the mouth of the newborn child), and with the loss of tone and the atrophy resulting from age, the relief of these philtral ridges decreases, and the philtrum becomes less well outlined and flattened.

Depressor Labii Inferioris (DLI)

Quadrilateral in shape, its inferior base arises at the anterior third of the external oblique line of the mandible, just above the line of attachment of the depressor anguli oris muscle. The DAO thus covers the DLI at this level and is therefore more superficial (very important when understanding the depth and the level of injection needed for botulinum toxin). As with the DAO, its fibers criss-cross and entwine with the anterior fibers of the platysma before inserting on the skin and the red edge of the mucosa on nearly the entire lower lip. As a transformer of the lower lip, its free edge widens. It expresses disgust and irony.

Risorius Muscle

According to some anatomists, the risorius, an inconstant, very thin and very superficial muscle, arises from fibers from the platysma. It extends horizontally in a triangle, with the posterior base on the middle part of the cheek, and attaches at the modiolus and the skin of the labial commissure. A superficial adjunct of the buccinator, it draws the commissure laterally and can deepen the dimple of the cheek by its mediojugal cutaneous insertion.

Signs of Aging in the Neck

To recap, the three signs of aging in the neck are:

1. Sagging, with loss of definition of the mandibular edge and the cervicomental angle, with cervical cutaneous ptosis.
2. Atrophy, in the form of platysmal bands.
3. Horizontal cervical wrinkles (also referred to as horizontal necklace lines).

We have already discussed these first two points in the preceding section.

Sagging, Ptosis of the Musculocutaneous Integument

This explains the loss of definition of the mandibular edge, with jowl formation, and the loss of definition of the cervicomental angle with ptosis of the integument. It concerns the skin, subcutaneous fatty tissue, and the platysma, and also explains the shrivelled skin, jowls, and "turkey neck" (Figure 15.2).

The Platysmal Bands

The genesis of platysmal bands was described in the preceding chapter: the result of changes

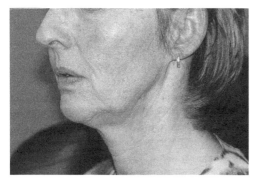

Figure 15.2 Jowl formation. Loss of definition of cervicomental angle and loss of definition of jaw line. Courtesy Dr. K. De Boulle, Belgium.

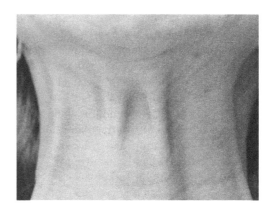

Figure 15.3 Prominent platysmal bands. Courtesy Dr. K. De Boulle, Belgium.

in the platysma over time, with some fibers among them forming clusters and shortening of the muscle at rest. Atrophy over time, along with the persistent platysmal activity to support the sagging neck and mouth floor structures leads to a more prominent appearance (Figure 15.3).

Horizontal Cervical Wrinkles

The first question to ask is whether horizontal cervical wrinkles are expression wrinkles. If they were, we would expect botulinum toxin to be effective, as with frontal wrinkles. But in fact botulinum toxin is not effective in any way, because these horizontal cervical wrinkles are not expression wrinkles. As a reminder, there are four types of wrinkles in the neck: superficial photodamage wrinkles, dynamic expression lines, deep crumpling lines, and tissue accumulation wrinkles (Figure 15.4).

Superficial Photodamage Wrinkles

These are superficial epidermal lines: perioral wrinkles on the upper lip are another example. This "barcode" is due to elastolysis of the superficial stratum papillaris, which loosens and becomes too baggy, compared to the underlying dermis. It creases and it is this fine creasing that creates the superficial wrinkles, as can also be noted in the neck area.

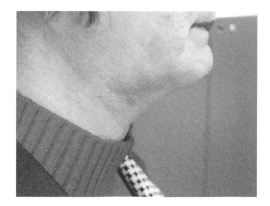

Figure 15.4 Deep crumpling horizontal lines and superficial photodamage wrinkles. Courtesy Dr. K. De Boulle, Belgium.

Dynamic Expression Lines

These are due, as is well known, to the influence of the cutaneous muscles on the skin to which they are attached; however, the platysma is attached very low on the skin that covers the acromion, and the deltoid and subclavicular regions. Above, although some fibers attach at the inferior edge of the mandible on the anterior part of its external oblique line, it is essentially inserted at the skin of the cheek and the labial commissure. At the neck therefore, the platysma covers only the anterolateral region of the neck in a split superficial fascia, and without inserting in the cervical skin as such. Thus, on the neck itself, one can hardly expect to find real expression wrinkles, which would have been the main reason for recommending botulinum toxin treatment [10, 11].

Deep Crumpling Lines

Horizontal cervical wrinkles are in fact permanent elastic creases, as are mediojugal wrinkles and vertical frontal wrinkles. These are "accordion wrinkles" caused by positional constraints of the neck and multiple flexion–extension movements of the head on the neck. The head is raised and lowered many times each day, folding the cervical skin like an accordion in a horizontal direction. These folds become perennial with the loss of cutaneous plasticity as the cervical skin loosens

with age, and becomes stretched compared to the subjacent neck. It also becomes less elastic, less plastic, thinner, more pliable, and more prone to creasing. The skin thus remains fixed in the position in which it is folded: it is a false fold, a permanent elastic wrinkle. These effects are exacerbated by the weight of this cutaneous tissue, which has loosened with age, and the fixed night-time position, often with the head slightly bent, which fixes these folds like a nearly-closed accordion. It thus becomes clear why botulinum toxin cannot have an effect on these wrinkles, which are elastic creases and not dynamic expression lines of muscular origin.

Neck Rejuvenation

From the earlier text, we could state that four signs characterize the aging neck are:

- Platysmal bands
- Loss of definition of the cervicomental angle with laxity and cervical cutaneous ptosis
- Loss of definition of the mandibular edge
- Horizontal cervical wrinkles.

So, is botulinum toxin effective on these four clinical signs? And, at this time, is there competition between botulinum toxin and the other techniques, especially surgical ones, for these four indications [11, 12]?

We have just seen in the Chapter 14 that:

- Horizontal cervical wrinkles are elastic creases and not dynamic expression lines of muscular origin; consequently, botulinum toxin is not effective and there is no indication for its use [13–16].
- Concerning cervical sagging with cutaneous ptosis, it is completely unrealistic to expect a real facelift effect. The "Botulinum Toxin Facelift" is a dream today.

Injections with botulinum toxin are completely ineffective in patients presenting with cervical sagging and cutaneous ptosis. This has been stated in many publications and most of the authors experienced in their practices no real evidence of lifting, and it is definitely not a substitute for long-term surgical results. Current thought is that botulinum toxin can be effective on hyperactive muscle lines (i.e., platysmal bands) in the appropriate patient, though there has been no well-described, proven effect on facial contour or improving horizontal neck wrinkles or laxity [15, 17, 18].

Phillip Levy deserves all the credit for having described the "Nefertiti Neck" concept and brought it to the forefront [16, 18]. For improving the jaw line contour and more or less providing a visual effect of a "mini-lift", this procedure has been considered to be helpful (Figure 15.5); however, results can be highly variable and for that reason Levy highlights the importance of proper patient selection. The treatment is likely to create a successful result when the patient has retained the integrity of their skin elasticity and their ligaments [16]. For this reason, younger patients, as well as those patients who have undergone a surgical neck lift are ideal candidates. But a real lifting of the lower face by means of injections of botulinum toxin in a platysmal band and submandibular area as a substitute for a surgical neck lift is impossible [10, 17, 19].

It was of course tempting to try, since "the art of succeeding is the art of sometimes being very daring". But, although the art of

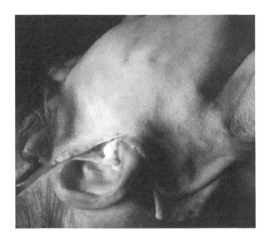

Figure 15.6 Example of a surgical cervicofacial facelift to restore definition of the cervicofacial oval.

succeeding is "the art of sometimes being very daring", it is even more true to say "the art of succeeding is the art of being sometimes very daring, sometimes very careful".

Only the classic surgical cervicofacial facelift can tighten the skin and the platysmal muscular-fascia system and restore good definition of the cervicofacial oval by resorbing the cutaneous-fatty surplus and redetermining the platysma muscular edge in a superoposterior tension vector [9, 11, 17] (Figure 15.6).

When the different mechanisms of aging and the different techniques are understood, it becomes clear that these techniques are complementary and not competitive. Surgery addresses ptosis and cutaneous surplus, filling addresses depressions, loss of volume, and the facial contours, lasers, and peelings address signs of photodamage, and toxin addresses the dynamic wrinkles. It is necessary to know how to combine these techniques since although they can all be used alone, and in some rare cases may be competitive, their evolution leans towards their tremendous complementarities, and their combination enables us to obtain results that are increasingly complete and increasingly convincing [3, 12, 20].

The first and the third characterizing signs of the aging neck remain, that is, the

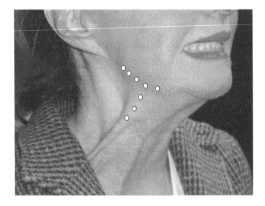

Figure 15.5 Position of injection points with 2U onabotuliumtoxin per point for the so called "Nefertiti lift". Courtesy Dr. K. De Boulle, Belgium.

appearance of platysmal bands and the loss of definition of the mandibular edge.

This is certainly the best indication at the neck for botulinum toxin. As described earlier, the platysma, a flat muscle, loses its homogeneity with age and its fibers assemble into clusters to form platysmal bands. Between these bands, empty spaces or loosely dense fibers are found, creating gaps in the flat surface of the platysma. Understanding these changes with aging is the basis for understanding the treatment with botulinum toxin and mastery of the technique [3, 10, 11].

Relaxation of the muscle fibers of the platysma bands enables their reduction or even disappearance, as they no longer congregate in bands, barring the neck vertically, but on the contrary, integrate with the relief and the slope of the neck, softening the cervical line.

The indications are:

- Necks with mild sagging but with new or marked bands, whether at rest or with movement.
- Another excellent indication is as a complement to a facelift.

In fact, with cervical cutaneous-fatty tissue sagging – the first indication for a surgical facelift – interventions targeting the platysma bands may be incomplete even in the hands of talented surgeons, and even if the result on the cutaneous ptosis itself is excellent.

This is where the role for botulinum toxin lies, in relaxing these bands and thereby reducing them or even making them disappear. This surgery–botulinum toxin combination is the demonstration of our adage "Optimization not Opposition" between techniques [3, 12, 20].

The literature on treating platysmal bands is quite divergent on techniques of injecting, dosing per platysmal band, total dosing for the neck, and patient outcome and overall satisfaction [10, 13, 17, 18, 21–24].

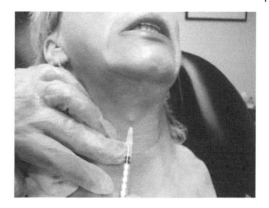

Figure 15.7 Injecting botulinum toxin for platysmal bands perpendicular to the skin and raising a bleb. Courtesy Dr. K. De Boulle, Belgium.

The technique of treating the platysmal bands is simple:

1. Visualize and mark the platysmal bands at rest and in the dynamic state by a forced cervical contraction.
2. In stages, inject a small dose of botulinum toxin (e.g., 2 U of onabotulinumtoxin or an equivalent of abobotulinumtoxin or incobotulinumtoxin [15, 16, 19, 25, 26]) or every 2 cm along the length of these cords, being careful to begin very high near the bony mental or mandibular edge.
3. The injection must be strictly subcutaneous so that the diffusion occurs in the muscle. To avoid deep diffusion, the injection should under no circumstances be submuscular. The best option is to raise a bleb upon injection, as in an intradermal test. If injecting by pinching the cord between the thumb and index finger, be careful not to inject between the two muscular sheets folded as a sandwich (since in this case, there will be five layers: skin–muscle on the thumb side and submuscular space–muscle and skin on the index finger side) (Figures 15.7 and 15.8).
4. The injection must cover the entire length of the platysmal band, with an injection every 2 cm [13, 16, 18, 21].
5. Preferably relax all the platysmal bands, because if only some bands or a part of some bands are relaxed, the non-relaxed

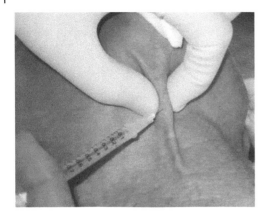

Figure 15.8 Alternative injection technique: beware of submuscular injection.

Keep in mind what we described earlier. There may be empty gaps at intervals of muscular fibers, since the fibers are clustered together to form the bands. In this instance, the injection is bound to occur deep in the submuscular spaces, with all the adverse effects and dangers that this can engender. In any case, injecting between the cords has no benefit, since the toxin is ineffective on the other signs (cutaneous sagging of the neck and horizontal cervical wrinkles) [4, 5, 8] (Figure 15.9a, b).

8. The follow-up is generally uncomplicated, with the odd bruising or ecchymosis [17].

areas can become hypertonic and hyperactive in a reflex manner, attempting to compensate for the relaxed parts. This is true for all muscles (the frontalis muscle provides the best example: when only the median part is relaxed, the lateral part can become hypertonic, producing a "Mephisto effect") [3, 7, 11].

6. Refrain from using massive total doses in the neck area (e.g., a total of 40–60 U of onabotulinumtoxin or an equivalent of abobotulinumtoxin or incobotulinumtoxin) [13, 14, 19, 27]. Several recent publications have recommended a maximal dose of 50 U for the global neck treatment [15, 16].

7. Be careful if injecting between the platysmal bands in the middle of the platysma.

Loss of Definition of the Mandibular Edge

This is the first sign of cervicofacial sagging. The oval of the face is less well outlined due to a mild ptosis at the mandibular edge that comprises the horizontal branch of the lower jaw and the angle of the jawbone. A hint of jowls also begins to form. The mandibular edge is thus not as well covered by the integument, which then covers its bony relief, namely the muscular plane of the platysma and the cutaneous fatty tissue, due to their displacement by gravity [4, 11, 19].

A beneficial effect on the definition of the mandibular edge can only be obtained in very moderate cases, and it is essential to distinguish muscular looseness from sagging of the integument. In the early stages, a result

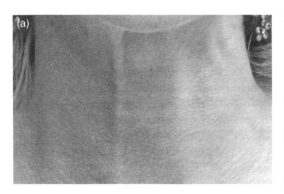
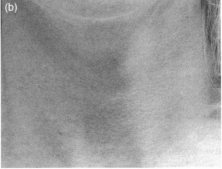

Figure 15.9 (a) Unilateral platysmal band before treatment at max contraction. (b) Result 1 week after injection of 12 U onabotulinum toxin in unilateral platysmal band. Courtesy Dr. K. De Boulle, Belgium.

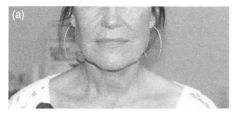
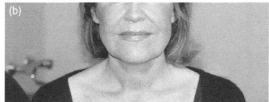

Figure 15.10 (a) Before treatment at rest. (b) After treatment with onabotulium toxin at rest. Courtesy Dr. K. De Boulle, Belgium.

that is certainly an improvement may be obtained, but it results from the relaxation of the platysma muscle by the botulinum toxin (Figure 15.10 and Figure 15.11).

In the moderate or marked forms, however, a facelift effect can never be achieved, since the cutaneous fatty tissue sagging dominates. For cases of more advanced definition loss and more sagging, this technique can only be considered for individuals not ready nor eligible for neck surgery, requesting an adjuvant to previous neck surgery, or requesting minimal or no downtime [10, 17, 24, 27].

How can this beneficial effect be explained? There are two possible explanations:

- The posterior and lateral fibers of the platysma cover the mandibular edge and are inserted higher up at the labial commissure, the skin of the mid-cheek, and also entwine with the fibers of the risorius muscle. The increased resting tone related to aging therefore lowers these cutaneous insertion areas and consequently results in a depressant effect on the lower part of the face. This depressant effect associated with

cutaneous sagging due to aging will also lower the area relative to the mandibular edge, leading to the loss of definition of the oval at this level. Relaxation by botulinum toxin will have the opposite effect: by lifting these cutaneous insertion sites, the cutaneous area at the mandibular edge will also rise and consequently this mandibular edge will be better outlined through a better application of the muscular-cutaneous cover on the bony relief, providing a better definition of the oval of the face [12, 19].

- The second explanation also starts with the principle of the increased resting tone and consequent shortening of the vertical muscle fibers. The muscular-cutaneous cover, which is made up of the skin and the platysma, integrates the natural curve of this anatomical area of the upper neck, that is, opposite and below the mandibular edge. Shortening of the platysma tightens it like the string on a bow, preventing this muscle from applying itself to the relief of the curve and submandibular space. Therefore, by relaxing the platysma muscle at this level, its fibers are lengthened, allowing

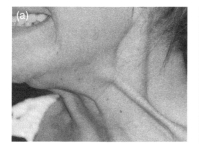
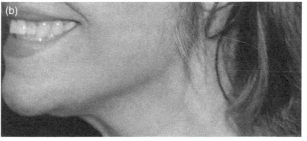

Figure 15.11 (a) Before treatment at max contraction. (b) After treatment with onabotulium toxin upon max contraction. Courtesy Dr. K. De Boulle, Belgium.

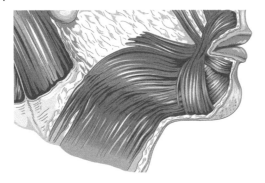

Figure 15.12 The posterior and lateral fibers of the platysma cover the mandibular edge and are inserted higher up at the labial commissure.

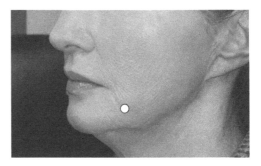

Figure 15.13 Injection point for m. depressor anguli oris with botulinum toxin. Courtesy Dr. K. De Boulle, Belgium.

better integration of the relief of the curve and space of this submaxillary depression (Figure 15.12).

The injections are made every 2 cm on a line situated 1 cm below the horizontal branch of the mandible. The injection must be very superficial, subdermally, without ever injecting through the platysma, to avoid deep diffusion. Somewhere between three and six injection points of a small dose of botulinum toxin (e.g., 2 U of onabotulinumtoxin or an equivalent of abobotulinumtoxin or incobotulinumtoxin [21, 25, 26]) are generally sufficient for each side. The platysma generally stops at the angle of the jaw, so there is no need to inject behind this point.

Why is it often beneficial to combine the relaxation of the depressor anguli oris with that of the platysma? Because they have certain synergistic actions. As discussed, the fibers of the platysma are inserted midcheek but also extend to the labial commissure and entwine with the DAO fibers (Figure 15.14). Thus, the platysma is a depressor for the inferior part of the face, as well as for the angle of the mouth in synergy with the DAO. Therefore, it is better to relax all the muscles that are responsible for a function, to avoid an increased reactive tone in muscles that were not or only partially relaxed.

Inject twice the dose of botulinum toxin per point compared to the platysmal band injections (e.g., 4 U of onabotulinumtoxin or an

equivalent of abobotulinumtoxin or incobotulinumtoxin [21, 25, 26]):

- subcutaneously and superficial to the DAO, avoiding excess depth, so as not to pass through the DAO risking to address the depressor labii inferioris
- 1 cm above the mandibular edge, avoiding going too high and then risking diffusion towards the orbicularis labii muscle
- 2 cm behind its anterior edge, that is, 2 cm behind the line of the labial commissure, so as not to risk diffusion medially, beyond the anterior edge of the DAO, towards the depressor labii inferioris muscle (Figure 15.13).

Patient Selection

Although there are no clear guidelines on proper patient selection to ensure a successful outcome with neurotoxin injection to the neck, most experts in the field agree on a few key principles [15, 16, 28, 29]:

- Treatment should be considered only for patients with satisfactory skin elasticity of the neck. Therefore, younger patients tend to see more improvement with the treatment.
- Patients with minimal drooping of submental fat see more marked improvements (Figure 15.15).
- Patients should have retained laxity in the platysma muscle. To assess this feature, the

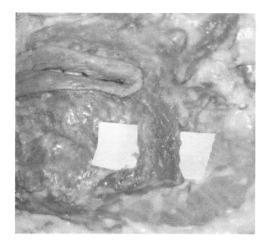

Figure 15.14 Dissection by L. Belhaouari and F. Lauwers., Department of Anatomy Toulouse University, France. *Source*: Reproduced from Ref. [3] courtesy L. Belhaouari; © 2013.

patient is asked to contract the platysma muscle; an ideal candidate will have loss of the mandibular border with platysma contraction [15].

Preventing Complications and Side Effects

The follow-up is uncomplicated, and ecchymosis is very rare. Side effects are minimal and are related to the motor function of the platysma muscle with exertion, particularly during forced inspiration. The resulting discomfort can be avoided by being cautious in initial treatment and thus reducing on the total quantity of toxin injected. Complications to the neck are essentially the risks of diffusion in deeper layers. Diffusion beneath the platysma muscle may be related either to

the mere fact of injecting too deeply, or to a too high total dose. [13–16, 24].

Overdose

The total must not exceed 40–60 U of onabotulinumtoxin or an equivalent of abobotulinum or incobotulinumtoxin for an entire neck [13–16, 21, 30]. We have learned that the first indication for botulinum toxin in the neck is the relaxation of platysmal bands, and to a lesser degree the beginning of loss of definition of the mandibular edge. There is therefore, at least to our knowledge, no need to strive to treat confirmed cervical sagging (the "Botulinum Toxin Facelift" does not exist), or horizontal "accordion" wrinkles on the neck. Doing so would be completely useless, and would risk increasing the injected doses and inflicting the risk of overdose.

Injecting too Deeply

This is obviously a technical error. We should recall the two items described earlier. First, between the platysma bands in the middle of the platysma muscle, there may be open gaps of muscular fibers since the fibers are clustered together to form the bands. An injection at this level does not meet the muscular barrier and is mandatorily deep in the submuscular spaces. Second, if injecting the platysma bands from laterally by pinching between the thumb and index finger, be careful not to inject between the two muscular sheets folded as a sandwich (since in this case, there will be five layers: skin–muscle on the thumb side and submuscular space–muscle and skin on the index finger side). The

Figure 15.15 *Source*: Reprinted courtesy L. Belhaouari from Ref. [1]; © 2006, L. Belhaouari.

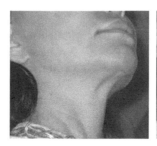
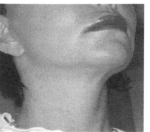

injections thus must be very superficial, sub-dermally, without ever passing through the platysma.

What are the Risks of Deep Diffusion?
[10–14, 16, 18, 21, 24, 27, 30, 31]

- Posture and static cervical support defect from weakening of the muscle tone, particularly in the case of diffusion towards the sternocleidomastoid. This can lead to neck tightness and difficulties in bending the neck.
- On the other hand, the platysma is contributing to bending the head forward. Too aggressive relaxation might result in the inability to bring the head forward.
- Smile discomfort.
- Risks of dysphagia, salivary insufficiency, from diffusion to the infra-hyoid muscles.
- Difficulty swallowing.
- Respiratory function disorders.

Serious Adverse Events are Extremely Rare

Rare cases of dysphagia, swallowing difficulties, speech disorders, false alimentary routes or respiratory disorders resulting in potentially fatal inhalation pneumonia have been described. These cases were reported in medical treatments, therefore at high therapeutic doses after injection in points other than the platysmal cervical musculature, in patients presenting with excessive muscular weakness. It is therefore not a risk in aesthetic indications and at doses used in cosmetic treatment. As such, we should not provide cosmetic treatment to patients with any suspicion or history of this type of disease [16, 31].

Conclusion

There are multiple techniques for addressing the signs of cervicofacial aging, and the development of techniques increasingly clearly favors the mildest treatments, keeping in mind their efficacy and their safety. A subtle mix of these factors will direct our indications for treatment. For the neck, botulinum toxin currently has benefits, but does not have the level of efficacy that can be seen in other areas in the face. It is nevertheless fantastic to treat platysmal bands and early loss of the mandibular edge without having to resort to more invasive surgical procedures, and to complement these surgical procedures, which remain the first indication for sagging and ptosis of the neck integument. Our art is to be audacious while remaining cautious, to maintain our credibility and the trust of our patients.

References

1 Noel S. La Chirurgie Esthétique: Son Rôle Social. Masson: Paris, 1926

2 Nahai F. The Art of Aesthetic Surgery. Quality Medical Publishing: Saint Louis, MO, 2005.

3 Belhaouari L, Gassia V. L'art de la toxine botulique et des techniques combinées en Esthétique; éditions Arnette Wolters Kluwer, France, 2013.

4 Hoefflin S. Anatomy of the platysma and lip depressor muscles. A simplified mnemonic approach. Dermatol Surg 1998;24: 1225–1231.

5 Hoefflin S The platysma aponeurosis. Plast Reconstr Surg 1996;97:1080.

6 Mitz V, Peyronie M. The superficial musculo-apeuronotic system (SMAS) in the parotid and cheek area. Plast Reconstr Surg 1976;58:80–88.

7 Belhaouari L, Gassia V, Lauwers F. Muscular balance and botulinum toxin. Ann Chir Plast Esthet 2004;49:521–526.

8 Cardoso de Castro C The value of anatomical study of the platysma muscle in cervical lifting. Aesthetic Plast Surg 1984; 8:7–11.

9 Mejia J, Nahai F, Nahai F, Momoh A. Isolated management of the aging neck. Semin Plast Surg 2009;23:264–273.

10 Gassia V, Beylot C, Béchaux S, Michaud T. Botulinum toxin injection techniques in the lower third and middle of the face, the neck and the décolleté: the "Nefertiti lift". Ann Dermatol Venereol. 2009;136(Suppl 4): S111–S118.

11 Kane M. The functional anatomy of the lower face as it applies to rejuvenation via chemodenervation. Facial Plastic Surg 2005;21:55–64.

12 Sclafani A, Kwak E Alternative management of the aging jawline and neck Facial Plastic Surg. 2005;21:47–54.

13 Fagien S, Raspaldo H. Facial rejuvenation with botulinum neurotoxin: an anatomical and experiential perspective. J Cosmet Laser Ther 2007;9(Suppl 1):23–31.

14 Lowe N, Yamauchi P. Cosmetic uses of botulinum toxins for lower aspects of the face and neck. Clin Dermatol 2004;22: 18–22.

15 Levy PM. Neurotoxins: current concepts in cosmetic use on the face and neck–jawline contouring/platysma bands/necklace lines. Plast Reconstr Surg 2015 Nov;136(5 Suppl): 80S–83S.

16 Raspaldo H, Niforos FR, Gassia V, et al. Lower-face and neck antiaging treatment and prévention using onabotulinumtoxin A: the 2010 multidisciplinary French consensus – part 2. J Cosmet Dermatol 2011 Jun;10(2):131–149.

17 Kane M. Nonsurgical treatment of platysmal bands with injection of botulinum toxin A. Plast Reconstr Surg. 1999;103(2):656–663.

18 Carruthers J, Fagien S, Matarasso S, et al. Consensus recommendations on the use of botulinum toxin type A in facial aesthetics Plast Reconstr Surg 2004;114:1S–22S.

19 Levy PM. The 'Nefertiti lift': a new technique for specific re-contouring of the jawline. J Cosmet Laser Ther 2007;9(4): 249–252.

20 Prado AS, Parada F, Andrades P, et al. Platysma chemical dénervation with botox

before neck lift. Plast Reconstr Surg 2010 Aug;126(2):79e–81e.

21 Asher B, Talarico S, Cassuto D, et al. International consensus recommendations on the aesthetic usage of botulinum toxin type A (Speywood Unit – part II: wrinkles on the middle and lower face, neck and chest. J Eur Acad Dermatol Venereol. 2010;24:1285–1295.

22 Brandt FS, Bellman B. Cosmetic use of botulinum A exotoxin for the aging neck. Dermatol Surg. 1998;24(11):1232–1234.

23 Brandt FS, Boker A. Botulinum toxin for rejuvenation of the neck. Clin Dermatol 2003;21:513–520.

24 Carruthers J, Carruthers A. Botulinum toxin A in the mid and lower face and neck. Dermatol Clin 2004;22:151–158.

25 De Boulle K. Botulinum neurotoxin type A in facial aesthetics Expert Opin Pharmacother 2007;8:1059–1072.

26 De Boulle K, Fagien S, Sommer B, Glogau R. Treating glabellar lines with botulinum toxin type A-hemagglutinin complex: A review of the science, the clinical data, and patient satisfaction. Clin Intervent Aging 2010;5:101–118.

27 Dayan SH, Maas CS. Botulinum toxins for facial wrinkles: beyond glabellar lines. Facial Plast Surg Clini North Am 2007; 15(1):41–49

28 Prager W, Bee EK, Havermann I, et al. IncobotulinumtoxinA for the treatment of platysmal bands: a single-arm, prospective proof-of-concept clinical study. Dermatol Surg 2015 Jan;41 Suppl 1: S88–S92.

29 Liew S. Discussion: microbotox of the lower face and neck: évolution of a personal technique and its clinical effects. Plast Reconstr Surg 2015 Nov;136(5 Suppl): 101S–103S.

30 Atamoros F. Botulinum toxin in the lower one third of the face. Clin Dermatol 2003 Nov–Dec;21(6):505–512.

31 Klein A. Complications, adverse reactions and insights with the use of botulinum toxin. Dermatol Surg 2003;29:549–556.

16

Correction of Facial Asymmetry

Scott Rickert, MD (FACS),[1] Lesley F. Childs, MD,[2] and Andrew Blitzer, MD (DDS, FACS)[3]

[1]Attending Physician, Assistant Professor of Otolaryngology, Pediatrics, and Plastic Surgery, NYU Langone Medical Center, New York, USA
[2]Attending Physician, Assistant Professor of Laryngology, Neurolaryngology, and Professional Voice, UT Southwestern, Dallas, TX
[3]Director, NY Center for Voice and Swallowing Disorders; Senior Attending Physician, St. Luke's/Roosevelt Hospital; Professor of Clinical Otolaryngology, Columbia University College of Physicians and Surgeons, New York, USA

Introduction

The facial nerve is the most commonly paralyzed nerve in the human body [1]. This impairment can be significant, as the seventh cranial nerve is not only responsible for facial expression, but also eye protection, lacrimation, oral competence, salivation, taste, and sensation. The constancy of facial expression is universal and cross-cultural. Without the ability to make meaningful facial expression, individuals can become socially isolated and emotionally unwell. The list of possible etiologies for facial nerve paralysis is extensive and most commonly include trauma, Bell's palsy, and iatrogenic and idiopathic causes [1].

Assessment

Several different methods exist for assessment of facial nerve impairment. None of the current instruments have been shown to sufficiently and reliably assess all the different types of facial asymmetry, including facial paralysis, focal partial facial weakness, and synkinesis. Thus, in assessing facial asymmetry, one must use the appropriate instruments for the condition of the patient.

The House–Brackmann system is the most widely used [2] (Table 16.1).

While the House–Brackmann scale is useful for gross quantifications of facial function, it does not reliably assess synkinesis or partial facial function well.

The Facial Clinimetric Evaluation (FaCE) scale is a 15-item instrument used to assess facial impairment and disability. It has been deemed a reliable and valid instrument for most facial asymmetries, but does not address synkinesis adequately.

The Synkinesis Assessment Questionnaire (SAQ) [3] is a nine-item instrument found to be valid and reliable for the assessment of synkinesis but does not adequately address more global facial asymmetries (Figure 16.1).

Question 9 is not used in the scoring of SAQ.

Treatment

In caring for patients with facial nerve weakness, protection of the eye is of the utmost importance. Specifically, the goal is to protect the cornea from irreversible complications that could lead to blindness. Lubrication strategies such as ophthalmic drops, ophthalmic ointment, taping the eyelid at night, and the use of a moisture chamber help to prevent ocular complications.

There are many surgical procedures that are used to address the asymmetric face. The

Table 16.1 The House–Brackmann system.

Grade	Description	Characteristics
I	Normal	Normal facial function in all nerve branches
II	Slight	*Gross:* Slight weakness on close inspection, slight synkinesis *At rest:* Normal tone & symmetry *Motion:* Forehead: Good to moderate movement Eye: Complete closure with minimum effort Mouth: Slight asymmetry
III	Moderate	*Gross:* Obvious but not disfiguring facial asymmetry. Synkinesis is noticeable but not severe. May have hemi-facial spasm or contracture *At rest:* Normal tone & symmetry *Motion:* Forehead: Slight to moderate movement Eye: Complete closure with effort Mouth: Slight weakness with maximum effort
IV	Moderately severe	*Gross:* Asymmetry is disfiguring and/or obvious facial weakness *At rest:* Normal tone & symmetry *Motion:* Forehead: No movement Eye: Incomplete eye closure Mouth: Asymmetrical with maximum effort
V	Severe	*Gross:* Only slight, barely noticeable, movement *At rest:* Asymmetrical facial appearance *Motion:* Forehead: No movement Eye: Incomplete closure Mouth: Slight movement
VI	Total	No facial function

procedures generally are aimed at creating a balanced face at rest and in motion. At rest, upper eyelid gold weight placement and/or lower eyelid canthoplasty can help to address the asymmetric orbital region, and prevent drying of the cornea. Static facial slings as well as a standard rhytidectomy can help to provide static correction of lower and midface gross asymmetries at rest.

More dynamic solutions can help provide correction at rest and with motion. Muscle transposition using the temporalis or masseter muscle is one example of a dynamic sling. Nerve grafting and neurorrhaphy via end-to-end nerve anastomosis (typically great auricular or hypoglossal), jump grafting (typically as hypoglossal with sural or great auricular), interposition grafting, or cross-facial grafting can provide long-term

nerve innervation to areas lacking current innervation.

The recent advent and use of botulinum toxin as well as cosmetic fillers has provided a promising avenue for nonsurgical treatment of facial asymmetry, both major and minor.

With the vast variety of presentations of facial asymmetry, it is important to formulate a solution that is specific to the patient. The goal of creating a balanced face at rest and in motion must always be the essence of the treatment. This can be through a single modality treatment or a combination of surgical and/or nonsurgical treatments. An example of combination therapy can be shown in rehabilitation after acoustic neuroma resection with disturbance of the facial nerve function at surgery. The combination of a hypoglossal-facial nerve anastomosis

Synkinesis Assessment Questionnaire (SAQ)

Date:

Please answer the following questions regarding facial function, on a scale from 1 to 5, according to the following scale:

1 = seldom or not at all
2 = occasionally, or very mildly
3 = sometimes, or mildly
4 = most of the time or moderately
5 = all the time or severely

	Question	Score
1	When I smile, my eye closes	
2	When I speak, my eye closes	
3	When I whistle or pucker my lips, my eye closes	
4	When I smile, my neck tightens	
5	When I close my eyes, my face gets tight	
6	When I close my eyes, the corner of my mouth moves	
7	When I close my eyes, my neck tightens	
8	When I eat, my eye waters	
9	*When I smile, my lower lips are matched in position*	
10	When I move my face, my chin develops a dimpled area	

Total Synkinesis Score: Sum of Scores 1 to 9/45 × 100

Figure 16.1 The Synkinesis Assessment Questionnaire.

with botulinum toxin injections for synkinesis optimized the facial symmetry at rest and in motion [4].

Synkinesis

Botulinum toxin has proven to be most useful in those patients who develop aberrant regeneration of fibers after facial nerve injury. Synkinesis, which is the presence of unintentional motion in one area of the face produced during intentional movement in another area of the face, represents one of the most troubling sequelae of facial nerve paralysis. Synkinetic movements are not only socially debilitating, but also can be quite painful, with simultaneous spasm of multiple muscle groups. Commonly, synkinesis is oculo-oral, involving involuntary oral commissure movement with voluntary eye closure, or vice versa. Surgical intervention for synkinesis is extremely challenging due to the aberrant reinnervation, and yields mixed results at best.

The etiology of synkinesis is thought to be multifactorial, with evidence supporting the role of aberrant axonal regeneration as well as central involvement of facial nucleus hyperexcitability. Two types of synkinesis are typically described [5]. First is a synergistic synkinesis where movement on the affected side is similar to but more excessive than that on the unaffected side. Secondly is a paradoxical synkinesis, in which the secondary facial movement is in a direction antagonistic to normal facial movement [5]. Bajaj-Luthra *et al.* [6] quantitatively analyzed the patterns of synkinetic facial movements on both the affected and unaffected sides. One of the major focuses of facial movement revolves around an area known as the modiolus, where several facial muscles converge just lateral to the buccal angle and form a three-dimensional fibromuscular mass. Patients with oculo-oral synkinesis were noted to have increased modiolar motion during eye closure relative to controls. This motion was noted to be asymmetry with increased intensity in both the horizontal and vertical plane [6].

As mentioned earlier, most facial grading systems focus on facial impairment and disability (House–Brackmann system, FaCE scale), but do not reliably assess synkinesis as part of facial impairment. The recent advent of a validated SAQ [3], the patient-graded nine-item questionnaire focused on assessment of facial synkinesis, has allowed for more consistent and reliable evaluation of patients with synkinesis.

Several different nonsurgical therapies have been used to treat synkinesis. One of the earliest reported physiotherapy programs with consistent positive results for synkinesis rehabilitation has been mime therapy. This technique was originally developed in the Netherlands as a collaboration between clinicians and mime actors [7]. Today, the most common therapeutic modalities for the treatment of facial synkinesis include facial neuromuscular retraining and botulinum toxin administration, which can augment the retraining.

When initially evaluating a patient with synkinesis, it is crucial to note atypical features of synkinesis such as facial weakness, facial numbness, a decreased corneal reflex or any other cranial nerve abnormalities. In these clinical scenarios, a space-occupying lesion should be excluded with an imaging study, typically magnetic resonance imaging and/or angiography. If such a lesion is identified, neurosurgical consultation and further workup is warranted.

When botulinum toxin is used to help treat synkinesis, the goal is to weaken the abnormally stimulated facial musculature to allow for more symmetrical movement as well as postures at rest. The upper and lower face is treated at the same initial setting. Optimal dosing is decided on an individuated basis based upon the patient's active and passive facial symmetry. A thorough understanding of facial anatomy is crucial for a proper treatment technique. The zygomaticus muscles, levator angli oris, depressor angli oris, risorius, and the platysma are the most often injected muscles under electromyographic control [8].

The zygomaticus major muscle arises from the zygomatic bone in front of the zygomaticotemporal suture. The muscle descends obliquely and inserts into the angle of the mouth. This muscle draws the angle of the mouth backward and upward, as in laughing. The zygomaticus minor originates from the malar bone and inserts into the outer portion of the upper lip. It draws the upper lip backward, upward, and outward.

The levator angli oris arises from the canine fossa, just below the infraorbital foramen. These fibers insert into the angle of the mouth. The depressor angli oris arise from the oblique line of the mandible and insert into the angle of the mouth. The action of this muscle depresses the angle of the mouth, acting antagonistically to the action of the levator.

The risorius arises in the fascia over the masseter and passes horizontally forward, superficial to the platysma. It then inserts into the skin at the angle of the mouth. Its action retracts the angle of the mouth.

The platysma is a broad sheet arising from the fascia covering the upper parts of the pectoralis major and deltoid. The fibers cross the clavicle and proceed obliquely upward and medially along the side of the neck. The anterior fibers interlace, below and behind the symphysis menti, with the fibers of the muscle of the opposite side; the posterior fibers cross the mandible, some being inserted into the bone below the oblique line, others into the skin and subcutaneous tissue of the lower part of the face, many of these fibers blending with the muscles about the angle and lower part of the mouth. The platysma retracts and depresses the angle of the mouth [9].

Botulinum toxin is typically effective for 3–4 months after the injection. Patients receive follow-up treatment and injections as needed, typically on a 3- to 4-month schedule. To minimize side effects and adequately gauge response, additional or 'touch-up' treatments are typically deferred until the patient's following visit when a higher total dose can be used [5].

Asymmetry of Smile

Asymmetry of facial features can be balanced using strategically well placed injections of botulinum toxin. An asymmetrical smile, where the musculature on one side contracts at a different force than the other side, has a significant and overlooked impact on the patient's quality of life. Subtle differences are frequently noticed in the overall appearance of an unbalanced face. Similarly a 'gummy' smile, with too much lip retraction can make patients self-conscious as well. The elevators of the upper lip include the levator labii superioris, the levator labii superioris alaeque nasi, the zygomaticus major and minor, the levator anguli oris, and the risorius. The depressors of the lower lip include the depressor labii inferioris, mentalis, and platysma. Depending on the asymmetry, botulinum toxin injections to individual muscles can help balance the smile and decrease excess pull of the upper or lower lip. These injections are all carried out under electromyographic control [5] to minimize complications of poor injection placement.

Furthermore, if there appears to be a hollowing or flattening effect of the smile unable to be corrected by balancing injections on the opposing side, directed filling injections (calcium hydroxylapatite, fat) can be used to balance the asymmetry as well.

Asymmetry of Eyelids

Asymmetry of the eyelids or 'drooping' eyelids can be addressed with nonsurgically with small doses of botulinum toxin. Careful injection in the lower lid lateral to the mid-pupillary line helps to prevent the excess activity of the orbicularis oculi causing 'drooping' eyelids. This allows the lower lid to 'tighten' and correct minor asymmetries. When the 'drooping' is excessive, combination therapy of lower blepharoplasty with adjunctive botulinum toxin has been shown to be an effective treatment. It is important to perform a snap test of the lower eyelid prior to any intervention and ensure there is adequate tone of the eyelid. If the tone is inadequate, intervention may lead to blepharitis and/or epiphora.

Masseter Hypertrophy/ Reshaping of Face

Masseteric hypertrophy is commonly caused by bruxism, temporomandibular joint disorders, or a misaligned jaw and presents with local mandibular discomfort and a boxy facial appearance. Initial treatments of masseteric hypertrophy were surgical, but botulinum toxin is a very effective way to systematically decrease the hypertrophy. But chemically deinnervating the muscle under electromyographic control [8], over time the muscle begins to decrease in size – relieving local discomfort and correcting facial appearance. Unless the underlying cause of the hypertrophy muscle is fully addressed, repeated treatments of botulinum toxin are necessary to prevent further hypertrophy.

Paresis of the Face

Patients with unilateral facial weakness frequently note frustration in their inability to have a balanced face. Many physicians are reluctant to treat them symptomatically as they frequently recover their nerve function and the timeline for potential recovery is not always consistent. Although these patients are a "moving target" as they potentially recover, injections in the healthy (nonparetic) side of the face to balance the face are very effective and provide a great deal of relief to the patient while they wait for their recovery. It is recommended that the injections are not too aggressive but they should balance the asymmetry as seen on exam. The advantage of botulinum toxin is its effective time frame of 3–4 months – if there had been some interval recovery in the 3- to 4-month time frame, the facial balancing injections can be adjusted accordingly to continue to have a balanced, symmetric face. In conjunction with botulinum toxin injections, local filling materials (calcium hydroxyapatite, or polylactic acid) can help balance the face. Particular areas of need include the naso-labial crease on the more functional side as well as minor corrections in symmetry of the mouth and eyebrows.

Disorders of Lipodystrophy

Disorders of lipodystrophy include congenital and acquired disorder of lipodystrophy. Currently, the predominant cause of lipodystrophy is associated with the use of highly active antiretroviral therapy (HAART) in the treatment of HIV. It typically presents with loss of fat from the face and can give an appearance of sunken eyes and prominent cheekbones. While changing the HAART regimen has been shown to improve symptoms in some patients [10], most need treatment for their change in facial appearance. Local filling materials such as calcium hydroxylapatite, or poly-L-lactic acid can be used to help careful address of the area of wasting. It is important to attempt to create adequate facial symmetry while individualizing each patient's treatment.

Complications of Facial Botulinum Toxin Injections

Several complications can arise from facial musculature administration of botulinum toxin. As always, it is important to have an experienced medical professional who has an excellent grasp of facial anatomy to obtain the best results from administration of botulinum toxin. Since the toxin is typically effective for 3–4 months, any complications will last a similar amount of time but will dissipate as the toxin does.

Injection of botulinum toxin below the orbital rim can lead to diffusion of the toxin into the levator muscle of the upper lid leading to upper lid ptosis. It is possible to help stimulate Muller's muscle with a sympathomimetic eye drop such as Apraclonidine 0.5% or 1.0% drops (1 drop tid) while waiting for the toxin to dissipate.

Excessive toxin in the musculature around the eye may result in muscular weakness and a decreased blink. If untreated, an exposure keratitis may develop over time. Treatment of exposure keratitis is typically frequent use of ophthalmic artificial tear solution, ointment, and/or a temporary patch over the eye for protection.

Injection of botulinum toxin in the lower face superficially may lead to local diffusion into the nasolabial fold and cause a local flattening of the fold. If this effect is strong enough, it may lead to an asymmetric smile. This is correctable over time by using smaller doses on future visits and/or balancing the facial asymmetry by injecting toxin into the unaffected side. Also, one can inject filling materials such as hydroxyapatite crystals or fat to correct localized facial asymmetry and remedy contour variations that may result from injection of botulinum toxin [8].

Excessive toxin in the perioral region may result in lip weakness or oral incompetence. This would manifest itself as intermittent drooling or escape of food and drink during meals. Injection deep to the platysma in the anterior neck may result in dysphagia or hoarseness. Dietary modification may be needed in cases of severe dysphagia.

There have been reported cases of immune resistance to botulinum toxin (either A or B). This can be tested in individuals by injecting a small dose in the glabellar region and seeing if it effectively smooths the horizontal rhytids in the area. If there is no noted effect from the initial injection, one should try the other type of botulinum toxin (A or B). Frequently those with some immune resistance to one type of botulinum toxin do not have resistance to the other type.

Case Presentations

The two cases presented below illustrate some of the challenges of each case and the need to individualize treatment, whether it is single modality or combination treatment.

Case 1

A 66-year-old woman presents after a hemorrhagic midbrain cerebrovascular accident

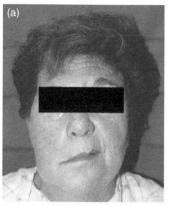 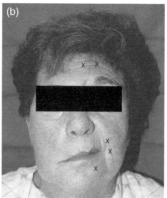 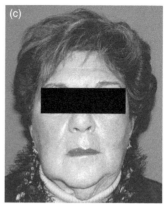

Figure 16.2 (a) Preoperative photograph; (b) planned intervention overlaying photograph (black x, botulinum toxin injection sites); (c) 2-month postoperative photograph.

with right facial paralysis. To treat her appropriately she underwent a combined treatment of surgical and nonsurgical interventions. She first underwent static reconstruction with a gold weight to the right upper eyelid, a right sided static sling, and a right sided browlift. She also underwent a hypoglossal-facial nerve anastomosis. This was followed botulinum toxin injections to the left face (left frontalis, left levator anguli oris, left zygomaticus, and left depressor anguli oris) to create symmetry to the face (Figure 16.2).

paralysis. To treat her appropriately she underwent a combined treatment of surgical and nonsurgical interventions. She first underwent surgical reconstruction of the facial nerve with a sural nerve interposition graft. This was followed by injection of botulinum toxin into the three grossly asymmetric muscles – right risorius, right levator anguli oris, and right zygomaticus. A small amount of local filling material (calcium hydroxapatite) is also used to equilibrate the asymmetric nasolabial folds (Figure 16.3).

Case 2

A 50-year-old woman presents after blunt trauma to the left face with left facial nerve

Conclusion

Correction of facial asymmetry is a complicated issue and depends greatly on the

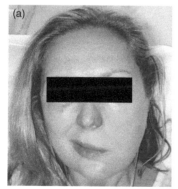 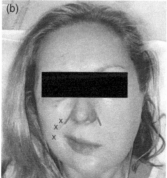 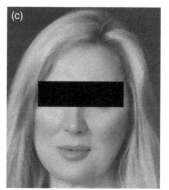

Figure 16.3 (a) Preoperative photograph; (b) planned intervention overlaying photograph (black x, botulinum toxin injection site; blue areas. area of placement of filling material); (c) 6-month postoperative photograph after further botulinum toxin injection/filler.

condition of the individual patient. Each patient must be thoroughly evaluated and include aspects of facial symmetry, weakness, wasting, synkinesis, and potential recovery. Each patient's treatment should be individualized as monotherapy or combination therapy (surgical and/or nonsurgical) and handled by professionals with excellent knowledge of facial anatomy. Above all the goal in cases of facial asymmetry is to create a balanced, symmetric face at both rest and in motion.

References

1 Clark JM, Shockley WW. Management and reanimation of the paralyzed face. facial plastic and reconstructive surgery. In Papel ID (Ed.) *Facial Plastic and Reconstructive Surgery* (pp 660–685). New York, NY: Thieme Medical Publishers, Inc., 2002.

2 House JW, Brackman DE. Facial nerve grading system. Otolaryngol Head Neck Surg. 1985;93:146–147.

3 Mehta RP, WernickRobinson M, Hadlock TA. Validation of the Synkinesis Assessment Questionnaire. Laryngoscope 2007 May;117(5):923–926.

4 Laskawi R. Combination of hypoglossal-facial nerve anastomosis and botulinum toxin injections to optimize mimic rehabilitation after removal of acoustic neurinomas. Plast Reconstr Surg 1997 April;99(4):1006–1011.

5 Neely JG, Cheung JY, Wood M, *et al.* Computerized quantitative dynamic analysis of facial motion in the paralyzed and synkinetic face. Am J Otol 1992 Mar; 13(2):97–107.

6 Bajaj-Luthra A, VanSwearingen J, Thornton RH, *et al.* Quantitation of patterns of facial movement in patients with ocular to oral synkinesis. Plast Reconstr Surg 1998 May;101(6):1473–1480.

7 Beurskens CH, Heymans PG. Positive effects of mime therapy on sequelae of facial paralysis: stiffness, lip mobility, and social and physical aspects of facial disability. Otol Neurotol 2003 Jul;24(4): 677–681.

8 Blitzer A, Brin MF. Management of hemifacial spasm and facial synkinesis with local injections of botulinum toxin. Oper Tech Otolaryngol-Head Neck Surg 2004 June;15(2):103–106.

9 Gray H. *Anatomy of the Human Body*, 20th edn. New York, Bartelby.com, 2000.

10 Peterson S, Martins CR, Cofrancesco J Jr. Lipodystrophy in the patient with HIV: social, psychological, and treatment considerations. Aesthet Surg J 2008 Jul–Aug;28(4):443–451.

17

Complications and Diffusion

Matteo C. LoPiccolo, MD,[1] Farhaad R. Riyaz, MD,[1] and David M. Ozog, MD (FAAD, FACMS)[2]

[1] Henry Ford Health System, Department of Dermatology, Detroit, USA
[2] Chair, Department of Dermatology; C.S. Livingood Chair in Dermatology; Director of Cosmetic Dermatology, Henry Ford Hospital, Detroit, MI, USA

Introduction

Major or persistent unwanted effects from cosmetic botulinum toxin injection are extremely rare. This is due to the relatively short duration of action and natural reversal of the toxin effect. However, the practitioner who administers botulinum toxin for both on-label and off-label indications must still be extremely familiar with potential side effects and discuss them with his or her patient prior to treatment [1].

In general, complications can be categorized as those caused by an unintended direct pharmacologic effect of the toxin (a true side effect), those caused by improper technique when administering the toxin (such as improper placement or amount of the medication), and effects secondary to spread of the field effects of the toxin; termed "diffusion" by many clinicians. Injection-related and minor adverse events, major and systemic reactions, and lastly site-specific complications from injection of onabotulinumtoxinA (Botox®, Allergan, Irvine, CA), abobotulinumtoxinA (Dysport®, Medicis, Scottsdale, AZ), incobotulinumtoxinA (Xeomin®, Merz Pharma, Raleigh, NC) and rimabotulinumtoxinB (Myobloc®, Solstice, San Francisco, CA) will be discussed.

It is important to document any complications that arise after toxin injection for future dose and placement location adjustment, whether the patient or healthcare provider notices the undesired result. This strategy can improve patient satisfaction and over time will refine your injection technique.

Diffusion

Diffusion will be addressed comprehensively in a separate chapter, but due to its implication in many adverse events caused by botulinum toxin, it is briefly explained here.

Many clinicians have adapted the term diffusion to describe the field of muscular and eccrine gland effects exerted by an injection of botulinum toxin. Field effect spread occurs both horizontally to adjacent structures, and vertically to tissues superficial and deep to the original placement of toxin. The degree of diffusion seen with the injection of botulinum toxin may be influenced by several factors. Dilution of toxin and volume of injection may affect the area of toxin effects. While one study failed to show a difference in safety or efficacy with larger volume dilutions [2], other investigators observed up to a 50% greater area of effect on forehead lines with a fivefold greater dilution of toxin [3]. Higher dilutions have also been shown to lead to a greater incidence of adverse effects (such as eyebrow ptosis when treating glabellar

Botulinum Toxins: Cosmetic and Clinical Applications, First Edition. Edited by Joel L. Cohen and David M. Ozog.
© 2017 John Wiley & Sons Ltd. Published 2017 by John Wiley & Sons Ltd.
Companion Website: www.wiley.com/go/cohen/botulinum

rhytides), suggesting an increased diffusion of toxin with increased dilutions [4]. A recent study of abobotulinumtoxin effects on sweat glands suggests that the type of skin, location of injection, and increased activity of sweat glands all appeared to influence the field of effect [5]. Depth or volume of injection did not affect field size. Some authors suggest that manual manipulation of the treatment area may increase the extent of toxin diffusion [6].

Lastly, the scope of field effects cannot be directly generalized across all types of botulinum toxins. While there appears to be no difference in diffusion between onabotulinumtoxinA and abobotulinumtoxinA at a dose ratio of 1 : 2.5 U [7], a greater degree of diffusion with abobotulinumtoxin has been observed with 1 : 3, 1 : 4, and greater dosing ratios [8–11]. Additionally, botulinum toxin B has been shown to have a larger radius of effect compared to onabotulinumtoxinA in treating forehead wrinkles [12].

Complications and Adverse Reactions

Common Minor and Injection Site Reactions

The most common adverse events reported with the use of both botulinum toxin A (BoNTA) and botulinum toxin B (BoNTB) are injection-related, local, and self-limited. Localized pain, erythema, swelling, tenderness, bleeding, and bruising can be experienced at the injection site, with resolution occurring in minutes to days following the procedure (Figure 17.1). The degree of these effects varies with site and number

of injections. Pain can be minimized with intrafollicular orifice injection technique, use of bacteriostatic saline for toxin preparation, smaller gauged needles, and pretreatment with topical anesthetic or cryoanalgesia [13, 14]. Avoidance of nonsteroidal anti-inflammatory drugs, vitamin E, and aspirin 10–14 days prior to injection may decrease the extent of bruising [14]. For patients that are particularly susceptible to bruising, ice can be used before treatment as a vasoconstrictor. If bleeding occurs from an injection site, immediate pressure should be applied before continuing with the treatment. If bruising occurs, it can be treated with 595 nm pulsed dye laser with 10 mm spot, 10 ms pulse duration and 7 J/cm^2 [47].

Brief, self-limited headaches are also common following injections of the facial muscles [6, 15–17]. In one series, approximately 1% of 320 patients receiving BoNTA) injections experienced severe, debilitating headaches [18]. These are thought to be a result of immediate muscle spasm from injection prior to paralysis from toxin [39]. It may be helpful to avoid touching the needle to the deeper periosteal structures, keeping the injections more superficial just above or into the superior aspect of the muscle. Other minor reactions rarely reported include nasopharyngitis, skin tightness, respiratory illness, and flu-like symptoms.

Local injection site infections are exceedingly rare despite various reconstitution protocols and millions of injections annually. Reactivation of herpes simplex virus infection has rarely occurred, and herpes zoster virus reactivation after injection of botulinum toxin type A has also been reported [46].

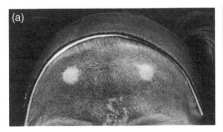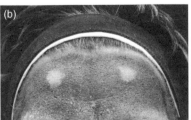

Figure 17.1 (a) Injection site erythema and (b) hematoma formation immediately following onabotulinumtoxin injection. Photograph courtesy of D. Hexsel, MD.

Fever, chest pain, chills, anxiety, dysgeusia, tinnitus, and peripheral edema have also been observed, although currently no evidence exists that these reported effects are conclusively linked to botulinum toxin [15, 16, 19]. Additionally, rimabotulinumtoxinB is associated with dry mouth, throat, and eyes, even in instances of injection at distant anatomic areas [19, 20].

Severe and Systemic Complications

As mentioned earlier, the therapeutic and cosmetic use of BoNTA and BoNTB has been generally safe and well tolerated, and most adverse effects are local and self-limited [6]. Systemic effects, while rare, have also been reported. Generalized muscle weakness known as asthenia, diplopia, blurred vision, ptosis, dysphagia, dysphonia, dysarthria, urinary incontinence, and dyspnea have been reported following the administration of both BoNTA and BoNTB [15, 16, 19].

Hypersensitivity reactions including urticaria, soft-tissue edema, and anaphylaxis leading to death (at a dose of 100 U onabotulinumtoxinA for cervical dystonia) have been reported with the use of onabotulinum toxin [48]. In the case of death from anaphylaxis, lidocaine was used as a diluent, and thus the causative agent cannot be conclusively identified. In patients with pre-existing cardiovascular disease being treated for noncosmetic purposes, death from arrhythmia and myocardial infarction have occurred [49]. In addition, new onset and recurrent seizures, syncope, and acute angle closure glaucoma have also been reported following onabotulinumtoxinA administration, although a direct causal relationship cannot be determined. Importantly, these severe and life threatening events have not been observed with the dermatologic use of up to 100 U at a time [15].

A variety of neuromuscular adverse events have ensued with the use of botulinum toxin as well. These symptoms may begin within days following the procedure and may persist up to 6 months. After the injection of 1400 U of abobotulinum toxin for axillary and palmar

hyperhidrosis, a case of "botulism-like syndrome" followed in which generalized muscle weakness, distant EMG muscle jitters, decreased cardiovascular reflex following deep breathing, diffuse asthenia, diplopia, mild bilateral ptosis, as well as decreased lacrimation, salivation, and sweating arose [21]. Generalized muscle weakness subsequent to injection of 250 U of abobotulinum toxin for cervical dystonia has also been reported [22, 23]. In both cases, large doses were used and generalized diffusion likely caused the reported effects. Pre-existing neuromuscular disorders including myasthenia gravis, amyotrophic lateral sclerosis, and Lambert–Eaton syndrome may increase the risk of developing botulism-like syndrome, and are thus contraindications to the use of botulinum toxin [17]. Should a patient experience botulism-like syndrome, intravenous anti-toxin should be administered as soon as toxicity is suspected. Multiple anti-toxins are available and dosing varies among preparations [24]. These treatments are not commercially available; they are reportedly kept frozen in discreet nationwide stockpile locations and must be approved for release by federal health officials.

Severe dysphagia has followed abobotulinumtoxinA administration for cervical dystonia. Aspiration may result from severe dysphagia and is a particular risk when treating patients in whom swallowing or respiratory function is already compromised [16]. This adverse outcome can persist for several weeks and may require the use of a feeding tube to maintain adequate nutrition and hydration. The adverse systemic effects seen with rimabotulinumtoxinB are similar to those seen with BoNTA, including botulism-like syndrome, severe respiratory compromise, and dysphagia [19].

Site Specific Complications

Forehead

Before injecting the forehead with botulinum toxin, it is best to examine the frontalis muscle in its full range of motion and map out any desired injection sites. This will help avoid improper placement of the toxin and associated adverse outcomes.

The most substantial complication encountered when treating the frontalis muscle for forehead lines is brow ptosis. This outcome is not only aesthetically unfavorable, but may produce a visual impairment that is temporarily debilitating to the patient. This commonly results from placement of the toxin too close to the eyebrow or when diffusion of the toxin occurs to the inferior portion of the frontalis. Thus, injections should be placed at least 2 cm above the brow or orbital rim and simultaneous paralysis of the brow depressors should be considered to minimize this risk [25]. Patient selection is also important in the avoidance of this effect; younger patients are preferred candidates for the treatment of upper forehead lines. Following injection of the frontalis, older patients and men may develop a redundant pocket of skin beneath the brow, termed pseudoptosis. If ptosis occurs, chemodenervation of the glabellar complex may reduce depressive forces and elevate the medial brow by 1–2 mm [25]. If the glabellar complex has already been treated with toxin, 1–2 U of onabotulinum toxin in the lateral orbicularis oculi may also elevate the lateral brow (Figure 17.2).

Care must also be taken that a "cockeyed" brow is not created when treating forehead lines. This occurs when the lateral fibers of the frontalis are not adequately paralyzed in relation to the medial aspect of the muscle, leading to cephalad movement of the lateral portion of the brow. This effect may be seen unilaterally or symmetrically, where it is termed the "Nicholson" brow for its similarity to actor Jack Nicholson's naturally elevated lateral brow. This is best avoided by ensuring that the lateral forehead injections are placed lateral to the iris. If it occurs, a small amount of toxin (1–3 U onabotulinum) may be injected into the lateral fibers of the frontalis to lower the brow to an even position. This should be injected 2 cm above the brow as the original medial injections should have been. Larger amounts of toxin may overcorrect the defect, leading to an overly depressed or "hooded" lateral brow, which may partially cover the eye [25].

Glabella

The most concerning complication of BoNTA and BoNTB injection of the glabellar complex is upper eyelid ptosis, which in early studies occurred in 0.8% to 9.0% of injections (Figure 17.3) [4, 25–29]. The current rate of this complication is much lower than 1%, due to both lower amounts of toxin used in these areas and more superficial injection techniques. This occurs because of diffusion of the toxin through the orbital septum leading to paralysis of the upper eyelid levator palebrae superioris and superior tarsal

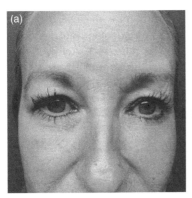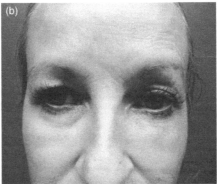

Figure 17.2 (a) Right eyelid ptosis following onabotulinumtoxin injection of the right frontalis muscle. (b) Partial resolution following 2 U onabotulinumtoxin to the lateral orbicularis oculi.

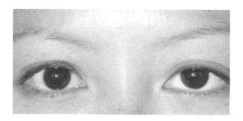

Figure 17.3 Left eyelid ptosis following onabotulinumtoxin to the glabella. Photograph courtesy of A. Carruthers, MD.

muscle [6]. It is more commonly caused when injecting the lateral corrugator just above the pupil in some patients. This effect may be avoided by keeping the injection medial to the mid pupillary line. As this portion of the corrugator inserts directly into the dermis, injections of only 1–2 mm deep are sufficient for desired treatment effect, and are unlikely to cause spread to the deeper structures in the orbit.

In the rare instance that lid ptosis develops, it begins between 2 and 10 days following injection, and may persist for 2–4 weeks. The degree of ptosis may be mild upon awakening but becomes progressively more pronounced throughout the day, eventually causing visual impairment. Such events are more common in older individuals, as the orbital septum may be thin or absent. It has also been reported in patients with a history of surgery in this area including brow lifts. Any prior surgery in this area may change predictable patterns of diffusion. Patients with a baseline ptosis or redundant eyelid skin may depend on frontalis action to fully open the eye and should be identified prior to treatment. Caution is warranted when considering glabellar injection for these patients.

A patient complaining of "heavy eyebrows" is likely experiencing eyebrow ptosis. This is another commonly reported complication. Interestingly, the incidence of brow ptosis has been shown to decrease with successive treatments of the glabella [28, 29]. Injections should be placed at least 1 cm above the orbital rim for corrugator treatment and 2 cm above the rim for frontalis treatment. Small

volumes should be used to minimize diffusion. It is also important to avoid injecting toxin into the eyebrow lateral to the inner canthus, as this may also increase the likelihood of ptosis. Additionally, patients should be instructed to avoid manipulation of the injected area and to actively contract the glabellar complex [6].

Patients who choose to apply ice to the treated area to minimize potential bruising should do so by holding pressure in an upward direction rather than massaging the area, which promotes diffusion. Alpha-adrenergic agonist eye drops including apraclonidine 0.5% and phenylepherine 2.5% may be used to treat eyelid ptosis should it occur. These agents cause contraction of the adrenergic Muller's muscle of the upper eyelid, leading to 1–2 mm of elevation of the lash margin [25]. Drops should be applied at three times daily for symptomatic improvement until the ptosis resolves, which is usually in 1–6 weeks [30]. Bruising may occur from injections in this region, but much less commonly than bruising in the peri-orbital area. Rarely, lid swelling, forehead rigidity, and forehead muscle spasms occur from administration of botulinum toxin into the glabella [4, 26, 28, 31–33]. Diagonal lines along the nasal sidewall (bunny lines) may also develop, which can easily be treated with 3–5 U of (onabotulinum) toxin in the medial aspect of the proximal nasal sidewall.

Compared to injections of botulinum toxin into other facial sites, headaches may be more common with injections into the glabella. Unlike the previously mentioned 1% overall rate of postinjection headache, 11% of botulinum patients and 20% of placebo patients reported headache in the Botox Glabellar Lines II Study Group [34].

Periorbital Lines

Several untoward affects may occur when administering BoNTA for cosmetic improvement of periocular rhytides. This region is the most likely to develop bruising following injection, as numerous superficial veins in the area are susceptible to injury [25, 33, 35].

The injections in this area should be kept superficial similar to a bleb from a PPD injection, thus avoiding deeper structures which may not be visible to the naked eye. Adequate lighting is key, and vein imaging may be considered to decrease the risk of vessel puncture [50].

Treatment of crow's feet lines may also lead to excessive skin folding atop the zygomatic arch. While itself aesthetically unpleasing, this may also lead to an exacerbation of zygomaticus lines as the redundant skin gravitates downward. Pre-assessment of skin laxity prior to injecting this area is key, and patients with considerable scleral show, excessive skin beneath the eye, or a slow snap test of the lower eyelid may be more likely to have an unfavorable result. Festooning, or bagginess of the infraorbial skin, has been reported after treatment of this area perhaps due to inhibition of the lymphatic muscle pump [51]. Bruising may be avoided by minimizing the number of injection sites, and injecting the toxin in a series of superficial blebs [25]. Icing the area pre- and postinjection will also constrict vessels and minimize bruising. If an early bruise is visible, the application of direct pressure and treatment with a 595-nm vascular laser may be used to minimize spread and expedite resolution [36]. In instances where the patient has a history of significant bruising or cannot tolerate any bruise, for example due to an upcoming social commitment, a small bleb of lidocaine with epinephrine may be placed at the site 10 minutes prior to injection to induce vasoconstriction.

Diffusion of toxin is also of concern in this periorbit. Diffusion inferiorly to the zygomaticus major may interfere with lip upturning and lead to an asymmetric smile and flaccid cheek. Likewise, diffusion inferior-medially to the orbicularis oculi may cause a lower ectropion. Lastly, medial diffusion may lead to paralysis of the lateral rectus muscle, producing a temporary but debilitating diplopia [25]. The above complications are best eluded by placement of injections no less than 1 cm beyond the orbital margin, staying superficial as the zygomaticus muscle lies deep to the orbicularis oculi, and avoiding the inferior margin of the zygoma. If diplopia occurs, patching of the affected eye can provide symptomatic relief and is needed for 7–10 weeks following symptom onset [37]. Other options include prismatic lenses or intentional paralysis of the contralateral medial rectus. An ophthalmology referral should be considered.

In addition to the adverse effects discussed above, the use of botulinum toxin B for periocular rhytides has been reported to cause mild to severe dry mouth and dry eyes. The average onset is roughly 12 days from injection, with symptoms persisting for nearly a month [38].

Upper and Lower Lip

While lip rhytides respond well to botulinum toxin treatment, clinicians should be cautious with its use in this area. Incompetence of the oral sphincter, flaccidity of the cheek, asymmetry of the smile and difficulty with speech may easily result from over dosage and diffusion of toxin, and overtreatment of the orbicularis oris muscle (Figure 17.4). Patients should be warned regarding these potential issues. Injections should be placed superficially and in a symmetrical pattern. Some authors recommend using a large-volume dilution to assure uniformity in toxin spread [25]. Treatment should be initiated at a low dose (0.5–1 U abobotulinum toxin per injection site, to a maximum of 4 sites), which may

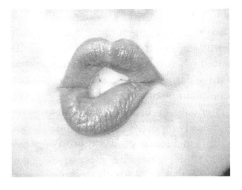

Figure 17.4 Asymmetric lower lip following perioral onabotulinumtoxin injection. Photograph courtesy of A. Carruthers, MD.

then be titrated up to the desired effect during subsequent sessions if necessary. Despite these techniques, some individuals find difficulty in whistling and forming "s" and "p" sounds for days-to-weeks following the injection. Singers, musicians, and others who rely on fine perioral muscle dexterity should be counseled on these effects and are not good candidates for this procedure. Lastly, flattening of the upper vermillion may occur, which is easily corrected with the addition of dermal filler [25].

Cheek and Chin

Treatment of the depressor anguli oris (DAO) to elevate the corners of the mouth may be complicated by diffusion of toxin to the obicularis oris, leading to an incompetent oral sphincter or flaccid cheek. Injections of the DAO should be made at the angle of the jaw posterior to the nasolabial fold and small doses should be used to best prevent these effects [25]. The depressor labii inferioris (DLI) may also be affected, leading to an asymmetric smile (Figure 17.5). When this occurs, 2 U of (onabotulinum) toxin may be injected into the opposite DLI to restore symmetry.

The mentalis is also commonly treated to alleviate chin clefts, folds, and lines. One must avoid injecting directly into the mental fold in these cases, as this may easily produce an incompetent mouth or asymmetric

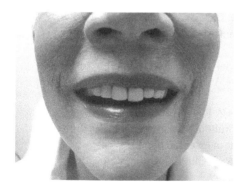

Figure 17.5 Asymmetric smile following 2 U of onabotulinumtoxin to the depressor anguli oris, with inadvertent toxin affects to the left depressor labii inferioris.

smile. Injections that are placed too laterally or superficially also can cause this issue [39]. Dosing should rarely exceed 6 U of onabotulinum toxin in this area [25, 40].

Platysmal Bands and Horizontal Neck Lines

The platysma may be treated with botulinum toxin to alleviate prominent vertical bands and horizontal neck lines [24]. Initially it was felt that large doses of toxin were needed for successful chemodenervation of this relatively large muscle: some authors reported the use of up to 200 U per session [41]. Such high doses of botulinum toxin in this area may have significant, potentially life-threatening adverse effects. The spread of toxin A or B to the deep muscles of deglutition in the larynx can lead to dysphagia [24]. Neck weakness may develop as a function of direct injection of the sternocleidomastoid, trapezius, or splenius capitus muscles, diffusion of toxin to the strap muscles, or a combination of these effects [42]. Uncommonly, respiratory distress and death have been reported following botulinum toxin injection in the neck [15, 16, 19, 25]. It has been found that lower doses are equally effective as the initially reported high doses, with a lower incidence of side effects. Superficial injection and the use of smaller doses of toxin (starting with 6–8 U of onabotulinum per platysmal band, and titrating upward to effect) are advised to decrease the risk of these complications [25, 40].

Less common sequelae from injecting in this area include edema, erythema, ecchymosis, muscle soreness, and neck discomfort. Bruising was the most common side effect in one series of BoNTA use, occurring in less than 20% of the patients. Less than 10% of patients reported transient, mild neck discomfort occurring 2–5 days after the treatment [24].

Hyperhidrosis

Treatment of palmar hyperhidrosis with 50–100 U of onabotulinum (and respective equivalents of abobotulinumtoxinA and rimabotulinumtoxinB) has been associated with decreased handgrip strength and finger power [10, 43]. This likely occurs secondary to diffusion of the toxin to the underlying musculature. This effect is transient, with subjective grip strength and finger power reductions lasting approximately two weeks. A small study comparing onabotulinum to abobotulinum in a 1 : 4 dosing ratio for palmar hyperhidosis suggests that this effect may be more frequently experienced with the latter preparation [10]. No direct comparison has been made at alternate dosing ratios, however. Dry mouth and dry throat are adverse events experienced with botulinum toxin B for palmar hyperhidrosis, but not routinely with BoNTA [20]. Some clinicians regard injection with botulinum toxin B in the palm to be more painful to their patients than injection with BoNTA, although a recent study found the injection of rimabotulinumtoxinB to be as painful as placebo [20].

Superficial placement of toxin may help prevent these effects when treating the palm. Treatment should be limited to one hand per session due to these risks-bilateral loss of grip strength may cause significant disability [25]. In patients who have experienced this effect, decreasing the injected dose placed directly above the thenar eminence should be considered during subsequent treatments [43]. Other common adverse reactions seen with injection of BoNTA and BoNTB into the palms include self-limited and localized tingling, pain, and numbness [44].

Patients treated for axillary hyperhidrosis have experienced localized itching with a mean duration of two to three weeks, and compensatory sweating in other areas lasting up to 12 weeks [43, 45]. Compensatory sweating is comparatively less severe than the preceding condition as it generally does not deter patients from seeking future treatments.

In summary, adverse effects from botulinum toxins are infrequent and can be minimized with careful injection technique and knowledge of the local anatomy. Fortunately, most events are transitory in nature and can be easily managed by the astute clinician.

References

1 Korman JB, Jalian HR, Avram MM. Analysis of botulinum toxin products and litigation in the United States. Dermatol Surg 2013;39(11):1587–91.

2 Hankins CL, Strimling R, Rogers GS. Botulinum A toxin for glabellar wrinkles. Dose and response. Dermatol Surg 1998; 24(11):1181–83.

3 Hsu TS, Dover JS, Arndt KA. Effect of volume and concentration on the diffusion of botulinum exotoxin A. Arch Dermatol 2004;140(11):1351–54.

4 Carruthers A, Carruthers J, Cohen J. Dilution volume of botulinum toxin type A for the treatment of glabellar rhytides: does it matter? Dermatol Surg 2007; 33(1 Spec No.):S97–S104.

5 Hexsel DM, Soirefmann M, Rodrigues TC, do Prado DZ. Increasing the field effects of similar doses of *Clostridium botulinum* type A toxin–hemagglutinin complex in the treatment of compensatory hyperhidrosis. Arch Dermatol 2009;145(7):837–40.

6 Carruthers A, Kiene K, Carruthers J. Botulinum A exotoxin use in clinical dermatology. J Am Acad Dermatol. 1996; 34(5 Pt 1):788–97.

7 Hexsel D, Dal'Forno T, Hexsel C, Do Prado DZ, Lima MM. A randomized pilot study comparing the action halos of two commercial preparations of botulinum toxin type A. Dermatol Surg. 2008;34(1): 52–9.

8 Nussgens Z, Roggenkamper P. Comparison of two botulinum-toxin preparations in the treatment of essential blepharospasm. Graefes Arch Clin Exp Ophthalmol. 1997; 235(4):197–9.

9 Ranoux D, Gury C, Fondarai J, Mas JL, Zuber M. Respective potencies of Botox and Dysport: a double blind, randomised, crossover study in cervical dystonia.

J Neurol Neurosurg Psychiatry. 2002;72(4): 459–62.

10 Simonetta Moreau M, Cauhepe C, Magues JP, Senard JM. A double-blind, randomized, comparative study of Dysport vs. Botox in primary palmar hyperhidrosis. Br J Dermatol. 2003;149(5):1041–5.

11 Trindade de Almeida AR, Marques E, de Almeida J, Cunha T, Boraso R. Pilot study comparing the diffusion of two formulations of botulinum toxin type A in patients with forehead hyperhidrosis. Dermatol Surg. 2007;33(1 Spec No.): S37–S43.

12 Flynn TC, Clark RE, 2nd. Botulinum toxin type B (MYOBLOC) versus botulinum toxin type A (BOTOX) frontalis study: rate of onset and radius of diffusion. Dermatol Surg. 2003;29(5):519–22; discussion 22.

13 Lewis T, Jacobsen G, Ozog D. Intrafollicular orifice injection technique for botulinum toxin type A. Arch Dermatol. 2008;144(12):1657–8.

14 Carruthers J, Fagien S, Matarasso SL. Consensus recommendations on the use of botulinum toxin type a in facial aesthetics. Plast Reconstr Surg. 2004;114(6 Suppl): 1S–22S.

15 Allergan. [9/5/2010]. Available from: http://www.allergan.com/assets/pdf/botox_cosmetic_pi.pdf.

16 Medicis. [9/5/2010]. Available from: http://www.dysport.com/prescribinginformation.html.

17 Hexsel D, Spencer JM, Woolery-Lloyd H, Gilbert E. Practical applications of a new botulinum toxin. J Drugs Dermatol. 2010; 9(3 Suppl):S31–S7.

18 Alam M, Arndt K, Dover J. Severe, intractable headache after injection with botulinum A exotoxin: report of 5 cases. J Am Acad Dermatol 2002;46:62–5.

19 Solstice. [9/5/2010]. Available from: http://www.myobloc.com/hp_about/PI_5–19–10.pdf.

20 Baumann L, Slezinger A, Halem M, Vujevich J, Mallin K, Charles C, et al. Double-blind, randomized, placebo-controlled pilot study of the safety and efficacy of Myobloc (botulinum toxin type B) for the treatment of palmar hyperhidrosis. Dermatol Surg. 2005;31(3): 263–70.

21 Tugnoli V, Eleopra R, Quatrale R, Capone JG, Sensi M, Gastaldo E. Botulism-like syndrome after botulinum toxin type A injections for focal hyperhidrosis. Br J Dermatol. 2002;147(4):808–9.

22 Bakheit AM, Ward CD, McLellan DL. Generalised botulism-like syndrome after intramuscular injections of botulinum toxin type A: a report of two cases. J Neurol Neurosurg Psychiatry. 1997;62(2):198.

23 Bhatia KP, Munchau A, Thompson PD, Houser M, Chauhan VS, Hutchinson M, et al. Generalised muscular weakness after botulinum toxin injections for dystonia: a report of three cases. J Neurol Neurosurg Psychiatry. 1999;67(1):90–3.

24 Matarasso A, Matarasso SL, Brandt FS, Bellman B. Botulinum A exotoxin for the management of platysma bands. Plast Reconstr Surg. 1999;103(2):645–52; discussion 53–5.

25 Klein AW. Complications, adverse reactions, and insights with the use of botulinum toxin. Dermatol Surg. 2003; 29(5):549–56; discussion 56.

26 Ascher B, Zakine B, Kestemont P, Baspeyras M, Bougara A, Santini J. A multicenter, randomized, double-blind, placebo-controlled study of efficacy and safety of 3 doses of botulinum toxin A in the treatment of glabellar lines. J Am Acad Dermatol. 2004;51(2):223–33.

27 Carruthers A, Carruthers J. Botulinum toxin type A for the treatment of glabellar rhytides. Dermatol Clin. 2004;22(2): 137–44.

28 Klein AW, Carruthers A, Fagien S, Lowe NJ. Comparisons among botulinum toxins: an evidence-based review. Plast Reconstr Surg. 2008;121(6):413e–22e.

29 Moy R, Maas C, Monheit G, Huber MB. Long-term safety and efficacy of a new botulinum toxin type A in treating glabellar lines. Arch Facial Plast Surg. 2009;11(2): 77–83.

30 Beer K, Cohen JL, Carruthers A. Cosemetic uses of botulinum toxin A. In: Ward AB, Barnes MP, editors. Clinical uses of botulinum toxins. Cambridge: Cambridge University Press; 2007. p. 328–248.

31 Carruthers A, Carruthers J, Flynn TC, Leong MS. Dose-finding, safety, and tolerability study of botulinum toxin type B for the treatment of hyperfunctional glabellar lines. Dermatol Surg. 2007; 33(1 Spec No.):S60–S8.

32 Sadick NS, Faacs. Botulinum toxin type B for glabellar wrinkles: a prospective open-label response study. Dermatol Surg. 2002;28(9):817–21.

33 Lew H, Yun YS, Lee SY, Kim SJ. Effect of botulinum toxin A on facial wrinkle lines in Koreans. Ophthalmologica. 2002;216(1): 50–4.

34 Carruthers JD, Lowe NJ, Menter MA, Gibson J, et al. Botox Glabellar Lines II Study Group. Double-blind, placebo-controlled study of the safety and efficacy of botulinum toxin type A for patients with glabellar lines. Plast Reconstr Surg 2003;112:1089–98.

35 Lowe NJ, Lask G, Yamauchi P, Moore D. Bilateral, double-blind, randomized comparison of 3 doses of botulinum toxin type A and placebo in patients with crow's feet. J Am Acad Dermatol. 2002;47(6): 834–40.

36 Karen JK, Hale EK, Geronemus RG. A simple solution to the common problem of ecchymosis. Arch Dermatol. 2010;146(1): 94–5.

37 Aristemodeu P, Watt L, Baldwin C, Hugkulstone C. Diplopia associated with the cosmetic use of botulinum toxin A for facial rejuvenation. Ophthal Plast Reconstr Surg 2006;22:134–6.

38 Baumann L, Slezinger A, Vujevich J, Halem M, Bryde J, Black L, et al. A double-blinded, randomized, placebo-controlled pilot study of the safety and efficacy of Myobloc (botulinum toxin type B)-purified neurotoxin complex for the treatment of crow's feet: a double-blinded, placebo-controlled trial. Dermatol Surg. 2003;29(5):508–15.

39 Vanaman M, Fabi SG, Carruthers J. Complications in the Cosmetic Dermatology Patient: A Review and Our Experience (Part 1). Dermatol Surg. 2016; 42(1):1–11.

40 Carruthers JD, Glogau RG, Blitzer A. Advances in facial rejuvenation: botulinum toxin type a, hyaluronic acid dermal fillers, and combination therapies—consensus recommendations. Plast Reconstr Surg. 2008;121(5 Suppl):5S–30S; quiz 1S–6S.

41 Brandt FS, Bellman B. Cosmetic use of botulinum A exotoxin for the aging neck. Dermatol Surg. 1998;24(11):1232–4.

42 Jankovic J, Brin MF. Therapeutic uses of botulinum toxin. N Engl J Med. 1991; 324(17):1186–94.

43 Schnider P, Moraru E, Kittler H, Binder M, Kranz G, Voller B, et al. Treatment of focal hyperhidrosis with botulinum toxin type A: long-term follow-up in 61 patients. Br J Dermatol. 2001;145(2):289–93.

44 Lowe NJ, Yamauchi PS, Lask GP, Patnaik R, Iyer S. Efficacy and safety of botulinum toxin type a in the treatment of palmar hyperhidrosis: a double-blind, randomized, placebo-controlled study. Dermatol Surg. 2002;28(9):822–7.

45 Naumann M, Lowe NJ. Botulinum toxin type A in treatment of bilateral primary axillary hyperhidrosis: randomised, parallel group, double blind, placebo controlled trial. BMJ. 2001;323(7313):596–9.

46 Graber EM, Dover JS, Arndt KA. Two cases of herpes zoster appearing after botulinum toxin type a injections. J Clin Aesthet Dermatol. 2011;4(10):49–51.

47 Morton LM, Smith KC, Dover JS, Arndt KA. Treatment of purpura with lasers and light sources. J Drugs Dermatol. 2013; 12(11):1219–22.

48 Li M, Goldberger BA, Hopkins C. Fatal case of BOTOX-related anaphylaxis?. J Forensic Sci. 2005;50(1):169–72.

49 Stähli BE, Altwegg L, Lüscher TF, Corti R. Acute myocardial infarction after botulinum toxin injection. QJM. 2011; 104(7):615–6.

50 Lowe NJ, Halliday D. Vein imaging laser reduces bruising in bruise-prone botulinum toxin injected patients. J Cosmet Laser Ther. 2016:1–3.

51 Goldman MP. Festoon formation after infraorbital botulinum A toxin: a case report. Dermatol Surg. 2003;29(5): 560–1.

18

Combination Therapy of Botulinum Toxin with other Nonsurgical Procedures

Amy Forman Taub, MD[1,2] and Lauren Fine, MD (FAAD)[3,4]

[1]*Director, Founder, Advanced Dermatology, LLC, Lincolnshire, USA*
[2]*Assistant Clinical Professor/Northwestern University Medical School, Chicago, USA*
[3]*Associate Dermatologist & Cosmetic Fellow, Advanced Dermatology, LLC, Chicago, USA*
[4]*Associate Dermatologist, Chicago Cosmetic Surgery and Dermatology, Chicago, USA*

Introduction

Most aesthetic practitioners combine treatments to achieve the best results for their patients. These combinations are myriad and difficult to study. In the medical world, it is rare for more than one drug to be studied concurrently, unless they have been combined into one drug (or are both made by the same company). In dermatology, the ingredients are often combined into one drug to increase compliance, reduce cost, and make it possible for the drug to be approved. In the aesthetic world things are no different. While there are many patients who only have one type of laser treatment, filler or toxin, it has become common for two or more to be performed simultaneously. Since botulinum toxin (BoNT) is the most commonly performed aesthetic treatment, it stands to reason that it would also be the most commonly combined with other treatments. One study combined BoNT with five different hyaluronic acid (HA) fillers into 13 areas of facial zones and resulted in 92.6% patient satisfaction 6 months after therapy [1]. Although it is intuitive that combining therapies will achieve better results, many investigators have attempted to understand and quantify these benefits. Herein we attempt to present the data on these combinations and try to put them into clinical perspective.

Fillers and Botulinum Toxin

Aging of the face is a complex, multifactorial process that results in rougher skin texture, increased laxity, decreased elasticity, dyschromia, telengiectasias, and the development of fine lines and wrinkles. Volume loss and muscle hyperactivity are also contributing factors to the aging process, resulting in concavities, and static and dynamic rhytides. Since dermal fillers restore volume while BoNT reduces muscle movement, combining therapies is an appealing option for rejuvenation of the aging face. Not all studies included in this chapter were performed with the same form of BoNT. It will be referred to throughout this chapter as BoNT, unless specifically referred to by their generic names (onabotulinum, abobotulinum or incobotulinum).

In one of the first studies examining the combined use of BoNT and soft tissue augmentation, Faigen and Brandt [2] found that patients who had BoNT injected 1 week prior to filler in deep glabellar furrows or lips experienced increased longevity of the hyaluronic acid. Two hypotheses for the cause of this increased longevity were suggested: (i) BoNT causes a reduction in the dynamic muscular component of wrinkle formation preventing attenuation of the material via repetitive muscular activity, and/or (ii) by inhibiting repetitive movement, the milieu for creating new collagen surrounding the implanted material was improved [3].

In another study focused on the glabellar area, 16 patients with severe glabellar rhytids at rest treated with both BoNT and a hyaluronic acid filler responded better than those treated with BoNT alone [4]. 94% of subjects injected with combination therapy had mild rhytides after therapy, whereas 0% of subjects treated with BoNT monotherapy achieved no or mild rhytides (Table 18.1). In a prospective randomized single-blinded study of 38 patients with moderate to severe glabellar rhytides, BoNT plus HA filler combination treatment improved outcomes both at rest and on maximum frown compared to HA filler alone [5]. Furthermore, the

Table 18.1 Combination treatments with toxins and fillers.

Authors	Study design/Methods	Evaluation schedule	Clinical results	Comments
Carruthers, Carruthers, & Maberley 2003 [4]	Retrospective study of 16 subjects treated with BoNT-A & Hylan B versus BTZ-A alone for glabellar rhytids; Responses assessed clinically and photographically	Before (Baseline) & After BoNT-A/ Hylan B treatment photographs	After BoNT-A alone none (0%) had achieved no or mild rhytids. After BoNT-A & Hylan B only 1 of 16 (6%) had moderate glabellar rhytids with the remainder (94%) being mild.	
Carruthers & Carruthers 2003 [5]	Prospective, randomized study of 38 subjects receiving BoNT-A & Restylane or Restylane alone for glabellar rhytids; Responses assessed clinically and photographically	Baseline and every 2 weeks for 32 weeks	Combined group showed better response at rest and maximum frown; response maintained for significantly longer (32 vs.18 wks). At week 16 response rates 95% vs. 83% (combination vs. BoNT-A alone)	Study limitations-no BoNT-A only arm.
Patel, Talmor, & Nolan 2004 [7]	Prospective, randomized study of 65 subjects receiving BoNT-A (22), Zyderm (20), or both (23) for glabellar rhytids; responses assessed using patient satisfaction scores and independent physician evaluation	Baseline, 1 week, 1 month, and 3 months	At all posttreatment visits combination group had greater improvement in wrinkle severity than either group alone (79% vs 56% & 50% at 1month)	

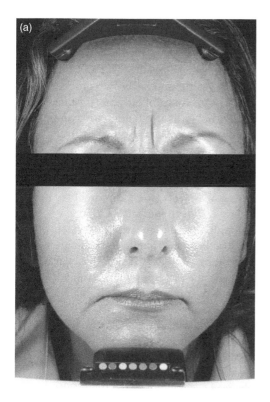 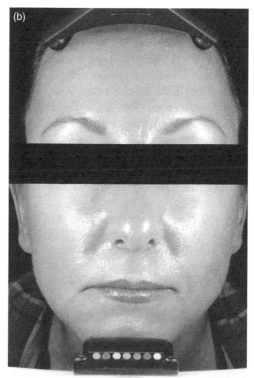

Figure 18.1 (a) Before treatment; (b) 3 weeks after one syringe HA to vertical glabellar furrows and 45 units of BoNT to glabella. *Source:* Courtesy of Amy Forman Taub, MD.

combination treatment nearly doubled the median duration of response compared with treatment with HA filler alone (32 weeks versus 18 weeks). Of note, this study did not include a BoNT only arm, so the effect of BoNT alone compared with combination treatment cannot be assessed (Table 18.1). In yet another split-face randomized control trial of 20 patients, half received BoNT in the glabella and the other half received BoNT and hyaluronic acid filler; 24 weeks after treatment, glabellar rhytides showed more improvement on the combination side than in the toxin only side [6]. Patel *et al.* found similar results [7]; 65 patients with moderate to severe glabellar rhytides received BoNT, collagen, or a combination of the two. After 1 month, subjects in the combination group demonstrated significantly greater improvement in furrows (79% versus 56% in BoNT alone and 50% in the filler group alone;

$p < 0.05$). Furthermore, the clinical effects were longer-lasting and patient satisfaction was higher in the subjects receiving both BoNT and collagen (Table 18.1).

The glabellar folds appear to be the most common area of the face to be treated with a combination of BoNT and filler (Figure 18.1). Monotherapy with BoNT alone is very effective in younger patients with primarily dynamic rhytids. With increasing photodamage and laxity, glabellar lines can become "etched" at rest and BoNT alone may be insufficient for full correction. If the number "1 or 11" vertical rhytid is obvious in the glabella without contraction, combination treatment (filling the vertical depressions 1–2 weeks after relaxing the muscles with BoNT) is usually necessary for full correction [8, 9]. In one experienced injector's experience [8, 10], about 15% of patients treated with the aforementioned protocol require maintenance with BoNT only and do not require further filling for 1–2 years. Pretreatment with BoNT allows for assessment of residual static rhytides after the toxin takes effect. According to the consensus recommendations put forth by the Facial Aesthetics Consensus Group (FACG) in 2008, BoNT is used in combination with filler in the glabellar area about 25 percent of the time [9]. In 73% of faculty combining treatments and staging treatments were reported in new patients, first injecting with BoNT and then with filler.

Although there is clear and ample evidence that combination of HA and BoNT in the glabellar area results in superior correction and longevity, extreme caution should be taken with filler injection in this area due to potential complications such as vascular occlusion leading to skin and tissue necrosis. These rare but serious complications can occur from inaccurate needle placement or applying too much pressure during injection [11–14]. Material should flow easily through the needle during injection of the glabella. Robust fillers (increased particle size or concentration used mainly for deep volume restoration), permanent or semi-permanent fillers should not be used here to avoid this complication. Injections should be relatively superficial. Hyaluronic acid fillers only are recommended in the glabella because hyaluronidase can be administered at the first sign of occlusion (blanching, pain or a sense of significant pressure on the part of the patient) and may alleviate the blockage and prevent ischemic necrosis of tissue. Injection of filler into the glabella is not FDA approved.

Shaping of the brow is another area particularly well suited for combination therapy with BoNT and filler. It is useful to view the brow region as a three-dimensional area. Brow ptosis is a common manifestation of the aging face and can inadvertently convey fatigue or disinterest. BoNT alone in the glabella of younger women will raise the brow approximately 1–2 mm [15]. Placement of BoNT in the lateral brow depressor will help lift the lateral brow, restoring a more defined arch [16]. Injection of filler into the lateral brow fat pad at the superior orbital rim will further augment the lateral brow lift and will anteriorly project the lateral brow contour, resulting in a more youthful brow. According to the FACG, BoNT is used alone to shape the brow area about 50% of the time [9]. Over 90% of this expert faculty group use filler in a subset of patients to replace volume in this area.

In the crow's feet area a combined approach has also been studied. In an open-label, nonrandomized pilot study by Beer, et al. [17], 20 subjects with mild to moderate temporal volume loss as well as glabellar and/or periorbital rhytids were studied. They received a combination of BoNT in the glabellar or periocular area as well as hyaluronic acid filler in the glabellar or temporal area. Although improvement declined at 3–9 months depending on whether toxin or filler were used, 64% of patients who had previously used toxin alone stated the results were superior with the combination. While all FACG faculty members continue to treat this area with BoNT, 80% of faculty members now use it in combination with filler to enhance malar volume [9]. Subcutaneous injection of filler inferior and lateral to the lateral canthus can augment a flat zygoma; combining BoNT to the crow's feet area simultaneously can further lift and reshape the upper cheek, ultimately achieving a more youthful zygoma [16]. Compared to the perioral region, filler in the cheek area lasts significantly longer since there is much less movement [17, 18]. When smile lines around the eyes extend medially to the malar cheek, BoNT alone should be avoided due to risk of affecting the infraorbital nerve and asymmetric smile, as well as lower lid ptosis. For the treatment of more medial malar smile lines all FACG faculty members use primarily hyaluronic acid fillers alone; fewer than 20% report occasional combination treatment in this area. The midportion of the obicularis oculi is a difficult area to treat. A small dosage of BoNT can be used to soften the palpebral part of the orbicularis oculi at the mid-pupillary line providing a prior snap test reveals good elasticity of the muscle. This can result in a more open eye, with the shape of the eye changing slightly from almond to round. This change in shape should always be discussed with the patient first. This is sometimes the first area that women in their twenties and early thirties notice rhytids. These rhytids cannot currently be corrected with available fillers due to the area being too superficial to get a natural looking result and the risk of Tyndall effect. Using toxin here for full relaxation of the muscle would lead to ectropion; however, use of filler in the tear trough may improve some infraorbital rhytides via stretch, analogous to the improvement in zygomatic cheek rhytides from cheek augmentation.

Another application of BoNT and filler combination is reshaping of the nasal dorsum and tip. The contour of the nasal tip can be affected by loss of volume as well as surgical depression or previous injury. Filler injection can result in elevation of the bridge of the nose and recontour of the tip. Injection of filler at the base of the columella can elevate the nasal tip. Small amounts of of BoNT to each side of the nasal spine area (levator labii superioris) and each lower nasalis (depressor septi nasi) can further improve the aesthetics of the nasal tip [9, 19]. Care must be taken in this area, as well as in the glabellar area, due to

reports of blindness after filler injections [20]. Although not limited to these areas alone, the highest risk of blindness is from the glabella, nose, and nasolabial fold.

The lower face is another area amenable to combination therapy. A helpful approach in treatment of this area is to view the area as a whole rather than as isolated regions [9]. While photodamage, textural changes, and loss of elasticity contribute to aging in this area, it is volume loss in the melomental folds and lips and the muscular contraction of the orbicularis oris that make this area so well suited for combination therapy. Repetitive contraction of the orbicularis oris is responsible for radiating perioral rhytides. The combined injection of BoNT into the depressor anguli oris, mentalis, and platysma removes the muscular depressor action of the lower face, thereby elevating the lateral oral commissures to a more relaxed, neutral position [21]. BoNT injection of the mentalis also ameliorates dimpling of the chin. The simultaneous addition soft tissue filler to buttress the mouth corners and prejowl sulcus will result in a more youthful appearance than with BoNT alone. The addition of volume to the prejowl sulcus softens the perception of jowls and gives the face a more oval and less rectangular orientation (Figure 18.2). Treating in multiple sessions on different days can be advantageous to reassess needs. To address vertical lip rhytides, injection of 4–8 U of onabotulinumtoxin in the upper lip

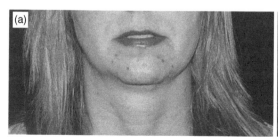
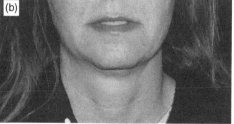

Figure 18.2 (a) Melomental folds mouth frown and puckered chin prior to BoNT to depressor anguli oris and chin hyaluronic acid filler to melomental folds and chin. (b) Postcombined treatment with BoNT and filler. *Source:* Courtesy of Amy Forman Taub, MD.

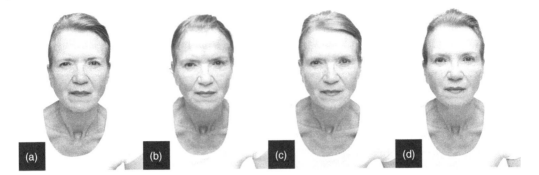

Figure 18.3 Cumulative effects of treatments on one woman's face. (a) Pretreatment; (b) after incobotulinumtoxinA; (c) after incobotulinumtoxinA + CaHA; and (d) after incobotulinumtoxinA + CaHA HA. *Source:* Fink 2014 [22]. Reproduced with permission of Matrix Medical Communications.

and 3–8 units in the lower lip can be used along with HA filler to enhance volume and help shape the vermillion border. Lastly, an important use of BoNT in the lower face is to treat asymmetric smiles. There may be different timing strategies for accomplishing this combination. Some may do on the same day, but it would be important then to inject the filler first and complete any manual massage before injecting BoNT. Once injected, toxin should not be manipulated as it may be spread to more distant areas and cause inadvertent effects.

A multiple treatment program with incobotulinumtoxin, calcium hydroxylapatite (CaHA) (Radiesse® Merz Pharmaceuticals GmbH, Frankfurt, Germany), and HA (Belotero®, Merz Pharmaceuticals GmbH, Frankfurt, Germany) was undertaken for 10 women to determine if their apparent age was reduced. The photographs were rated by each of 50 naïve judges based on age, health and attractiveness. The apparent age of all 10 women was statistically significantly improved in a stepwise fashion over the four-step treatment protocol [22] (Figure 18.3).

In late 2009, injectable poly-L-lactic acid (Sculptra®, Valeant) was approved by the US Food and Drug Administration (FDA) for the correction of shallow to deep nasolabial fold contour deficiencies and other facial wrinkles. Currently, there are no clinical trials examining the combination of BoNT with poly-L-lactic acid. In our experience, combining procedures has yielded similar results as compared with combined BoNT and HA filler (Figure 18.4). although there are no formal studies looking at this combination.

Current aesthetic thinking leads one to analyze the face as a complex 3-dimensional object: not only at rest but also in motion. It is a mistake to think of eradication of lines and creases as the end goal of aesthetic treatments. It appears that in selected areas of the face, a combination approach leads to a better and more lasting result for our patients. Neutralizing the rhytidogenic and/or depressor action of selected facial muscles while simultaneously or sequentially restoring lost volume are currently the primary tools the aesthetic surgeon has to create a balance that looks natural and harmonious in the aging face. Recent consensus recommendations confirm this vision [23].

Broadband Light Sources/ Nonablative Light-based Treatment and BoNT

Pulsed light (IPL) is a nonablative light-based technology used to effectively treat the dyschromia and telengiectasis associated with photoaging. Previous studies have

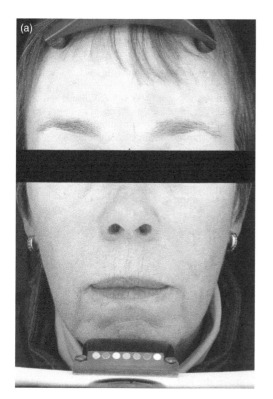 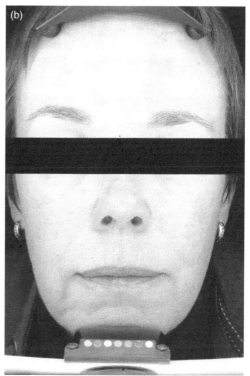

Figure 18.4 (a) Before treatment; (b) 6 weeks after one vial Sculptra® injections to cheeks, nasolabial folds, and melomental folds, and 4 U BoNT in vertical upper lip lines (as well as glabella and forehead). *Source:* Courtesy of Amy Forman Taub, MD.

shown that IPL alone can improve the appearance of facial rhytides [24–28]. The rationale behind combination broadband light therapy and BoNT chemodenervation is to more effectively and permanently treat facial rhytides commonly treated by either modality alone. There was also concern regarding energy-based devices potentially inactivating toxin when used in combination.

In 2004, Carruthers & Carruthers published the first prospective, randomized study of 30 patients comparing IPL treatment alone or in combination with BoNT for facial aging [29]. All subjects received full-face broadband light treatment; subjects assigned to the combination group also received 15 units of BoNT to the crow's feet of each side of the face. Compared with the IPL-only group, patents receiving both BoNT and IPL demonstrated improvements in crow's feet rhytides at rest and on maximum smile, as well

as a slight improvement in the appearance of telengiectasias, lentigines, apparent pore size, and skin texture. Their responses were assessed both clinically and photographically. These results suggest that both treatments may act synergistically to produce optimal facial rejuvenation [29, 30] (Table 18.2). Khoury *et al.* examined the effects of full-face IPL combined with intradermal injection of BoNT of the cheeks [31]. Patients in this study were treated with IPL plus eight 0.1-ml intradermal injections of onabotulinumtoxin in one cheek (8 U total) and eight injections of saline in the contralateral cheek. A significantly higher number of patients showed improvements in small wrinkles and fine lines with IPL plus toxin than IPL plus saline (93% vs 29% at week 4). A greater improvement in erythema was also noted on the combination side. Other factors such as hyperpigmentation, apparent pore size, texture, and overall

Table 18.2 Combinations of broad-band light or non-ablative laser with BoNT.

Authors	Study design/Methods	Evaluation schedule	Clinical results	Comments
Khoury, Saluja, Goldman 2008 [31]	Prospective, randomized, double-blind, split face study of 14 females all receiving standard IPL treatment along with BoNT injections to one cheek & saline in the other cheek; responses assessed photographically.	Baseline, 1 week, 4 weeks, 8 weeks	A significantly higher proportion of subjects showed improvement in small wrinkles and fine lines with IPL +BoNT than IPL+saline (93% versus 29%) at week 4.	BoNT-A & IPL side also achieved a greater degree of improvement in erythema. Other efficacy measures (hyperpigmentation, pore size, skin texture) showed comparable improvements with both regimens.
Carruthers & Carruthers 2004 [29]	Prospective randomized study of 30 women with crow's feet rhytids treated with BoNT-A & Broadband Light (BBL) versus BBL alone; responses assessed clinically and photographically.	Baseline, 3 wks, 6 wks, 9 wks, 12 wks, 18 wks, 26 wks	BoNT-A/IPL group experienced better response to treatment, both at rest and on maximum smile; combined group also had slightly improved response in associated lentigines, telangicatasia, pore size, facial skin texture.	Skin biopsies showed an increase in dermal collagen in each group. While BBL alone produced remarkable improvements in telangictasias, lentigines, and skin texture, the BoNT-A co-treatment increased these results by 15%.
Semchyshyn & Kilmer 2005 [32]	19 subjects received BoNT-A injections to either glabellar or crow's feet areas. One side of the treated area was treated with either VBeam Laser, SmoothBeam laser, CoolGlide laser, or an IPL or RF device within 10 min of BoNT-A injections; responses assessed photographically.	Baseline and 2–3 weeks posttreatment	No evidence of decrease in efficacy of BoNT-A denervation observed when glabellar or perioral areas were treated with VBeam Laser, SmoothBeam laser, CoolGlide laser, or an IPL or RF device within 10 min of BoNT-A injection.	First and only study to explore effects of combining BoNT-A and various non-ablative lasers and RF.

appearance were also measured, and showed no difference between the arms (Table 18.2). The idea that you would put an area "at rest" while you are "fixing it" is similar to a bone mending a fracture [29]. It is intuitive and one that patients understand when you explain it. These two studies, although small, suggest that there is a real scientific construct to this principle, but these results may be short-lived. According to the graphs presented in the Caruthers's paper, at 26 weeks the broadband light alone group seemed to have better resting results for rhytides (71% moderate and 29% mild) versus the combination group (92% moderate and 8% mild), with the success rate of 21% in rhytides at 26 weeks in IPL alone group and 0% improvement in the combo group [29]. In Khoury *et al*'s studies, the effect remained statistically significant into the eighth week when the study ended [31]. At the very least, one could use BoNT combination to get faster results with fine rhytides while the patient has to wait for the collagen production resulting from the heated fibroblasts takes place. The patient perception of better results in the early phases of treatment with nonablative photorejuvenation may encourage them to complete their series of treatments as well as continue any adjunctive skin care. It would be interesting to perform a study on patients who completed a series of nonablative treatments and had half of them continue their BoNT throughout one year then let it wash out versus those who discontinued it after the first treatment.

Semchyshyn & Kilmer evaluated whether the use of IPL immediately after BoNT injections had any effect on the efficacy of the chemodenervation [32]). Subjects received BoNT immediately prior (within 10 minutes) to laser rejuvenation. Pretreatment and 2-week posttreatment photos were compared, and no signs of decreased BoNT efficacy were demonstrated. Of note, this study also included subjects treated with BoNT and pulsed dye laser, long pulsed infrared laser, Nd:YAG 1064 long pulsed laser and monopolar radiofrequency device and found similar results (Table 18.2). More recently a retrospective study looking at combining microfocused ultrasound with BoNT and fillers affirmed the safety of the combinations [33].

To date, this is the only published work exploring BoNT in combination with these latter devices, their purpose being to demonstrate that energy based systems when applied immediately after BoNT does not inactivate the toxin nor increase side effects of either device. When combining energy based treatment and BoNT injections it is still probably better to treat with the energy based device first because the puncture wound and slight bit of dried blood may cause an area of increased absorption in the skin and hence an injury that could lead to a complication. One of the authors (AFT) typically waits 30 minutes after an energy based device treatment to allow the skin to cool, prior to injecting BoNT.

BoNT and Laser Resurfacing

Since the mid-1990s, laser resurfacing of the skin has revolutionized cosmetic dermatology. Ablative lasers such as the carbon dioxide and erbium:YAG laser selectively target water as the chromophore, precisely vaporizing the epidermis and superficial dermis, leading to profound wound healing and dermal remodeling. Besides improving skin texture and dyschromia, resurfacing addresses static rhytides by stimulating new collagen formation. Since BoNT treats dynamic rhytides, a combination of the two yields a global reduction of all rhytides. Combining BoNT denervation with laser resurfacing also prevents disruption of newly deposited dermal collagen due to a reduction of dynamic muscle activity [34].

There are numerous anecdotal reports of the benefits of combination therapy. Fagien reported "enhanced" laser results, particularly in the crow's feet region, in patients pretreated with abobotulinumtoxin before resurfacing [34, 35]. He theorized that BoNT pretreatment may improve the smoothing of newly resurfaced skin long enough to affect "more permanent eradication of wrinkles" [2, 34, 35]. West & Alster first reported on the effects of BoNT injections on movement-associated rhytids after CO_2 laser resurfacing [37]. Compared to a control group of patients receiving laser resurfacing alone, those receiving BoNT immediately following laser resurfacing were found to have greater and longer lasting improvement of the forehead, glabellar, and canthal rhytides (Table 18.3). Carruthers & Carruthers treated four female patients asymmetrically with BoNT-A before CO_2 laser resurfacing and found that patients were more satisfied overall with the pretreated side, however the degree of improvement and satisfaction was not quantified (Table 18.3). Furthermore, the recurrent crow's feet tended to be coarser, thicker, and more obvious in the non-pretreated side [37, 38]. Regular postoperative injections given every 6–12 months may prolong the effects of resurfacing [37–39].

Zimbler and colleagues went on to examine the effect of BoNT injection one-week prior to laser resurfacing with either CO_2 or erbium dual-mode laser [41]. In a prospective, randomized split-face trial of 10 patients, the pre-injected sites were found to have statistically significant greater improvement over the untreated sites. The results were clinically most significant in the crow's feet area (Table 18.3). For optimal results, the authors recommended continued maintenance with BoNT injections post –resurfacing. Lask *et al.* performed a split-face study on periorbital rhytides; one side received Er:YAG laser resurfacing with BoNT versus the contralateral side with Er: YAG resurfacing and saline injection [42]. At 12-week follow-up, the side treated with combination therapy demonstrated significantly greater improvement in the appearance of periorbital rhytides, texture, pigmentation, and other features of periorbital skin aging than the control side (Table 18.3).

As is the case with soft-tissue augmentation, BoNT should be given 1–3 weeks prior to resurfacing, thereby allowing the toxin to prevent muscle activity at the time of resurfacing [37, 39, 40]. By treating dynamic muscles prior to resurfacing, they will have less influence on the deposition and organization of newly remodeled collagen and elastic fibers and ultimately helps the remodeled dermis heal with a smoother surface topography [29, 41].

In recent years, fractional ablative and non-ablative resurfacing for skin rejuvenation has gained popularity due to fewer risks and reduced downtime compared to traditional resurfacing. The only published literature on this combination is a case report. Beer and Waibel reported on the synergism of BoNT and fractional resurfacing of rhytides in the cheek area in a single patient [43]. One day prior to laser treatment with a 1,540-nm fractional nonablative laser four injections of 1 U abobotulinum toxin into each cheek. Three treatments were conducted at 3-week intervals. Significant improvement of the radiating rhytides was noted after each treatment (Figure 18.5). Since this was not a split-face study, it is unclear what contribution was made by either component, although the accompanying photo demonstrates more improvement in cheek rhytides than would be expected with three nonablative resurfacing treatments, even with the highest energy settings.

Although there have been no large clinical double-blind studies performed comparing combination of laser resurfacing with and without BoNT, these cited studies point to an improvement in results of laser resurfacing with preceding BoNT, with the most proven effects observed in the periorbital area. In this author's experience, similar results using BoNT and other ablative resurfacing modalities such as the 2790 nm YSGG laser have been obtained (Figure 18.6). Although it seems intuitive that putting the skin to rest while it is creating new collagen would enhance and prolong the result, it would be beneficial to have more double-blind placebo controlled studies as well as clarification of the underlying molecular mechanisms.

Table 18.3 Combination of BoNT with laser resurfacing.

Authors	Study design/Methods	Evaluation schedule	Clinical results	Comments
West & Alster 1999 [37]	40 patients who had received full face CO_2 laser resurfacing were randomized to receive BoNT-A injections to glabella, forehead, or lateral canthal regions or no additional treatment; responses assessed clinically & photographically	Baseline and at 3, 6, & 9m	Enhanced and prolonged correction of movement-associated rhytids of the glabella, forehead, and lateral canthal region in the BoNT group vs non-BoNT treated pts.	
Zimbler *et al.* 2001 [41]	Prospective, randomized, blinded, split-face study of 10 female subjects comparing BoNT-A pretreatment (crows feet, forehead lines, glabellar frown lines) and laser resurfacing (CO_2 or erbium dual-mode laser) versus laser resurfacing alone; Responses assessed clinically and photographically	Baseline, 6 weeks, 3mo, 6mo	Sites pretreated with BoNT showed statistically significant improvement over the nontreated side, with crows feet region showing the greatest improvement.	For optimum results, continued Botox maintenance post-procedure is recommended. No difference between resurfacing modalities
Yamauchi, Lask, Lowe 2004 [42]	Prospective, randomized, placebo-controlled study comparing efficacy and safety of BoNT-A and periorbital Er:YAG resurfacing versus resurfacing alone in 33 subjects; responses assessed clinically and photographically	Baseline, 1 wk, 2 wks, 4 wks, 8 wks, 12 wks.	BoNT-treated side improved significantly more than placebo side in diminishing periorbital rhytids, textural, pigmentation, and other features of periorbital aging.	
Beer & Waibel 2007 [43]	Case report of fractional resurfacing of cheeks combined with BoNT-A to each cheek one day prior to first resurfacing session	3 treatment sessions, 3 weeks apart	Significant improvement of cheek rhytids noted after first laser treatment; improvement increased after second resurfacing session and was enhanced slightly after the third.	Specifically looks at cheek rhytids. Limitations – case report, no control

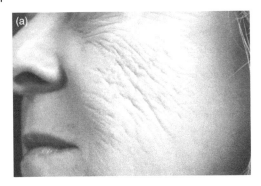 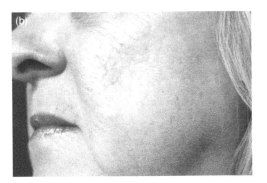

Figure 18.5 Left cheek (a) prior to and (b) following BoNT and fractional resurfacing. *Source:* Beer 2007 [43].

BoNT and Other Modalities – Chemical Peels, Chemabrasion, Cosmeceuticals

Chemical peels, topical medications, and various cosmeceuticals are additional options available for the aesthetic patient to improve their aging face. These are also frequently used in combination with BoNT, although again there are few controlled studies. In a multicenter clinical study led by Dr. Jody Comstock, 2,697 patients who were also undergoing various procedures such as abobotulinumtoxin, dermal fillers, nonablative and ablative laser treatments,

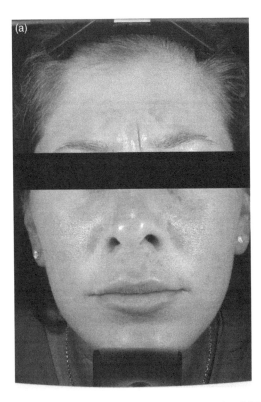 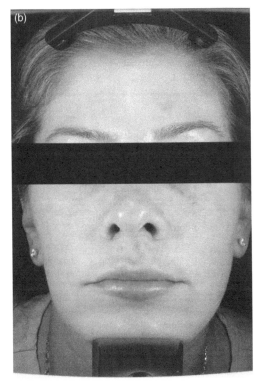

Figure 18.6 (a) Before treatment. (b) 2 weeks after full face Erbium:YSGG and 53 U of BoNT to glabella, forehead, and lateral brow depressors. *Source:* Courtesy of Amy Forman Taub, MD.

microdermabrasion, and chemical peels also applied a four-step tretinoin/hydroquinone treatment system for a mean of 4 weeks pretreatment and 6 weeks posttreatment [44]. Patient's demographics were typical of the antiaging market (95% females aged 35–65). Among the 239 patients that received BoNT and the topical regimen, improvements of at least 1 grade in sallowness, tactile roughness, hyperpigmentation, and fine periocular lines were observed in > 80% of patients. More than 30% of patients in the BoNT group experienced at least a 2-grade improvement in hyperpigmentation, tactile roughness, and periocular fine lines. They concluded that the complementary use of a tretinoin/hydroquinone based system may result in additional improvements in various signs of facial aging versus other treatments alone. A major limitation of this study is that both treatment options were not tested alone.

Marina Landau examined the combination of chemical peels with BoNT in three patients clinically and photographically [45]. All three patients experienced a significant improvement, however these results were not specifically quantified and they were not compared to either treatment alone. Landau speculates that the combination treatments create a synergistic rejuvenating effect that is likely more significant than either therapy alone.

Kadunc and colleagues looked at the effect of BoNT pretreatment of the orbicularis oris muscle for upper perioral vertical wrinkles with manual chemabrasion in 12 patients [46]. The BoNT was injected unilaterally at the vermillion border 1 week prior to chemabrasion (35% trichloroacetic acid followed by dermasanding). Two blinded observers at baseline, 30 days, 90 days, 180 days, and 3 years assessed wrinkle severity by using a four-point Facial Wrinkle Severity Scale (FWSS). From day 90 to year 3, the BoNT injected sides showed smaller grades in the FWSS than control sides ($p < 0.05$). Few other studies looking at BoNT combination therapy have been able to successfully demonstrate the potential long-term benefits of combined therapy.

BoNT and Monopolar Radiofrequency

Monopolar Radiofrequency (MRF) employs radiofrequency energy via capacitive coupling to provide volumetric tissue heating of the deep dermis and subcutaneous tissues while simultaneously cooling the epidermis (47–49). The result is dermal remodeling which takes place over a 3- to 6-month period. It is used as a lifting, tightening, and contouring procedure for treatment of the face, neck, brow, eyelid, and body areas. In the forehead and periocular area, both MRF and BoNT are used for brow elevation and reduction of periocular rhytides. Dr. Stephen Bosniak was one of the first aesthetic physicians who noted that pretreatment of the brow depressors with BoNT 2 weeks before MRF aids in relaxation of the muscles that depress the brow [50]. By eliminating the downward pull of the brow depressors, unopposed collagen remodeling can occur [50]. Although the final result may not be appreciated for 4–6 months, at the conclusion of the MRF procedure some degree of brow elevation should be apparent. In the lateral canthal area, pretreatment of the orbicularis oculi sphincter with BoNT will allow greater temporal lifting with MRF [8, 50]. Unfortunately, there are no quantitative studies to prove the synergy between these two procedures, just the anecdotal observations of numerous practitioners in the aesthetic arena.

BoNT and Muscle Stimulation (MS)

A device utilizing repetitive high-amplitude electrical stimulation of the muscles of the face and neck can be used to increase muscular volume. The goal is to induce muscular hypertrophy that will lead to a lift and firming of the brow, cheeks, jawline, and neck and is based on the "body building of the face" protocol described by Mulholland [52]. While proven to yield substantial 3-demensional improvements in facial volume by patients and physicians, this procedure remains relatively obscure in the

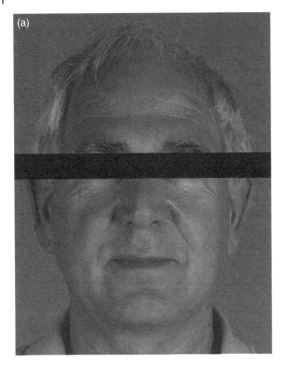 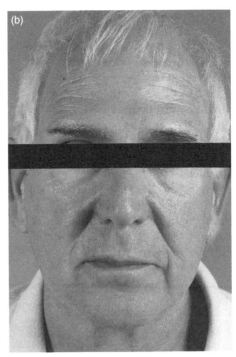

Figure 18.7 (a) Before treatment. (b) One year after 47 Pan G™ lift treatments and 3 weeks after BoNT to glabella, forehead, and crow's feet. *Source:* Courtesy of Amy Forman Taub, MD.

cosmetic market due to lack of marketing and promotion, and difficulty of training and implementation. However, one of the authors has used this procedure successfully for 14 years in their practice. This author completed a study of 17 adult women aged 50–56 years undergoing the 20 treatments over 10 weeks and monthly treatments thereafter followed up to 12 months. Most these subjects also had BoNT in the upper one-third of the face [51]. While the improvements in lift for the jowls, cheek, eye, and neck area from MS could be measured, the improvement in the brow area could not be assessed due to the confounding variable of the BoNT treatment. Since the MS therapy would enhance the movement of the frontalis muscle as well as the periocular muscles, this could both enhance lift and result in rhytidogenesis. However, in our experience, consistent indefinite high-voltage treatments in combination with BoNT in the upper one-third of the face results in an enhanced

cosmetic result over that of myofacial stimulation alone (Figure 18.7, Figure 18.8, and Figure 18.9). One theory is that BoNT injected into facial muscles that are antagonistic to facial elevators effectively "frees" the facial elevator muscles, allowing more complete hypertrophy to occur during the MS process. However, one could as easily argue that for the upper one-third of the face these two modalities are antagonistic more than synergistic, since stimulation of muscle could increase dynamic rhytides. Muscle stimulation enhances facial appearance through the increased volume that the "hypertrophied" facial elevator muscles occupy.

Conclusions

The combination of BoNT and other aesthetic procedures: fillers, lasers and light sources, and tissue tightening, along

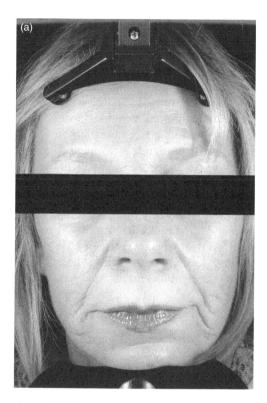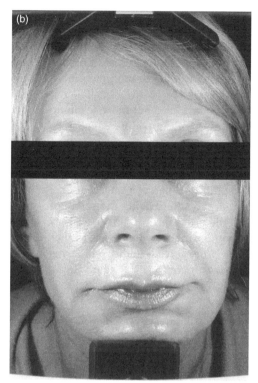

Figure 18.8 (a) Before treatment. (b) 2 years after 34 Pan G lift treatments and 3 weeks after 54 U BoNT to glabella and crow's feet and six syringes of juvedèrmUltra™ to nasolabial and melomental folds. *Source:* Courtesy of Amy Forman Taub, MD.

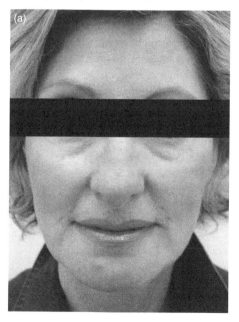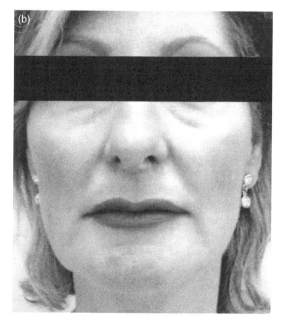

Figure 18.9 (a) Before treatment. (b) 5 months after 20 Pan G™ lift treatments and 60 U of BoNT in glabella, forehead, and crow's feet. *Source:* Courtesy of Amy Forman Taub, MD.

with chemical peels, cosmeceuticals, and microcurrent is a fact of life in almost all aesthetic clinics today. In our fast-paced life many patients desire reducing the number of visits required, leading to multiple procedures being performed at one visit [53, 54]. Three major factors have put most aesthetic providers at ease with providing concurrent treatments: (i) the burgeoning number of aesthetic tools; (ii) better understanding of the complexities of aging changes necessitating multiple different interventions; and (iii) studies demonstrating the safety of doing multiple procedures [54]. At the very least, the combination of BoNT with other rejuvenation procedures is additive in terms of combination therapy [22] (Figure 18.3).

There is much literature, albeit mostly small studies some of which are not placebo controlled, which indicate that there is a very real synergism between BoNT and fillers as well as intense pulsed light and possibly ablative and non-ablative lasers [55]. The best evidence exists for both efficacy and longevity for the BoNT and filler combination in the glabellar area, With newer technology that enables us to more easily study the 3-dimensional static and active components of the human face, we will no doubt discover new relationships between wound healing, metabolism and other molecular activities in the skin and facial muscle movement, leading to a deeper understanding of the scientific underpinnings of combination therapy.

References

1 Molina B, David M, Jain R, *et al.* Patient satisfaction and efficacy of full-facial rejuvenation using a combination of botulinum toxin type A and hyaluronic acid filler. Dermatol Surg 2015 Dec;41(Suppl 1): S325–S332.

2 Fagien S, Brandt FS. Primary and adjuvant use of botulinum toxin type A (BOTOX) in facial aesthetic surgery: beyond the glabella. Clin Plat Surg 2001;28: 127–148.

3 Fagien S. Botox for the treatment of dynamic and hyperkinetic facial lines and furrows: adjunctive use in facial aesthetic surgery. Plast Reconstr Surg 2003;112: 40S–53S.

4 Carruthers J, Carruthers A, Maberley. Deep resting glabellar rhytides responds to BoNT-A and Hylan B. Dermatol Surg 2003; 29:539–544.

5 Carruthers J, Carruthers A. A prospective, randomized, parallel group study analyzing the effect of BoNT-A (Botox) and nonanimal sourced hyaluronic acid (NASHA, Restylane) in combination compared with NASHA (Restylane) alone in severe glabellar rhytides in adult female subjects: treatment of severe glabellar rhytides with a hyaluronic acid derivative compared with the derivative and BoNT-A. Dermatol Surg 2003;29:802–809.

6 Dubina M, Tung R, Bolotin D, *et al.* Treatment of forehead/glabellar rhytides\ complex with combination botulinum toxin a and hyaluronic acid versus botulinum toxin A injection alone: a split-face, rater-blinded, randomized control trial. J Cosmet Dermatol 2013 Dec;12(4):261–266.

7 Patel M, Talmor M, Nolan W. Botox and collagen for glabellar furrows: advantages of combination therapy. Ann Plast Surg 2004;52(5):442–447.

8 Bosniak S. Combination therapies: a nonsurgical approach to oculofacial rejuvenation. Opthamol Clin N Am 2005; 18:215–225.

9 Carruthers J, Glogau R, Blitzer A, Facial Aesthetics Consensus Group Faculty. Advances in facial rejuvenation:botulinum toxin type A, hyaluronic acid dermal fillers, and combination therapies-consensus recommendations. Plast Reconstr Surg 2008;121(5S):5s–30s.

10 Bosniak S, Cantisano-Zilkha M, Purewal BK, Zdinak L. Combination therapies in oculofacial rejuvenation. Orbit 2006;25: 319–326.

11 Matarasso S, Carruthers J, Jewell M, Restylane Consensus Group. Consensus recommendations for soft-tissue augmentation with nonanimal stabilized hyaluronic acid (Restylane). Plast Reconstr Surg 2006;117:3s–34s.

12 Friedman PM, Mafong EA, Kauvar AN, et al. Safety data of injectable nonanimal stabilized hyaluronic acid gel for soft tissue augmentation. Dermatol Surg 2002;28:491.

13 Schanz, S, Schippert W, Ulmer A, et al. Arterial embolism caused by injection of hyaluronic acid (Restylane). Brit J Dermatol 2002;146:928.

14 Hanke CW, Higley HR, Jolivette DM, et al. Abscess formation and local necrosis after treatment with Zyderm or Zyplast collagen implant. J Am Acad Dermatol 1991;25:319.

15 Huilgol SC, Carruthers A, Carruthers JD. Raising eyebrows with botulinum toxin. Dermatol Surg 1999;25(5):373–375.

16 Carruthers J, Carruthers A. Facial sculpting and tissue augmentation. Dermatol Surg 2005;31(11):1604–1612.

17 Beer K, Julius H, Dunn M, Wilson F. Remodeling of periorbital, temporal, glabellar, and crow's feet areas with hyaluronic acid and botulinum toxin. Journal of Cosmetic Dermatology 2014;13:143–150.

18 Klein A, Fagien S. Hyaluronic acid fillers and botulinum toxin type A: rationale for their individual and combined use for injectable facial rejuvenation. Plast Reconstr Surg 2007;120(6S):81s–88s.

19 Dayan SH, Kempiners JJ. Treatment of the lower third of the nose and dynamic nasal tip ptosis with Botox. Plast Reconstr Surg 2005;111(6):1784.

20 Beleznay K, Carruthers JD, Humphrey S, Jones D. Avoiding and treating blindness from fillers: a review of the world literature. Dermatol Surg 2015 Oct;41(10):1097–1117.

21 Coleman K, Carruthers J. Combination therapy with BOTOX and fillers: the new rejuvenation paradigm. Dermatol Ther 2006;19:177–188.

22 Fink B, Prager M. The effect of incobotulinumtoxin a and dermal filler treatment on perception of age, health, and attractiveness of female faces. J Clin Aesthet Dermatol 2014 Jan;7(1):36–40.

23 Carruthers J, Burgess C, Day D, et al. Consensus recommendations for combined aesthetic interventions in the face using botulinum toxin, fillers, and energy-based devices. Dermatol Surg 2016. May;42(5): 586–597.

24 Goldman MP, Weiss RA, Weiss MA. Intense pulsed light as a nonablative approach to photoaging. Dermatol Surg 2005;31:1179–1187.

25 Goldberg MP, Cutler KB. Nonablative treatment of rhytids with intense pulsed light. Lasers Surg Med. 2000;26: 196–200.

26 Weiss RA, Weiss MA, Beasley KL. Rejuvenation of photoaged skin: 5 years results with intense pulsed light of the face, neck, and chest. Dermatol Surg 2002;28: 1115–1119.

27 Sadick NS, Weiss R, Kilmer S, Bitter P. Photorejuvenation with intense pulsed light: results of a multi-center study. J Drugs Dermatol 2004;3(1):41–49.

28 Hedelund L, Due E, Bjerring P, Wulf HC, Haedersdal M. Skin rejuvenation using intense pulsed light: a randomized controlled split-face trial with blinded response evaluation. Arch Dermatol 2006 Aug;142(8):985–990.

29 Carruthers J, Carruthers A. The effect of full-face broadband light treatments alone and in combination with bilateral crow's feet botulinum toxin type A chemodenervation. Dermatol Surg 2004;30:355–366; discussion 366.

30 Carruthers J, Carruthers A. Adjunctive botulinum toxin type A; fillers and light-based therapies. Int Ophthalmol Clin 2005 Summer;45(3):143–151.

31 Khoury J, Saluja R, Goldman M. The effect of botulinum toxin type a on full-face intense pulsed light treatment: a

randomized, double-blind, split-face study. Dermatol Surg 2008;34:1062–1069.

32 Semchyshyn N, Kilmer S. Does laser inactivate botulinum toxin? Dermatol Surg 2005;31:399–404.

33 Fabi SG, Goldman MP, Mills DC, *et al.* Combining microfocused ultrasound with botulinum toxin andtemporary and semi-permanent dermal fillers: safety and current use. Dermatol Surg 2016 May;42(Suppl 2):S168–S176.

34 Zimbler M, Nassif P. Adjunctive applications for botulinum toxin in facial aesthetic surgery. Facial Plast Surg Clin N Am 2003;11:477–482.

35 Fagien S. Botox for the treatment of dynamic and hyperkinetic facial lines and furrows. Plast Reconstr Surg 1999;103: 701–713.

36 Fagien S. Extended use of botulinum toxin A in facial aesthetic surgery. Aesthet Surg J 1998;18:215–219.

37 West T, Alster T. Effect of botulinum toxin type A on movement-associated rhytides following CO_2 laser resurfacing. Dermatol Surg 1999;25:259–261.

38 Carruthers J, Carruthers A. Combining botulinum toxin injection and laser resurfacing for facial rhytides. In: Coleman LW, ed. *Combined Therapy: BOTOX and CO_2 Facial Laser Resurfacing.* Baltimore, MD: Williams & Wilkins;1998:235–243.

39 Carruthers J, Carruthers A. Botulinum toxin and laser resurfacing for lines around the eyes. In: Blitzer A, Binder WJ, Carruthers A, eds. *Management of Facial Lines and Wrinkles.* Philadelphia, PA: Lippincott Williams & Wilkins;2000: 315–318.

40 Carruthers J, Carruthers A, Zelichowska A. The power of combined therapies: Botox and ablative facial laser resurfacing. Am J Cosmet Surg 2000;17:129–131.

41 Zimbler M, Holds J, Kokoska M, *et al.* Effect of botulinum toxin pretreatment on laser resurfacing results: a prospective, randomized, blinded trial. Arch Facial Plast Surg 2001;3:165–169.

42 Yamauchi P, Lask G, Lowe N. Botulinum toxin type A gives adjunctive benefit to periorbital laser resurfacing. J Cosmet Laser Ther 2004;6:145–148.

43 Beer K, Waibel J. Botulinum toxin type A enhances the outcome of fractional resurfacing of the cheek. J Drugs in Dermatol 2007;6:1151–1152.

44 Comstock J. Using a 4% hydroquinone/tretinoin-based skin care system in conjunction with facial rejuvenation procedures. Poster presented at the Americal Academy of Dermatology 66th Annual Meeting; February 1–5, 2008; San Antonio, TX.

45 Landau M. Combination of chemical peelings with botulinum toxin injections and dermal fillers. J Cosmet Dermatol 2006;5:121–126.

46 Kadunc BV, Almeida ART, Vanti AA, Chiacchio N. Botulinum toxin A adjunctive use in manual chemabrasion: controlled long-term study for treatment of upper perioral vertical wrinkles. Dermatol Surg 2007;33:1066–1072.

47 Sadick N. Radiofrequency Technology. Minimally Invasive Techniques of Oculo-Facial Surgery. New York:Thieme; 2005:12–21.

48 Sukal SA, Geronemus RG. Thermage: the noablative radiofrequency for rejuvenation. Clin Dermatol 2008;26(6):602–607.

49 Hodgkinson DJ. Clinical applications of radiofrequency: nonsurgical skin tightening (thermage). Clin Plast Surg 2009;36(2):261–268, viii.

50 Bosniak S, Cantisano-Zilkha M, Nestor M. Thermalifting of face, neck, and brows. Oper Tech Oculoplast Orbital Reconstr Surg 2001;4(2):113–117.

51 Mullholland, RS. The Pan G^{TM}:A non-surgical soft-tissue contouring of the face and alternative to face lifting. Presented at the 22nd Annual Meeting of the Rocky Mountain Plastic Surgery Association, Salt Lake City, March 15, 2003.

52 Taub AF. Evaluation of a nonsurgical, muscle-stimulating system to elevate soft

tissues of the face and neck. J Drugs Dermatol 2006;5(5):360–364.

53 Langelier N, Beleznay K, Woodward J. Rejuvenation of the upper face and periocular region: combining neuromodulator, facial filler, laser, light, and energy-based therapies for optimal results. Dermatol Surg 2016 May;42 (Suppl 2):S77–S82.

54 Cuerda-Galindo E, Palomar-Gallego MA, Linares-Garcíavaldecasas R. Are combined same-day treatments the future for photorejuvenation? Review of the literature on combined treatments with lasers, intense pulsed light, radiofrequency, botulinum toxin, and fillers for rejuvenation. J Cosmet Laser Ther 2015 Feb;17(1):49–54.

55 Molina B, David M, Jain R, Amselem M, Ruiz-Rodriguez R, *et al.* Patient Satisfaction and Efficacy of Full-Facial Rejuvenation Using a Combination of Botulinum Toxin Type A and Hyaluronic Acid Filler. Dermatol Surg 2015 Dec;41(Suppl 1): S325–S332.

19

Peri-Procedure Botulinum Toxin for Skin Cancer Patients and Scars

Timothy Corcoran Flynn, MD,[1,2] Molly C. Powers, MD,[3] and David M. Ozog, MD (FAAD, FACMS)[4]

[1] Clinical Professor of Dermatology, University of North Carolina at Chapel Hill, Chapel Hill, USA
[2] Medical Director, Cary Skin Center, Cary, USA
[3] Dermatology Senior Resident, Department of Dermatology, Henry Ford Hospital, Detroit, USA
[4] Chair, Department of Dermatology; C.S. Livingood Chair in Dermatology; Director of Cosmetic Dermatology, Henry Ford Hospital, Detroit, MI, USA

Introduction

There have been several reports of botulinum toxins being used to improve outcomes of facial reconstruction [1–6]. Making use of the principles of tissue immobilization as an aid to wound healing, botulinum toxin is employed to reduce the action of facial mimetic muscles. By reducing the movement of these muscles of facial expression, the overlying skin affected by the musculature has reduced movement, ultimately leading to lessened intensity of tensile forces on a healing wound. Additionally, the use of botulinum toxin in the treatment of pathogenic scars, such as hypertrophic scars and keloids, continues to be evaluated. Additional work suggests that there may be a direct effect of botulinum toxin on the fibroblasts and their cytokine expression involved in wound healing [7–9]. This chapter will explore how botulinum toxin can be used for reconstruction in traumatic wounds and skin cancer patients as well as a potential treatment for hypertrophic scars and keloids.

Botulinum Toxin for Facial Reconstruction

Patients are often disappointed in the appearance of their scars. Not only does pathological scar formation lead to functional limitations, but it also causes significant anxiety due to the cosmetic concerns of patients. It is well reported that patients are often troubled about the appearance of the reconstructed surgery site, just as much as they are about the removal of the cutaneous cancer. Appearance-related concerns may lead to increased self-consciousness and social anxiety, which may ultimately result in psychological and social dysfunction [10]. Minimizing the appearance of scars including those for skin cancers excisions, repairs, and traumatic scars remains a top priority among surgeons.

Wound healing is very complex, involving multiple intertwining processes including inflammation, proliferation, and remodeling. Any disruption in this complex process may result in pathological wound healing. Increased wound tension, for example, has been shown to prolong the inflammatory phase of wound healing [11]. Repetitive microtrauma leads to increased deposition of glycosaminoglycans and collagen within the wound [5, 12]. Given these principles of wound healing, surgeons have been adopting wound closure techniques to minimize tension and ultimately microtrauma with undermining, flap reconstructions, deep plicating sutures, etc. [13]. Exploiting the temporary paralytic effects of botulinum toxin continues to be evaluated in surgical and traumatic wound healing to reduce wound tension (and such microtrauma) to these healing wounds.

There have been several reported studies indicating the effects of botulinum toxin reducing the appearance of scars in the immediate surgical repair period. Most studies have demonstrated superior cosmesis as compared with placebo. The generally accepted mechanism of action is currently the reduction in wound tension attained by chemical denervation of surrounding muscles; however, some research has suggested direct effects on promoted wound healing through TGF-β1, collagen synthesis, CTGF, and other cytokines that will be addressed in the chapter.

There are several clinical reports on the benefits of botulinum toxins in wound healing. An early report by Choi, et al. in 1997 reported on the benefits of onabotulinumtoxin injected into blepharoplasty patients at risk for wound complications after eyelid reconstruction. Risk factors included prior radiation exposure, burns, scarring from previous surgeries, muscles spasms, etc. The dynamic musculature following eyelid reconstruction may lead to higher rates of dehiscence, scarring, and eventual eyelid malposition. Wound immobilization with onabotulinumtoxin in the eleven patients reports lead to promoted wound healing believed to be secondary to full wound immobilization that was achieved with chemical denervation as compared with partial wound immobilization by mechanical measures [14]. However, this was an uncontrolled study.

In 2000, Gassner et al. performed a double-blind, placebo-controlled trial with the use of botulinum toxin type A on lateral forehead sutured wounds in primates [2]. The molecule was used to immobilize tissue surrounding these wounds and was able to demonstrate improved cosmesis of facial scars, as determined by three blinded observers using the visual analogue scale (VAS). Final evaluation was conducted 12 weeks after treatment with toxin. Although these results could not be generalized to humans, proof of concept was obtained.

Further work by Gassner et al. was reported on chemoimmobilization for improving facial scars [5]. Of patients with either forehead lacerations or forehead excisions (non-melanoma skin cancers and other tumors), 31 completed all phases of the study. The patients were randomized to receive toxin or placebo into the musculature adjacent to the wound within 24 hours after closure. A blinded assessment of standardized photographs was undertaken by two experienced facial plastic surgeons at six months. The overall median visual analogue scale (VAS) score for the botulinum toxin treated group was 8.9 compared to 7.2 for the placebo group (p = .003) indicating improved cosmesis and enhanced wound healing. Doses of onobotulinumtoxinA used in these forehead wounds were 15 U for wounds up to 2 cm long, 30 U for wounds 2–4 cm long and 45 U for wounds > 4 cm.

Wilson in 2006 discussed the use of botulinum toxin type A to prevent widening of facial scars [4]. Given that immobilization is a basic therapeutic principle in wound healing, this study sought to achieve immobilization through chemical denervation ultimately leading to reduced tension on wounds lying with unfavorable orientation to the lines of Langer. The paper reported on 30 patients with revision surgery for unsightly and previously widened scars on the face and 10 patients who were undergoing excisional surgery of facial lesions. All wounds were perpendicular to the lines of Langer. OnobotulinumtoxinA was used to induce a temporary paralysis of the muscles during surgery. A dose of 1.5 U per linear cm was used. The average repair length was 9.8 cm. Using objective and subjective scales, 90% of patients had an improved outcome; however, there was no placebo arm for this study and scales were not validated.

Flynn in 2009 published a study using intraoperative botulinum toxin type A or B in patients following Mohs micrographic surgery for treatment of skin cancer [1]. Eighteen subjects were treated. They were considered for intraoperative treatment with either onobotulinumtoxinA or rimabotulinumtoxinB if the Mohs surgery defect was affected by skin movements of the underlying muscles of facial expression. These 18 patients had their defects repaired with either primary complex closures or adjacent tissue transfers. Immediately following the repair the patients were injected with either onobotulinumtoxinA or rimabotulinumtoxinB. Injections were placed within a 1–2 cm radius around the suture lines, to affect muscles directly pulling on the repair. If the movement of a facial muscle or muscle groups were found to affect the closure they were temporarily chemodenervated. For example, if a repair on the scalp was stretched with the actions of the frontalis muscle, the entire frontalis muscle was temporarily chemodenervated, as shown in the case in Figure 19.1. The doses of botulinum toxin were appropriate for those muscles with the goal being complete immobilization of the muscle unit. Figure 19.2 shows a case of a repair involving the base of the nose. The entire glabella complex was treated intraoperatively.

Nine patients received onobotulinumtoxinA and nine patients received rimabotulinumtoxinB. There was no difference in outcomes for patients treated with either toxin and no significant complications were noted with the botulinum toxins. The only complication noted was that one patient who received onobotulinumtoxinA had an epidermal slough in one area of the adjacent tissue transfer. Patients were seen in follow up at three months, and it was noted that no

patient had retained a significant effect of the botulinum toxins at that time. Cosmetic outcomes were excellent in most patients.

A previous paper by Flynn et al. has demonstrated that rimabotulinumtoxinB has a faster onset of action and an increased area of effect compared to onobotulinumtoxinA when dosed at a 100 : 1 ratio [15]. The faster onset of action of rimabotulinumtoxinB has been noted in clinical use, as well as the laboratory study [16]. Therefore, the faster onset of action of the type B toxin may be desirable in skin cancer reconstruction patients when the toxin is infiltrated at the time of the repair. It has also been noted that the duration of effect of the type B toxin is less than that of the type A toxins [17]. This may be desirable because the return of function may be achieved faster without longer-lasting residual effects; however, there is no clinical evidence to date that supports this hypothesis.

To investigate if botulinum toxin had a primary effect on wound healing in normal skin a separate study was designed. Healthy adult human volunteers were injected with 18 U of onobotulinumtoxinA on one side of their buttocks and saline on the other as a control. Three weeks later subjects underwent ablative laser resurfacing of the epidermis and upper dermis using an erbium-YAG laser with a wavelength of 2940 nm and a fluence of 6 J/cm^2. Wounds created areas of tiny, pinpoint bleeding and the sites were photographed daily for 6 days and every 3 days thereafter to 41 days. The botulinum toxin placed intradermally had no effect on wound healing, as the results for the onobotulinumtoxinA treated sites were identical to the results of the saline treated controls.

In 2009, Gassner et al. [5] reported two interesting cases of chemoimmobilization of lower facial wounds using onabotulinumtoxinA [6]. The first case involved a 26-year-old woman who sustained a crush injury to the lower lip from a motor vehicle. The irregular defect involved the vermillion border and complete transection of the orbicularis oris muscle was observed. They used

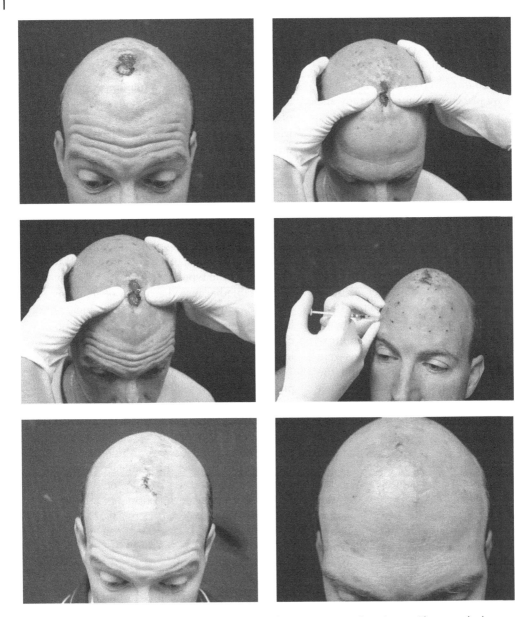

Figure 19.1 A 42-year-old male underwent Mohs surgery for a squamous cell carcinoma. The wound edges could be approximated with the surgeon's hands, but with frontalis contraction there was significant traction laterally widening the wound. The wound was repaired and his frontalis was treated immediately post-operatively with 3000 U of rimabotulinumtoxinB. Effect of the toxin is shown at 48 hours after the injection. Complete effect of the type B toxin is still present at 2 weeks following the repair.

a technique of dissolving 7.5 U of onobotulinumtoxinA per ml of 1% lidocaine containing 100,000 U epinephrine. The total dose given, using this technique was 40 U. Follow-up showed a flaccid paralysis of the injected portion of the lower lip, closely resembling the degree of paralysis shown from injection of the lidocaine. This dose of toxin resulted in their patient having a short-term, 1-month duration reduced oral sphincter function

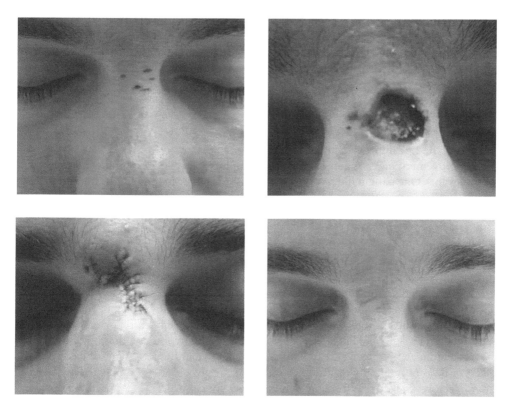

Figure 19.2 A 33-year-old male underwent Mohs surgery for a basal cell carcinoma on the root of the nose. His postoperative defect is shown and a rhombic transposition flap used for the repair. 24 U of onobotulinumtoxinA was placed intraoperatively into the entire glabellar complex (procerus, depressor supracilli, and corrugator supercilli muscles). The result at 4-month follow-up is shown.

with occasional spillage of liquids and mild dysarthria. The final surgical result was outstanding [5].

Their second case involved a scar revision on the left cheek, which resulted from incision and drainage of a recurrent facial abscess. In this case 30 U of onabotulinumtoxinA were injected into the buccinator and zygomatic facial muscles. The patient experienced a clinically significant paralysis without any dynamic tension or distortion of the wound clinically. At 10 weeks after surgery the muscle function had returned and an excellent result was seen. The authors have commented that to eliminate the tension on the healing tissue, paralysis of the muscle groups adjacent and subadjacent to the wound should be as complete as possible. These patients, who were concerned about the eventual appearance of their scars, were very accepting of the explained temporary functional deficits. This study differed from the study completed by Flynn in that greatly increased doses of botulinum toxin were used to affect a complete paralysis; however, these results may have been possible with lower doses of toxin. If this technique is used, the patient should be advised to expect a possible significant functional impairment of a large area around the reconstruction [5].

In 2013, Ziade *et al.* [18] conducted a blinded, randomized, placebo-controlled study of facial trauma patients who presented to the emergency room. Onabotulinum toxin or placebo was injected into the muscle groups, which were deemed to cause tension on the sutured wound at the time of closure. The mean dose of toxin injected was

20 U (range 15–40 U); 24 patients completed the study and 1 year follow-up. Their 1-year photographs were evaluated by six separate physicians. The median overall visual analog score (VAS) score was 8.25 in the toxin group and 6.38 in the control group, p < 0.001. The strengths of this study include length of time for follow-up (1 year), blinded nature, placebo control, and the 1.87 improvement in VAS score (an improvement of 1.5 is considered clinically relevant). One patient did have an asymmetrical smile after injections into zygomaticus minor and levator labii superioris alaeque nasi on day 7 follow-up [18].

The only split-scar, double-blind, randomized controlled trial to assess the safety and efficacy of botulinum toxin A (BTA) in operational scars was completed by Kim et al. in 2015. Fifteen patients who underwent open thyroidectomy by a single surgeon were included in the study. The right and left sides of the scar were randomized to receive treatment with BTA or 0.9% normal saline within 10 days of thyroidectomy, injected by a single dermatologist who was also blinded. Patient follow up was at 2 weeks, 1 month, 3 months, and 6 months postoperatively. The mean scar length was 8 cm, and mean 32.2 U of BTA were used. The modified Stony Brook Scar Evaluation Scale revealed a baseline score of the BTA-treated side of 4.07 before treatment and 6.70 six months after treatment and while the control group scores were 4.07 before treatment and 4.17 six months after treatment (p = 0.000). Clinical photographs demonstrated excellent results. The superior cosmetic outcomes are attributed to BTA's ability to reduce tension on the wound and through its direct inhibitory effects on fibroblasts and TGF-β1 expression [19].

Botulinum toxin has been used to improve results in wounded skin in other clinical scenarios. Treatment with onobotulinumtoxinA before and after laser resurfacing has been shown to diminish wrinkles and prevent reestablishment of facial lines [20, 21]. Yamaguchi found it helpful in periorbital laser resurfacing [22]. OnobotulinumtoxinA has been used with 35% TCA and dermasanding

to improve wrinkles in the lip [23]. These studies continue to demonstrate the beneficial effects of perioperative/periprocedural BTA use.

Botulinum Toxin in Keloidal and Hypertrophic Scars

Hypertrophic scars can be a significant problem due to pain, itching, and limitation of range of movement. Routine treatments include intralesional corticosteroids, laser and excisional therapy, radiation therapy, and compression treatment among many others. There are several interesting reports of the use of botulinum toxin for the treatment of pathologic scars such as hypertrophic and keloid scars. The primary effects of botulinum toxin have been reported by several authors. The hypothesis that botulinum toxin is effective in the treatment of keloidal and hypertrophic scars is supported by in vitro biochemical processes that will be discussed further throughout the chapter. The studies below discuss this clinical efficacy of the use of botulinum toxin.

In a prospective 2009 study to evaluate the effects of onobotulinumtoxinA in the treatment of keloids, Zhibo et al. injected intralesional toxin into 12 keloids [24]. The total dose used in the keloid sessions was 70–140 U. The treatment was given at 3-month intervals for a maximum of 9 months. Outcomes were assessed at 1 year and were judged as excellent in three patients, good in five patients, and fair in four patients. Importantly, none of the patients showed signs of enlargements or recurrence of the keloids.

Treatments of mature hypertrophic scars of greater than 2 years' duration were reported in 2009 by Xiao et al., who injected 19 patients using the type A toxin from China (Lanzou Biologic Company, Lanzou City, People's Republic of China) [8]. Intralesional injections of this botulinum type A (BTA) toxin were placed into the hypertrophic scars at a dose of 2.5 U/cm^3 of hypertrophic scars at 1-month intervals for 3 months. Doses ranged from 2 to 87 U/scar owing to the large difference in scar sizes. The follow-up conducted at 6 months showed improvement of the scars with a high therapeutic satisfaction. The authors noted that redness and itching had improved after the injections and the scars became softer. Patients and plastic surgeons were asked to rate the overall improvements in the hypertrophic scars. Possible grades were: no improvement, poor improvement (0–25% improvement), fair improvement (26–50% improvement), good improvement (51–75% improvement) or excellent improvement (76–100% improvement). Patients felt the treated hypertrophic scars reached the level of "good" in twelve cases and "excellent" in seven cases. Plastic surgeons evaluated the results rating fifteen cases deemed "good" and four "excellent." Limitations of this study included the lack of a control group and a relatively short follow-up duration [8].

In contrast, Gauglitz et al. in 2012 reported on four patients with steroid-resistant keloidal scars injected with BTA (70–120 U) every 2 months for up to 6 months. Height and volume measurements were obtained clinically and with a 3D optical profiling system. Additionally, the expression of collagen (COL)1A1, COL1A2, COL3A1, TGF-β1, TGF-β2, TGF-β3, fibronectin, laminin-β2, and α-SMA was obtained with real-time PCR. It was discovered that there was no difference between pre- and posttreatment appearance of keloids as well as expression of ECM, collagen synthesis or TGF-β. This study was limited by a very small sample size and a short treatment duration [25].

Robinson reported in 2013 on twelve patients with keloidal scars with BTA for a mean duration of 11 months (range 2–43 months). Nine patients had keloids on the central chest/sternum, and the remaining had scars on the neck, thigh, and cheek. Eight of these patients were alternating intradermal steroids with BTA therapy. The patients had between 20 and 100 U of BTA injected at any one time based on scar size and location. In nine patients, complete flattening of the keloidal scar in an average of 11 months

was noted using the Vancouver Scar Scale. Two patients developed recurrences adjacent to previously treated areas. One patient was concomitantly receiving intralesional steroids with BTA, and the other received intense pulse light therapy. This study was not randomized or controlled. While improvement of the scars was noted, delineating the role of BTA in their improvement is difficult because many patients were undergoing treatment with additional modalities [26].

Postexcisional treatment of keloids with intralesional BTA and 5-fluorouracil (5-FU) has been reported to have success. In 2013, Wilson et al. treated 80 patients with keloidal scars with 0.4 mL of 50 mg/mL of 5-FU every centimeter in addition to 0.4 mL of 50 IU/mL of BTA every centimeter for a maximum dose of <140 IU on the ninth day following excision of the keloids. Patients were followed for 17–24 months and recurrence rates were less than 3.75%. This is significantly less than previously reported studies assessing other therapeutic modalities, including but not limited to excision alone, pressure garments, intralesional steroids, radiation, brachytherapy, silicone sheeting, laser therapies, and cryotherapy. Although the study demonstrated marked reduced recurrence rates, the study was not controlled or randomized [27].

There are many reports suggesting the clinical efficacy of botulinum in the treatment of pathogenic scars. Further research has been conducted to help explain the beneficial results that are reflected clinically. For example, Xiao et al. have further researched the effect of the Lanzhou botulinum toxin type A on fibroblasts derived from hypertrophic scars [9]. They explored the effect of the toxin on transforming growth factor beta 1 (TGF-β1) in these fibroblasts. TGF-β1 is known to be the most potent growth factor involved in wound healing and is a key regulator in the pathogenesis of hypertrophic scars. After isolating the fibroblasts, the cells from the hypertrophic scar were treated with the type A toxin. The growth of the fibroblasts treated with toxin was slower than those without type A toxin treatment (p < 0.01). TGF-β1 was decreased in cells treated with botulinum toxin type A.

This work is similar to that of Lee *et al.* in 2009, who used botulinum toxin type A to relax adjacent muscles in the backs of rats [28]. Surgical wounds were created in the animals and left to heal by secondary intention. The botulinum toxin treated wounds showed larger diameters, but histology revealed decreased inflammation, fibrosis, number of fibroblasts, and TGF-β1 expression. The larger diameter of toxin-treated wounds was hypothesized to be secondary to decreased tension and fibroblast activity on wound edges.

Further work by Xiao's group involved connective tissue growth factor (CTGF) [7]. In hypertrophic scar formation, CTGF is an important factor that regulates cell growth and adhesion, as well as excessive deposition of collagen. It is mediated by TGF-β1 levels, which were previously shown to decrease after treatment with BTA. Their laboratory used the fibroblasts obtained from eight patients with hypertrophic scars. The cells were treated with BTA and untreated cells were the control. Again, the proliferation of fibroblasts treated with toxin was slower than those with no toxin treatment. The cells treated with BTA had a dose response to the toxin with increasing exposure to BTA reducing the expression of a CTGF protein. They plan to study the effects of toxins on keloid-derived fibroblasts.

Haubner *et al.* evaluated the effects of BTA on dermal fibroblasts and microvascular endothelial cells. After incubating the cells with varying concentrations of BTA, the expressions of fibroblast growth factor (FGF), interleukin-6 (IL-6), vascular endothelial growth factor (VEGF), and macrophage colony-stimulating factor (M-CSF) were not significantly different. Additionally, these normal cell lines did not show a difference in cellular proliferation [29]. The findings are interesting as this study used commercial cell lines for fibroblasts and endothelial cell, whilst the work of Xiao used fibroblasts from patient hypertrophic scars. This finding may suggest the selective effect of BTA on abnormal fibroblasts from hypertrophic scars.

Many studies evaluating the use of BTA in pathological scar treatment are very limited and not controlled or randomized. Additionally, these studies often demonstrate clinical improvement with the adjuvant therapy of intralesional BTA, but do not compare this treatment to other well-recognized treatments for hypertrophic and keloidal scars such as intralesional steroids, pressure garments, excisions, silicone sheeting, and radiation among other treatments. The effect of BTA on cytokine expression remains a topic of research and may continue to prove concept of treatment for these pathologic scars.

Conclusion

There are multiple reports by several investigations showing improved wound healing with intraoperative or pretreatment with botulinum toxins. Improved results have been shown in humans and across species. The use of intralesional botulinum toxin type A in mature hypertrophic scars and keloids has also shown improvement. The toxin is thought to work in these cases by affecting TGF-β1 and CTGF and ultimately collagen deposition. Additional studies are ongoing to delineate the mechanisms of action, dosing, and timing of injections.

References

1 Flynn TC. Use of intraoperative botulinum toxin in facial reconstruction. Dermatol Surg 2009;35(2):182–188.

2 Gassner HG, Sherris DA, Otley CC. Treatment of facial wounds with botulinum toxin A improves cosmetic outcome in

primates. Plast Reconstr Surg 2000;105(6):1948–1953; discussion 1954–5.

3 Gassner HG, Sherris DA. Chemoimmobilization: improving predictability in the treatment of facial scars. Plast Reconstr Surg 2003;112: 1464–1466.

4 Wilson AM. Use of botulinum toxin type A to prevent widening of facial scars. Plast Reconstr Surg 2006;117(6):1758–66; discussion 1767–8.

5 Gassner HG, Brissett AE, Otley CC, Boahene DK, Boggust AJ, Weaver AL, Sherris DA. Botulinum toxin to improve facial wound healing: A prospective, blinded, placebo-controlled study. Mayo Clin Proc 2006;81(8):1023–1028.

6 Gassner HG, Sherris DA, Friedman O. Botulinum toxin-induced immobilization of lower facial wounds. Arch Facial Plast Surg 2009;11(2):140–142.

7 Xiao Z, Zhang M Liu Y, Ren L. Botulinum toxin type a inhibits connective tissue growth factor expression in fibroblasts derived from hypertrophic scar. Aesthetic Plast Surg 2011;35(5):802–807.

8 Xiao Z, Zhang F, Cui Z. Treatment of hypertrophic scars with intralesional botulinum toxin type A injections: a preliminary report. Aesthetic Plast Surg 2009;33(3):409–412.

9 Xiao Z, Zhang F, Lin W, Zhang M, Liu Y. Effect of botulinum toxin type A on transforming growth factor beta1 in fibroblasts derived from hypertrophic scar: a preliminary report. Aesthetic Plast Surg 2010;34(4):424–427.

10 Lee SJ, Jeong SY, No YA, Park KY, Kim BJ. Combined treatment with botulinum toxin and 595-nm pulsed dye laser for traumatic scarring. Ann Dermatol 2015;27(6): 756–758.

11 Martel H, Walker DC, Reed RK, Bert JL. Dermal fibroblast morphology is affected by stretching and not by C48/80. Connect Tissue Res 2001;42(4):235–244.

12 Zheng Z, Yenari MA. Post-ischemic inflammation: molecular mechanisms and therapeutic implications. Neurol Res 2004; 26:884–892.

13 Sherris DA, Larrabee WF Jr, Murakami CS. Management of scar contractures, hypertrophic scars, and keloids. Otolaryngol Clin North Am 1995;28(5): 1057–1068.

14 Choi JC, Lucarelli MJ, Shore JW. Use of botulinum A toxin in patients at risk of wound complications following eyelid reconstruction. Ophthal Plast Reconstr Surg 1997;13(4):259–264.

15 Flynn TC, Clark RE, 2nd. Botulinum toxin type B (MYOBLOC) versus botulinum toxin type A (BOTOX) frontalis study: rate of onset and radius of diffusion. Dermatol Surg 2003;29:519–522; discussion 22.

16 Flynn TC. Myobloc. Dermatol Clin 2004;22(2):207–211, vii.

17 Carruthers A, Carruthers J, Flynn TC, Leong MS. Dose-finding, safety, and tolerability study of botulinum toxin type B for the treatment of hyperfunctional glabellar lines. Dermatol Surg 2007; 33(1 Spec No.):S60–S68.

18 Ziade M, Domergue S, Batifol D, Jreige R, Sebbane M, Goudot P, Yachouh J. Use of botulinum toxin type A to improve treatment of facial wounds: a prospective randomised study. J Plast Reconstr Aesthet Surg 2013;66(2):209–214.

19 Kim YS, Lee HJ, Cho SH, Lee JD, Kim HS. Early postoperative treatment of thyroidectomy scars using botulinum toxin: a split-scar, double-blind randomized controlled trial. Wound Repair Regen 2014;22(5):605–612.

20 Carruthers J, Carruthers A. The adjunctive usage of botulinum toxin. Dermatol Surg 1998;24(11):1244–1247.

21 Zimbler MS, Holds JB, Kokoska MS, Glaser DA, Prendiville S, Hollenbeak CS, Thomas JR. Effect of botulinum toxin pretreatment on laser resurfacing results: a prospective, randomized, blinded trial. Arch Facial Plast Surg 2001;3(3):165–169.

22 Yamauchi PS, Lask G, Lowe NJ. Botulinum toxin type A gives adjunctive benefit to

periorbital laser resurfacing. J Cosmet Laser Ther 2004;6(3):145–148.

23 Kadunc BV, Trindade DE, Almeida AR, Vanti AA, Di Chiacchio N. Botulinum toxin A adjunctive use in manual chemabrasion: controlled long-term study for treatment of upper perioral vertical wrinkles. Dermatol Surg 2007;33(9):1066–1072.

24 Zhibo, X, Miaobo, Z.; Intralesional botulinum toxin type A injections as a new treatment measure for keloids. Plast Reconstr Surg 2009; 124:275e–277e.

25 Gauglitz GG, Bureik D, Dombrowski Y, Pavicic T, Ruzicka T, Schauber J. Botulinum toxin A for the treatment of keloids. Skin Pharmacol Physiol 2012;25(6): 313–318.

26 Robinson AJ, Khadim MF, Khan K. Keloid scars and treatment with Botulinum Toxin Type A: the Belfast experience. J Plast Reconstr Aesthet Surg 2013;66(3):439–440.

27 Wilson AM. Eradication of keloids: Surgical excision followed by a single injection of intralesional 5-fluorouracil and botulinum toxin. Can J Plast Surg 2013;21:87–91.

28 Lee BJ, Jeong JH, Wang SG, Lee JC, Goh EK, Kim HW. Effect of botulinum toxin type a on a rat surgical wound model. Clin Exp Otorhinolaryngol 2009;2(1):20–27.

29 Haubner F, Ohmann E, Müller-Vogt U, Kummer P, Strutz J, Gassner HG. Effects of botulinum toxin a on cytokine synthesis in a cell culture model of cutaneous scarring. Arch Facial Plast Surg 2012;14(2):122–126.

20

Achieving a Natural Look

Dóris Hexsel, MD,[1] Camile L. Hexsel, MD (FAAD, FACMS),[2] and Carolina Siega, BSc[3]

[1] Dermatologist and Dermatologic Surgeon, Brazilian Center for Studies in Dermatology, Porto Alegre, Brazil
[2] Dermatologist and Dermatologic Surgeon, Madison Medical Affiliates, Mohs Surgery, Glendale and Waukesha, USA
[3] Biologist, Brazilian Center for Studies in Dermatology, Porto Alegre, Brazil

Introduction

The goal of botulinum toxin use is mainly to achieve a natural look and enhance beauty, while maintaining facial expressions and avoiding distortions. Combined procedures, proper techniques and doses of BoNTA have been discussed in the past decade, aiming to provide better cosmetic outcomes and more harmonious appearance.

The concept of natural beauty varies according to the culture and fashion, and its assessment is essentially subjective, varying among individuals from the same social groups. There is no scientific definition of what "natural" looks like [1]. But, the debate on this matter takes place very often on the aesthetic field, since patients typically want to avoid a "procedure-like" face. Dayan has recently discussed the issue and suggests that the three-dimensional and movement aspects of the face should be regarded when aiming to preserve the natural look of the face [1]. The frozen look might not be perceptible while facial muscles are not contracted, but may give an artificial look while talking or expressing feelings and emotions.

Botulinum Toxin Formulations

The most widely known botulinum toxin A (BoNTA) formulations are onabotulinumtoxinA (ONA; Botox/Vistabel®, Allergan, Inc., Irvine, USA), abobotulinumtoxinA (ABO; Dysport/Azzalure®, Ipsen Ltd, Maidenhead, UK), and incobotulinumtoxinA (INCO) (Xeomin®, Merz Pharmaceuticals, Frankfurt, Germany). They are also the most used commercial preparations of BoNTA. Following a huge series of well-referenced published papers, for both pathological and cosmetic indications, clinical conversion tables have been drawn up between the drugs: 1 unit of ONA and INCO is approximately equivalent to 2.5 units of ABO [2–4].

However, other toxins are currently available in markets outside the United States, as displayed in Table 20.1.

Storage and Reconstitution

To obtain effective and long-lasting results, certain precautions regarding the storage and reconstitution of BoNTA must be taken.

Table 20.1 Other toxins available on the market.

BoNT	Type	Manufacturer
Prosigne®	A	Lanzhou Institute of Biological Products, Lanzhou, China
Neuronox®	A	Medy-Tox Inc., South Korea
PurTox®	A	Mentor Corporation, Santa Barbara, USA
Neurobloc®/Myobloc®	B	Ellan Pharmaceuticals, Ireland

We recommended that reconstitution with preservative containing 0.9% saline solution (bacteriostatic saline) be carried out immediately prior to use. Benzyl alcohol, which is used as the preservative, has an immediate anesthetic effect, which makes injections more comfortable. Dilutions from 1 to 5 mL are currently being used for cosmetic purposes, according to the physician's choice or to attend the patients' needs.

Recently, a consensus on the storage and reuse of previously reconstituted neuromodulators has been published [5]. The authors stated that a vial of toxin appropriately reconstituted can be safely and effectively used to treat a single or multiple patients, even if refrigerated or refrozen for at least 4 weeks before injection, assuming appropriate storage and handling [5].

Patient Assessment, Preparation, Education, and Recommendations

A detailed knowledge and understanding of facial anatomy and a safe and effective individual therapeutic approach are the keys for successful results. These must meet doctors and patients' expectations, with safety, harmony, balance, and naturalness. An empathic and respectful attitude towards patients will make them feel comfortable in revealing their wishes, expectations, fears, and concepts regarding the procedure. The use of minimal effective dosing diluted in minimal volumes is recommended. This is specifically important in the lower face and seems to reduce the risks of complications of undesirable effects in adjacent muscles.

For the best natural results, patients must have realistic expectations and wishes. As an example, the look is not natural if patient want their muscles as paralyzed as possible. Patients with unrealistic expectations should be carefully managed or even avoided [6]. Physicians must also be aware of body dysmorphic disorder, whose prevalence in dermatology medical offices varies from 5 to 15% [7]. The goals of the BoNTA treatment and the expected cosmetic results must be discussed with patients. Botulinum toxins alone improve dynamic wrinkles, mainly superficial ones, offering better results in the upper face. Patients must be aware that some static and/or deep wrinkles may remain after the treatment. In this case, BoNTA may be combined with other procedures.

For some patients, it is important to keep a few wrinkles and/or avoid the treatment of some facial muscles, to obtain a natural look. It is also important to avoid side effects. These can be either cosmetic, such as asymmetries or excessive elevation of the tail of the brow, or medical, such as eyelid ptosis. Although side effects of BoNTA injections are usually transitory, when they happen the patient will look unnatural.

Patients with previous blepharoplasty and face lifts should be carefully evaluated, as well as those with brow tattoos. The tattoos are usually asymmetric, and this can become more evident after BoNTA injections. The patient must also be informed that BoNTA effects usually appear from 24 to 72 hours after the injections, reaching a maximum level at around 2 weeks [8]. The expected duration of the effects is limited and the treatment must be repeated at intervals of

4–6 months to maintain the results. For natural results, it is preferable to inject BoNTA every 4 months at lower effective doses than to overdoses every 6 months or at any interval. The use of effective doses avoids short-lasting effects.

Besides excellent injection technique and the choice of correct doses, additional recommendations are still considered important by many physicians to prevent undesirable BoNTA action in the adjacent muscles: patients should remain in the vertical position, avoid manipulation of the injected area, and avoid intense physical exercise for at least 4 hours after injections [9, 10].

Touch-ups can be carried out after 15–30 days to optimize the results by treating residual unwanted lines and correcting minor side effects, such as discrete asymmetries that can occur despite the use of a proper technique. Nevertheless, avoid performing frequent or repeated touch ups.

Injection Points, Doses and Techniques

For a natural look, symmetry is very important. Botulinum toxin injections should be symmetric regarding location and dosage, except for patients presenting previous asymmetries, when injection sites and doses should be customized.

In the following paragraphs, a series of recommendations for natural results are given, considering the main indications of BoNTA treatments.

Upper Face

Microinjections of BoNTA

The complete paralysis of the frontalis muscle gives an unnatural appearance, known as frozen look, and can sometimes lead to brow ptosis, which is not desired. To prevent the frozen look, as well as brow ptosis, low doses should be used to treat this area. On the other hand, the treatment of the corrugators and

procerus muscle usually requires a full dose established by consensus due to the strength of these muscles.

Despite the treatment of specific facial muscles, a new technique that uses microdoses of BoNTA is also being used to target a natural look. It differs from the traditional technique regarding dilution, doses per site, and number and depth of the injections. Larger volumes of saline are used, as reported by Steinsapir, who used 3 ml to dilute a 100 U-vial of ONA [11]. Doses of 0.33–0.66 U ONA/injection point and 2 U ABO/injection point have been reported [11, 12]. Several intradermal or subdermal points are injected in the face and/or neck [13]. Recent publications support that this technique promotes aesthetic improvement to the upper face – without the unnatural forehead paralysis associated with conventional doses – and resulting in high patient satisfaction [11, 12]. The latest consensus for ONA suggests that the microdroplet technique is beneficial for some indications [14].

Glabellar Lines

Treat the glabellar lines in safe and very effective ways Glabellar lines may be interpreted as portraying negative feelings, such as sadness, anger, and frustration [15]. Moreover, glabellar muscles are strong depressors, being also responsible for lowering the upper eyelid, giving patients an aged appearance of this region. Injections of BoNTA in the glabella may result in central, medial, and lateral brow elevation [16]. Two-fingered palpation of these muscles can be used to minimize the occurrence of side effects, especially eyelid ptosis (Figure 20.1) [9]. The usual recommended doses for the treatment of an average size glabella are 20 U of ONA/INCO [17] and the consensus of ABO recommends 50 U for this area [18]. The latest consensus for ONA indicate that the typical total dose range for glabellar lines is 12–40 U [14]. As a larger muscle mass requires a higher dose to achieve a similar effect, doses are usually adjusted accordingly [19]. Besides gender differences in muscle mass, large patient-to-patient

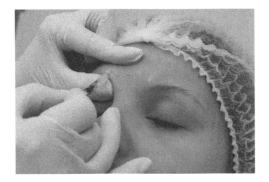

Figure 20.1 Technique of injection in the glabellar region.

variation in mass and other muscular features are observed [19].

Use combined approach to treat deep glabellar lines The improvement of deep glabellar lines may require combined procedures, such as Subcision® and/or fillers [9]. Fillers in the glabellar region should be carefully injected, due to the risk of vascular injuries with severe repercussions. Subcision® is a useful and safe technique that acts synergistically to BoNTA in the glabellar region [20].

Select the technique according to the patient's needs, avoiding side effects, including cosmetic side effects Injections in the glabella can change the brow shape and position. It is important to prevent a feminine look for men, with arched eyebrows. The male and female features differences have been described by de Maio [21], and are very

important when natural results are wanted. Eyebrows in a straight line look better and more natural and appropriate for men. The excessive elevation of the brow tail is another undesirable cosmetic side effect of glabellar injections of BoNTA.

Eyelid ptosis is the most feared complication related to BoNTA injections on the glabellar area. In this area, it is important to avoid injections of high doses and/or larger volumes of BoNTA, direct injection at the levator palpebrae superioris muscle and excessive manipulation of the injected sites after the application to prevent this side effect [22].

Follow-up and touch patients up, if needed Patients can be followed up 15–30 days after treatment with BoNTA. Excessive brow elevation, asymmetry or undesirable brow shape can be easily treated with a few units of BoNTA in the right sites, giving a more pleasant, natural look.

Periorbital Wrinkles

Tell patients about the expected results The treatment of periorbital wrinkles is effective in reducing hyperkinetic wrinkles, but it is not suitable for treating the static wrinkles caused by photoaging, skin redundancies or sleeping habits (Figure 20.2 and Figure 20.3) [18].

Use proper technique and doses The BoNTA is injected lateral and superficially

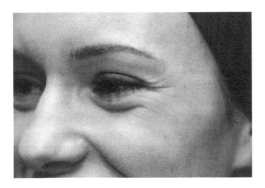

Figure 20.2 Periorbital area before BoNTA treatment.

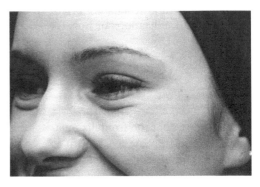

Figure 20.3 Same patient as shown in Figure 20.2 after BoNTA injections; no improvements in the skin redundancies in the lower eyelid were observed.

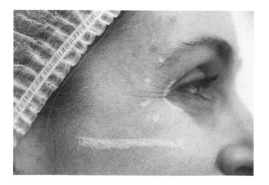

Figure 20.4 Injection points for the periocular area.

[18]. The first point is marked at the center of the maximum contraction area, usually located at the lateral canthus, at a minimum distance of 1 cm from the lateral orbital margin. Two or three additional points may be injected, 1–1.5 cm above and below the first marked, in a line that follows the orbital curvature (Figure 20.4). The recommended doses range from 4–15 U/side of ONA/INCO [14] or to 15–30 U/side of ABO distributed in two to five points on each side, according to the patients' needs [18].

Special attention to the crow's feet wrinkles located below the lateral cantus Injection points below an imaginary line between zygomatic arch and malar eminence (Figure 20.5) can reach the zygomatic muscles, resulting in an unnatural look. It is important to avoid the region of zygomaticus major

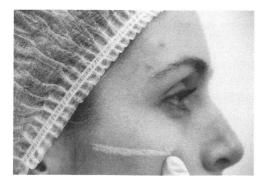

Figure 20.5 Safe injection sites should be above a line between the zygomatic arch and malar eminence. This is of particular importance for patients who underwent one or more face lifts.

muscle as it may also provoke the drooping at the corners of the mouth [17, 18].

Lower eyelid lines are also suitable for BoNTA injections Hypertrophy of the orbicularis occuli muscles, patients wishing to increase ocular aperture, and those presenting fine wrinkles in the lower eyelid can be treated with intradermal injections of 0.5 to 2 U of ONA/INCO or 2 to 5 U of ABO at the mid-pupillary line, about 2 mm below the lower eyelid border [14, 23]. Ideal patients are those who present a good snap test.

Bad candidates for BoNTA lower lid treatment Botulinum toxin injections must be avoided in patients presenting skin redundancies and laxity, eye bulging, static wrinkles or severe phodamage.

Combination regimes are also suitable for periorbital lines Since BoNTA relaxes muscles and treats hyperkinetic wrinkles effectively [18], wrinkles caused by other factors can be adjunctively treated with specific HA fillers (Figure 20.6 and Figure 20.7) [24], lasers [25], energy-based devices [26, 27], and chemical peels [28].

Horizontal Forehead Lines

Be conservative in treating the frontalis muscles Frontalis muscles are thin muscles that respond to small doses of BoNTA. The consensus papers recommend 10–30 U for ONA/INCO [17] and 20–60 U for ABO [18]. The latest consensus for ONA refer that the typical total dose for horizontal forehead lines is 8–25 U [14]. Low doses are recommended for a more natural look. For the treatment of horizontal forehead lines, four to eight points below the hairline are recommended (Figure 20.8) [14, 18].

Avoid frozen look or mask-like appearance Low doses, limited number of injection points, and partial treatment of frontalis muscle may be the best option for some patients. Treatment of the upper part of the frontalis muscle (Figure 20.8) gives a more natural look and maintains the patient's expressiveness.

Give patients an appropriate brow shape The injections can be marked in a slightly curved V-shape in women and a

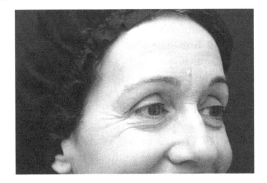

Figure 20.6 Periorbital area before BoNTA treatment combined with fillers.

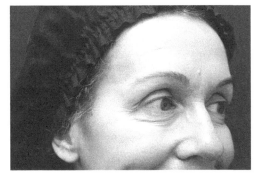

Figure 20.7 Same patient as shown in Figure 20.6 after combined treatment.

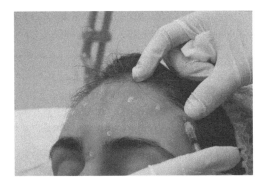

Figure 20.8 Injection points for the treatment of horizontal forehead lines.

straight line in men [18]. The injections must be applied 1–2 cm above the orbit, and superficially placed, to prevent brow ptosis, causing an appearance of tiredness [29]. To promote a natural look, excessive eyebrow elevation should be avoided, if possible, even when requested by patients (Figure 20.9 and Figure 20.10).

Treat asymmetries Special techniques are required for patients with asymmetries. This is discussed in detail in Chapter 16 Correction of Facial Asymmetry.

Mid and Lower Face

Use low doses for lower face indications Low doses are recommended to achieve the best desired effects and to prevent side effects in the lower face. If needed, touch up patients with additional doses after one month.

Attention to multiple treatments points It is important to avoid multiple treatment points in the lower face due to the risk of sum of effects and consequent side effects.

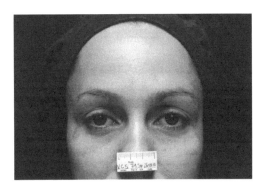

Figure 20.9 Patient before forehead treatment with BoNTA.

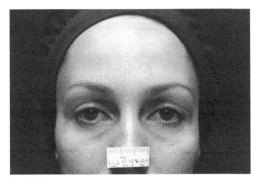

Figure 20.10 Same patient as shown in Figure 20.9 with brow lift effect after forehead treatment with BoNTA.

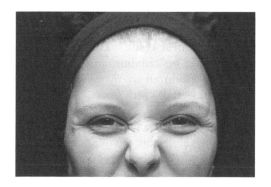

Figure 20.11 Presence of bunny lines before treatment with BoNTA in the upper third of the face.

Nasal Wrinkles

When present, always treat nasal ("bunny lines") wrinkles After the treatment of crow's feet and glabella, the nasalis muscles are usually more recruited when smiling. This is the reason why nasal wrinkles worsen after BoNTA injections in these indications, known as "bunny lines" or "Botox sign". To prevent and treat these wrinkles, it is important to also treat the nasalis muscles (Figure 20.11).

Inject BoNTA at the right sites Low doses of BoNTA must be applied in the high lateral nasal wall, below the angular vein [30] to avoid effects of the toxins in the levator labii superioris muscle.

Use the recommended doses The consensus papers recommend 2–4 U/point of ONA/INCO and 5–10 U/point of ABO [14, 23] for the treatment of nasal or bunny lines. These doses are not sufficient for some patients, who continue to recruit the nasal muscle. Considering that the size of the field of muscular effects (also known as "diffusion" halos) is dose dependent [2], it is preferable to avoid higher doses and touch up patients giving an additional dose 15–30 days later as this can avoid side effects.

Gingival Smile

Identify the type of gummy smile The smile is influenced by the proper proportion and arrangement of teeth, gums, and lips. The exposure of more than 3 mm of gum during smiling is known as gingival or gummy smile.

Based on the area of excessive gum displayed and the identification of the muscles involved, four different types of gingival smile (GS) were identified: anterior (the most frequent), posterior, mixed, and asymmetrical [31].

Treat the excessive gum exposure in the right sites and keeping mouth movements The use of BoNTA represents a simple, fast, and effective method for the aesthetic correction of GS [31, 32]. Botulinum toxin type A should be applied at two points on each side of the levator labii superioris alaeque nasi muscle in the nasolabial fold [30] to prevent the excessive anterior exposure of the gums while smiling, thus preserving the remaining mouth movements. For a more natural look, posterior gummy smile can also be treated. To reduce posterior gingival exposure BoNTA should be injected in two points at the malar region, one in the nasolabial fold, at the point of greatest lateral contraction during the smile, and the other point 2 cm lateral to the first point, at the level of the tragus [31]. The usual doses of BoNTA to treat gummy smile are 0.5–2 U of ONA/INCO per point [18] and 2.5–5 U per side of ABO [31]. Higher doses should be avoided due to the risk of a cosmetic side effect known as "joker's smile". Natural asymmetries should also be treated for a more harmonious and natural look.

Perioral Wrinkles

Low doses promote significant less side effects The perioral area has an important role in the aesthetic appearance of the face as well as in its function. Proper skills to inject low doses are extremely important to treat this indication and avoid the occurrence of side effects such as asymmetry, muscle dysfunction or temporary incapacity. Injections of BoNTA are applied at the superficial dermis, at the vermilion border or up to 5 mm from the border [9]. Select two or three sites in the perioral area and use the lowest effective dose to avoid complications such as muscle incompetence. The consensus recommended total doses are 1–5 U for ONA/INCO and from 4 to 12 for ABO, distributed in four points on the upper lip and two on the lower lip [14,23]. Cohen *et al.* suggest the use of 7.5 U of ONA to obtain significant reductions in perioral lines and high levels of subject satisfaction up to 16 weeks [33].

Combine procedures BoNTA is considered an adjuvant treatment for perioral wrinkles. For better and more natural results, the treatment of the perioral area is best managed by combining procedures, such as BoNTA, energy based treatments and fillers [23,34].

Marionette Lines

For safe and effective treatment, combine procedures Marionette lines give a sad and dissatisfied expression to the face and are primarily treated with fillers [23]. However, BoNTA can also be useful to treat marionette lines.

Use safe doses at DAO Botulinum toxin type A may be applied bilaterally into the depressis angulis oris (DAO). A total of 2–4 U of ONA/INCO per side and 5–10 U of ABO per side is recommended [14,23]. Loss of control of movement of the mouth corners should be avoided by using lower doses and keeping injections toward the lateral aspect of the muscle, away from the depressor labii inferioris.

Consider to treat the mentalis first. The mentalis muscle acts as an agonist of DAO (Figure 20.12). Injection of BoNTA at the mentalis imply in less recruitment of DAO.

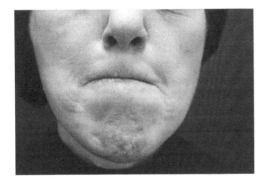

Figure 20.12 The mentalis muscle is an agonist and supports the contraction of the DAO muscle.

Dimpled Chin

Use BoNTA to improve more than wrinkles for better, natural results The treatment of the dimpled or "cellulitic" aspect of the chin can be optimized by the association of BoNTA injections with fillers, since the contraction of the mentalis muscle, and loss of collagen and subcutaneous fat in this region contributes significantly to this condition [22]. Subcision® can also be combined with good results. The technique and doses vary. Whereas the consensus for ONA suggests one to four points of injection [14], the consensus for ABO suggests two points of injection [23]. The typical total dose of 4–10 U of ONA [14] or 10–20 U of ABO is suggested and should be applied at the most distal point of the mentalis muscle at the prominence of the chin [23]. There can also be gender differences in total dose, with another study recommending 2–8 U of ONA for men and 2–6 U of ONA for women; it improves wrinkles and DAO movements as described earlier.

Face Lifting

The use of BoNTA can improve facial appearance by also promoting discrete a face lifting effect. It is important to notice that BoNTA cannot replace the surgical lift with similar cosmetic results.

Identify correctly if there is indication for BoNTA face lift Some of the platysma muscle fibers are located in the mandibular region, promoting the lowering of this area. To assess if the patient will respond positively to the treatment, the physician should ask the patient to pull down the platysma muscle. The disappearance of the mandibular border may indicate the potential success of the procedure [35].

Obtaining the lift effect For a lift effect and to improve the definition of the mandibular border or angle, BoNTA should be applied in two to four points along the lateral mandibular border [9]. The doses are divided into 1–2 U of ONA/INCO or 2–5 U of ABO per point [9].

Combine procedures Some procedures can be combined to improve the lifting effects, such as radiofrequency, infrared light, microfocused ultrasound, and fillers.

Neck and Chest

Treating neck and chest simultaneously to the face can provide a more harmonious and natural rejuvenation Neck usually presents more signs of aging than the face. Neck wrinkles are more frequently related to photoaging and skin laxity than platysmal bands, but BoNTA can be used in cases of visible contractions of this muscle [9].

Touch ups are usually needed in this area. Residual platysmal bands can be treated with additional doses of BoNTA.

Combined treatments can also be used to improve the appearance of these regions In general, wrinkles of the anterior midchest are caused by the position adopted during sleep (called "sleep wrinkles") and photodamage, but in some patients, they result from the action of the medial fibers of the pectoralis major muscle and the tail portion of the platysma muscle Therefore, BoNTA can be very effective in this case and more effective results can be obtained by combined procedures, such as lasers and peelings [23].

To be effective for chest wrinkles, the pectoralis major muscle must be involved The involvement of the pectoralis major muscle can be investigated by palpation of these muscles, while asking the patients to cross their arms [9]. If these muscles are involved in these wrinkles, BoNTA can be considered for the treatment, alone or in combination with other procedures.

Use proper, effective doses The recommended doses for the neck range from 6 to 12 U of ONA/INCO per band and maximum total of 60 U [14], and a total of 50–100 U of ABO [23]. The total number of injection points depends on the number and length of platysmal bands. The injections should start with the first point at the jaw line, and go down every 2 cm to at least the middle of the band [23]. The total maximum dose should not be exceeded as dysphagia, dysphonia, and neck weakness can appear; they are related to very high doses [23].

The recommended total doses for the chest range from 30 to 100 U of ONA/INCO and 75–120 U of ABO, and should be given in a "V" shape over the wrinkles, divided into three to six points on each side [9, 23].

Conclusion

The current goals of all cosmetic procedures are to achieve a natural look and improve beauty, avoiding distortions and keeping facial expressions. To reach these goals, each patient must be treated with a safe and effective individual therapeutic doses and approach, meeting doctors and patients' expectations, with harmony, balance, and naturalness.

The doses of botulinum toxins should be adjusted depending on the indications, mass, and anatomical location of the muscles being treated and on the wishes of the patient. The use of minimally effective dosing and volume are highly recommended in some areas to avoid unwanted side effects, since a larger field of effect or strong results can result in a frozen, unnatural appearance. Considering each patient's characteristics, needs, and expectations, as well as knowing the proper techniques, is essential to obtain optimal, safer, natural results.

References

1 Dayan SH, Ashourian N. Considerations for achieving a natural face in cosmetic procedures. JAMA Facial Plast Surg 2015;17(6):395.

2 Hexsel D, Brum C, do Prado DZ, *et al.* Field effect of two commercial preparations of botulinum toxin type A: a prospective, double-blind, randomized clinical trial.

J Am Acad Dermatol 2012;67(2): 226–232.

3 Hexsel D, Soirefmann M, Porto MD, *et al.* Fields of muscular and anhidrotic effects of 2 botulinum toxin-A commercial preparations: a prospective, double-blind, randomized, multicenter study. Dermatol Surg. 2015;41(Suppl 1):S110–S118.

4 Carruthers J, Fournier N, Kerscher M, *et al.* The convergence of medicine and neurotoxins: a focus on botulinum toxin type A and its application in aesthetic medicine – a global, evidence-based botulinum toxin consensus education initiative: part II: incorporating botulinum toxin into aesthetic clinical practice. Dermatol Surg. 2013;39(3 Pt 2):510–525.

5 Alam M, Bolotin D, Carruthers J, *et al.* Consensus statement regarding storage and reuse of previously reconstituted neuromodulators. Dermatol Surg. 2015;41(3):321–326.

6 Malick F, Howard J, Koo J. Understanding the psychology of the cosmetic patients. Dermatol Ther 2008;21:47–53.

7 Wilson JB, Arpey CJ. Body dysmorphic disorder: suggestions for detection and treatment in a surgical dermatology practice. Dermatol Surg 2004;30:1391–399.

8 Salti G, Ghersetich I. Advanced botulinum toxin techniques against wrinkles in the upper face. Clin Dermatol 2008;26: 182–191.

9 Hexsel D, Hexsel CL. Botulinum toxins. In: Robinson JK, Hanke CW, Siegel DM, Fratila A, eds. *Surgery of the Skin – Procedural Dermatology*, 3rd edn. Edinburgh: Elsevier 2015; 427–440.

10 Wollina U, Konrad H. Managing adverse events associated with botulinum toxin type-A: a focus on cosmetic procedures. Am J Clin Dermatol 2005;6(3):141–150.

11 Steinsapir KD, Rootman D, Wulc A, Hwang C. Cosmetic microdroplet botulinum toxin A forehead lift: A new treatment paradigm. Ophthal Plast Reconstr Surg 2015;31(4): 263–268.

12 Iozzo I, Tengattini V, Antonucci VA. Multipoint and multilevel injection technique of botulinum toxin A in facial aesthetics. J Cosmet Dermatol. 2014;13(2): 135–142.

13 Wu WT. Microbotox of the lower face and neck: Evolution of a personal technique and its clinical effects. Plast Reconstr Surg. 2015;136(5 Suppl):92S–100S.

14 Sundaram H, Signorini M, Liew S, *et al.* Global aesthetics consensus: botulinum toxin type a-evidence-based review, emerging concepts, and consensus recommendations for aesthetic use, including updates on complications. Plast Reconstr Surg. 2016;137(3):518e–529e.

15 Carruthers JA, Lowe NJ, Menter MA, Gibson J, *et al.* A multicenter, double-blind, randomized, placebo-controlled study of the efficacy and safety of botulinum toxin type A in the treatment of glabellar lines. J Am Acad Dermatol 2002;46(6):840–849.

16 Carruthers J, Carruthers A. Botulinum toxin in facial rejuvenation: an update. Dermatol Clin 2009:27(4):417–425; v. Review.

17 Carruthers JD, Glogau RG, Blitzer A. Advances in Facial Rejuvenation: Botulinum Toxin Type A, Hyaluronic Acid Dermal Fillers, and Combination Therapies-Consensus Recommendations. Plast Reconstr Surg 2008;121(5 Suppl): 5S–30S.

18 Ascher B, Talarico S, Cassuto D *et al.* International consensus recommendation on the aesthetic usage of botulinum toxin type A (Speywood unit)-part one: upper facial wrinkles. J Eur Acad Dermatol Venereol 2010:24(11):1278–1284.

19 Monheit G, Lin X, Nelson D, Kane M. Consideration of muscle mass in glabellar line treatment with botulinum toxin type A. J Drugs Dermatol. 2012;11(9): 1041–1045.

20 Hexsel D. Combining procedures with botulinum toxin in dermatology and dermatological surgery. In: Hexsel D, Almeida AT, eds. *Cosmetic Use of Botulinum Toxin*. São Paulo: AGE 2002; 211–215.

21 de Maio M. Ethnic and gender considerations in the use of facial injectables: male patients. Plast Reconstr Surg 2015;136(5 Suppl):40S–43S.

22 Hexsel C, Hexsel D, Porto MD, Schilling J, Siega C. Botulinum toxin type A for aging face and aesthetic uses. Dermatol Ther 2011;24(1):54–61.

23 Ascher B, Talarico S, Cassuto D et al. International consensus recommendations on the aesthetic usage of botulinum toxin type A (Speywood Unit)—Part II: Wrinkles on the middle and lower face, neck and chest. J Eur Acad Dermatol Venereol 2010;24(11):1285–1295.

24 Coleman KR, Carruthers J. Combination therapy with BOTOX and fillers: the new rejuvenation paradigm. Dermatol Ther 2006;19(3):177–188.

25 Semchyshyn NL, Kilmer SL. Does laser inactivate botulinum toxin? Dermatol Surg 2005;31(4):399–404.

26 Khoury JG, Saluja R, Goldman MP. The effect of botulinum toxin type A on full-face intense pulsed light treatment: a randomized, double-blind, split-face study. Dermatol Surg 2008;34(8):1062–1069.

27 Carruthers J, Carruthers A. The effect of full-face broadband light treatments alone and in combination with bilateral crow's feet Botulinum toxin type A chemodenervation. Dermatol Surg 2004;30(3):355–366.

28 Landau M. Combination of chemical peelings with botulinum toxin injections and dermal fillers. J Cosmet Dermatol 2006;5(2):121–126.

29 Flynn TC, Carruthers J, Carruthers A. Botulinum-A toxin treatment of the lower eyelid improves infraorbital rhytides and widens the eye. Dermatol Surg 2001; 27(8):703–708.

30 Carruthers J, Carruthers A. Aesthetic botulinum A toxin in the mid and lower face and neck. Dermatol Surg 2003;29(5):468–476.

31 Mazzuco R, Hexsel D. Gummy smile and botulinum toxin: a new approach based on the gingival exposure area. J Am Acad Dermatol 2010;63(6):1042–1051.

32 Polo M. Botulinum toxin type A in the treatment of excessive gingival display. Am J Orthod Dentofacial Orthop 2005;127:214–218.

33 Cohen JL, Dayan SH, Cox SE, et al. OnabotulinumtoxinA dose-ranging study for hyperdynamic perioral lines. Dermatol Surg 2012;38(9):1497–1505.

34 Carruthers J, Burgess C, Day D, et al. Consensus Recommendations for Combined Aesthetic Interventions in the Face Using Botulinum Toxin, Fillers, and Energy-Based Devices. Dermatol Surg 2016;42(5):586–597.

35 Levy PM. The "Nefertiti lift." J Cosmet Lasers Ther 2007;9:249–252.

21

Special Considerations in Darker Skin

Cheré Lucas Anthony, MD[1,2] and Marta I. Rendon, MD (FAAD, FACP)[1,3]

[1]*Medical Director, Rendon Center for Dermatology and Aesthetic Medicine, Boca Raton, USA*
[2]*Voluntary Faculty, Dermatology and Cutaneous Surgery, University of Miami, Miller School of Medicine, Miami, USA*
[3]*Voluntary Associate Clinical Professor, University of Miami, Dermatology Department, Miami, USA*

Introduction

As people embrace ethnic diversity, the ideal of beauty is changing. This shift has influenced the cosmetic approach for darker skin types. Successful outcomes hinge on understanding key differences in skin properties and facial shape and utilizing this knowledge in tailored regimens.

In 2015, 25% of all cosmetic procedures were performed on racial and ethnic minorities [1]. The rapidly growing ethnic population underscores the necessity for healthcare professionals to become familiar with the unique skin properties and aesthetic concerns in people of color. Dynamic rhytids often predominate in aging, making botulinum toxin an integral component of care for this expanding cosmetic population. We advocate for early intervention in patients with pigmented skin, since they have fewer treatment options to combat aging. In this chapter, we will discuss the unique characteristics of darker skin and special considerations in a treatment program utilizing botulinum toxin A.

Unique Qualities in Skin of Color and Facial Structure

While properties of skin and facial structure are more similar than different across ethnic backgrounds, there is some variability. Individuals with pigmented skin comprise a wide range of ethnic groups. Racial categories are somewhat arbitrary, and significant variability is seen within these groups. Latin Americans, black Caribbeans and African Americans often have diverse genetic backgrounds. The Latin American population in particular encompasses all skin types, which makes generalization difficult.

Understanding the complexity of this issue is important to evaluation and treatment. For the purposes of this chapter, we define darker skin types as Fitzpatrick III–VI in African Americans; black Caribbeans, Latinos and Hispanics; Asians; Pacific Islanders; Indians; Pakistanis; and persons of Middle Eastern descent.

Differences in skin of color are relevant to evaluation and treatment of the cosmetic patient. Current literature supports variance in melanin content, ultraviolet light penetration, dermal thickness, and elastic recovery, in addition to other properties.

The size and distribution of melanosomes vary among ethnic groups. It has been well documented that darker skin types have a greater number of melanosomes and that these melanosomes are more evenly distributed and larger. Szabo and colleagues [2, 3] were among the first to find that melanosomes are singly dispersed in black skin and more aggregated in white skin. As

Botulinum Toxins: Cosmetic and Clinical Applications, First Edition. Edited by Joel L. Cohen and David M. Ozog.
© 2017 John Wiley & Sons Ltd. Published 2017 by John Wiley & Sons Ltd.
Companion Website: www.wiley.com/go/cohen/botulinum

the skin type changes – or for skin in Asian or racially mixed people – the melanosome distribution becomes more complex. It can also change in sun-exposed skin [4, 5].

Melanin content also varies, and this becomes relevant in aging and in patient evaluation for cosmetic procedures. Melanin confers photoprotection by absorbing and deflecting ultraviolet light. Five times more ultraviolet A (UVA) and ultraviolet B (UVB) reaches the upper dermis of white people than black people. In fact, all wavelengths of light are filtered equally by melanin [6]. Thus, darker skin is less susceptible to acute and chronic actinic damage.

Histologically, the dermis of sun-damaged skin in white people shows lilac- and blue-stained elastic fibers, signifying significant elastosis [7], whereas the skin of black people demonstrates minimal elastosis and no lilac-stained elastic fibers. Superior inherent photoprotection secondary to increased melanin delays the signs of aging until the fifth or sixth decade in people with darker skin [8].

In Asians, the onset of skin wrinkle is also delayed. Studies of various Asian ethnic groups consistently show fewer signs of aging, when compared with age-matched non-Asians with light skin [9–11]. While wrinkling in photoaged Asian skin is less prominent, hyperpigmentation and solar elastosis are seen [12]. The frequency and extent of these changes in the skin of Asians varies and depends on sun exposure and proximity to the equator.

While inherent photoprotection and lack of elastosis are typical in skin of color, the dermis also exhibits unique properties. In the skin of black people and Asians the dermis is thicker and contains more collagen than in skin of white people [13, 14]. In addition, elastic recovery time has been found to be slightly higher in black people than in white people and Hispanics [15, 16]. These distinct characteristics account for variations in the appearance of aging and reinforce the general notion that skin of color appears less photodamaged, and signs of aging are delayed.

Differences also exist in facial structure, and maintaining these unique characteristics is important in preserving ethnic appearance. The shape of the face, particularly the angle and shape of the eye, are unique.

A review of facial structure among ethnic groups [17] revealed a great deal of variation, particularly among Latin Americans and African Americans, where racial mixture is common. Nevertheless, some generalizations have been noted. Asians, Latinos and African Americans tend to have rounder faces than white people [12, 18, 19]. Additionally, masseter muscle hypertrophy, primarily described in Asian populations, can lead to a more pronounced squareness in jaw shape.

In some people of Mexican descent, the length of the columnella is shorter [20, 21]. And fuller, more protuberant lips are seen not only in African Americans, but also in Asians [22, 23].

The eye and brow vary greatly among ethnic populations. The lack of a superior palpebral fold in Asians is often cited in contrast to other ethnicities; however, more subtle differences also exist.

Eyebrow shape and placement are similar in white people, Indians and Asians [24], with the apex (highest point of the brow) generally positioned between the lateral limbus and lateral canthus. The distance from the brow to the upper lid margin is greater in Asians [25]. In Indians, the distance from the end of the brow to the lateral canthus is shorter, possibly because of an upwardly slanted eye, or increased palpebral fissure inclination, a characteristic of Indian and Chinese populations.

Palpebral fissure inclination is sometimes referred to as the lateral canthal angle. It was recently postulated that the lateral commissure may be higher than the medial commissure to a greater degree in African Americans [26]. Africans and African Americans also have more prominent orbital proptosis, as compared with Caucasians. The unique eye shapes of Asians, Indians, and African Americans (and many Latin Americans) should be considered prior to cosmetic treatment to preserve normal ethnic appearance.

Cosmetic Implications

Special Considerations when Using Botulinum Toxin A

The unique skin and facial structure in persons of color cause them to age differently. These variations impact cosmetic treatment (see Table 21.1). We will discuss specific considerations in the preservation, restoration, and enhancement of the ethnic face with botulinum toxin A.

Upper Face

Increased melanin confers photoprotection, and thus, dynamic wrinkling predominates over superficial wrinkling caused by actinic damage. Therefore, it is not surprising that aging of the upper face in darker-skinned individuals is most commonly seen in the glabella area [27]. Multiple studies have evaluated the treatment of glabellar rhytids with botulinum toxin A in skin of color and have consistently shown a similarity in dosage and safety of botulinum toxin A across racial and ethnic groups [14, 28–30]. On average, the glabellar region was treated with 20 U of Botox® (onabotulinumtoxinA)/Xeomin® (incobotulinumtoxinA) and 40–50 U

Dysport® (abobotulinumtoxinA) at five injection points. Slightly more botulinum toxin A was used in men than in women.

Interestingly, a secondary finding of one Dysport® study was increased effectiveness and longer-lasting results in African Americans as compared with other patients [31]. The same study showed a slightly higher incidence of ocular adverse events in African Americans than in other ethnicities (6% versus 4%), but a lower incidence of injection-site reactions [31]. Similar findings of longer efficacy were seen in an analysis of pooled clinical data. Safety and time of onset was similar between skin of color and white patients; however, the response rate after 1 month was greater in skin of color patients [32].

Botulinum toxin A is placed midline into the procerus. Injections are performed bilaterally into the corrugator supercilii medially just above the eyebrow along the medial canthal line and just inside the lateral corrugator supercilii. Injection deep and just above the periosteum minimizes involvement of the inferior frontalis, minimizing brow droop and allowing upward pull as the brow depressors relax.

The first three injections are typically made with 4–5 U of Botox® and approximately 10 U of Dysport®. The final two injections into the lateral corrugator supercilii often require less product, and 2–3 U of Botox®

Table 21.1 Characteristics of ethnic groups and how these characteristics impact aging.

	Variations in darker skin types	Changes with aging
Facial shape	• Rounder in Asians, African Americans and Latin Americans • Masseter hypertrophy in Asians	• Loss of volume • Jowl formation/sagging • Mental crease
Brows	• Lateral apex • Shorter distance between end of brow and lateral canthus (Indians, Chinese)	• Medial apex • Descending brow
Eyes	• Lack of epicanthal fold, increased distance to brow, palpebral fissure inclination (Asians) • Increased lateral canthal angle (African Americans, Indians)	• Descending lateral canthal angle
Columella	• Shorter columella (some Mexicans)	• Lengthens with age
Lips	• Fuller lips (African Americans, Asians)	• Volume loss

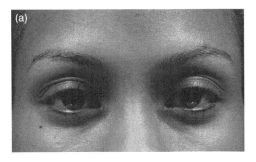 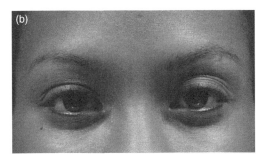

Figure 21.1 (a) Baseline. (b) Mild elevation of brow after treatment with BTA, preserving lateral apex.

or Xeomin® and 5 U of Dysport® are typically used. Because one side of the face is stronger than the other, we typically have patients return in 2 weeks for reassessment.

Improvement of forehead rhytids is more variable. We advocate for earlier treatment of darker skin to prevent persistent horizontal lines. Different techniques have been described in earlier chapters. A total of 8–12 U of Botox® or Xeomin® and 20–30 U of Dysport® is typically used, depending on the degree of movement the patient desires, the proximity of the brow to the upper eyelid, and the size of the forehead. In a narrow forehead, injection sites can be placed horizontally. In a fuller forehead, injections can be made in a V shape, or the products distributed through a single central injection site and two vertical sites on each side, with a possible small aliquot made laterally and higher. We stress careful evaluation of the face in a dynamic position and at rest prior to injection to account for ethnic variations and muscle strength.

Although the placement of botulinum is a relatively quick procedure, there is a definite art to tailoring the treatment. Women tend to have more shape to the brow, with a more obvious apex. In some ethnic women, particularly Asians, the distance from the brow to the eyelid is greater. It is important to stay well above the brow – approximately 2 cm – to avoid or minimize brow ptosis. In our practice, we inject botulinum higher and more centrally, which allows for some lateral upward pull, while conserving brow height.

In addition to improving forehead lines, botulinum treatment of the forehead can influence the shape of the brow. In youth, brow shape peaks laterally, whereas older people exhibit a more medial brow apex [33]. It is extremely important to evaluate brow placement and shape in skin of color. We typically ask patients to raise their forehead to make the apex of the brow more prominent. We then draw a diagonal line from the apex of the brow to the temporal hairline, where the lateral frontalis pulls superiorlaterally. Injection sites are kept medial to this line when treating the forehead. Relaxing the medial portion of the forehead confers additional lift to the lateral brow and places the apex to a more youthful, lateral position (Figure 21.1).

Because the distance from the brow to the eyelid is greater in Asian and African American faces, lifting the brow is important to restore a more natural look. Treating the glabellar frown lines will lift the brow, since the procerus and corrugator supercilii are brow depressors. Chemodenervation of the orbicularis oculi lateral and outside the location where the orbital rim curves inferiorly usually leads to modest elevation of the lateral brow [34]. We place 2 U of Botox® or Xeomin® in this location, being careful not to breach the orbital rim margin.

Periorbital/Eye Complex

As mentioned earlier, the lateral canthal angle tends to be greater in young African Americans as compared with young white people. While brow ptosis occurs later in African Americans, it is postulated that the lateral

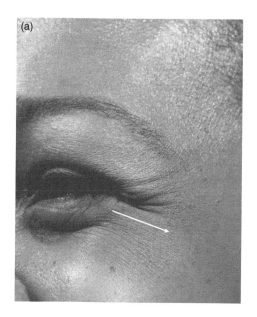 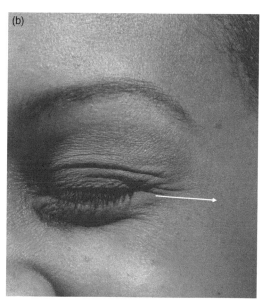

Figure 21.2 (a) Baseline: downward slanted canthus accentuated in dynamic position with rhytids along the orbital rim. (b) After: improvement of canthal angle in dynamic position with softening of rhytids and lateral position of brow apex.

canthal angle descends faster. Thus, aging of the upper face occurs primarily in the periorbital area. The mean lateral canthal angle in African Americans measures an average of 2.39° in youth and 1.05° after the age of 45 years. The angle is small, but a slight change in elevation can result in significant aesthetic improvement. Botulinum toxin can be used to subtly restore the lateral canthal angle to a more youthful position (Figure 21.2).

In our practice, approximately 2 U of Botox® or Xeomin® and 5 U of Dysport® are injected into the laterosuperior and lateroinferior superficial orbicularis oculi muscle to relax the downward pull on the lateral canthal complex. As small a volume as possible is utilized to avoid the diffusion that occurs with greater volume. We combine this procedure with shaping and lifting of the lateral brow as mentioned earlier, to enhance the appearance of an upwardly slanted lateral canthal complex.

Crow's Feet

The development of crow's feet is delayed in darker skin types, and in some people, may be minimal. This may be the result of photoprotection conferred by greater amounts of melanin and a thicker dermis, as discussed earlier; however, skin types III and IV, particularly in individuals who have had significant sun exposure, may develop crow's feet. Typically, 8–15 U of Botox® or Xeomin® and 15–30 U of Dysport® are used per side. Multiple injection sites in small aliquots with botulinum toxin A produce a smooth effect on lateral lines. Anecdotally, Dysport® may not require as many injection sites as Botox® or Xeomin®, but this may be more dependent on the end volume of the reconstituted product – more volume can lead to larger areas of diffusion. The product is injected in two to four sites placed intradermally lateral to the orbital rim along the curvature.

While crow's feet may not be as prominent in darker skin types, the eyes can appear smaller and less open with age, despite minimal superficial wrinkling. Treatment of the superficial orbicularis oculii not only softens crow's feet, but will open the palpebral aperture [35]. Results are particularly impressive in the Asian eye; however, we advise discussing this effect with the patient prior to injection, since widening may not be desirable in all ethnic groups. Upon agreement, we inject about 2 U of Botox® or 5 U of Dysport® to the infraorbital lid where the lower pretarsal orbicularis widens the eye. Because periocular skin is thin, creating a bleb ensures proper intradermal depth of injection. Appropriate smoothing of crow's feet and maintenance of the eyes' shape can be achieved by avoiding infraorbital injection.

Lower Face

Lower facial aging in darker skin types manifests as pronounced sagging or laxity. Melomental folds and mouth frown may be the most significant signs of aging in the lower face, as little or no superficial wrinkling will usually develop. Perioral wrinkles appear later and are rarer.

Downturned mouth corners can be softened by placing 2–3 U of Botox® or Xeomin® or 4–6 U of Dysport® into the depressor anguli oris (DAO). Concurrent treatment of the mentalis can augment the effect. Injecting small doses of botulinum toxin A to each lateral mentalis band lessens the potential of weakening the orbicularis oris. Similarly, melomental folds are improved by placing a minimal amount of product into the DAO 1 cm lateral to the oral commissure and at the angle of the mandible. Flattening of the lower lip contour can occur if the injection is placed too high. To find the proper injection point, we ask the patient to frown, and we follow the mental crease to the point where it intersects with the jawline. We then inject lateral to this point and deep, just above the bone.

Full lips are characteristic of darker skin types and have been culturally desirable in this country. Volume loss in the lips does occur over time, and although lip lines may be minimal, perioral injections can help restore fullness to the lips.

If vertical lip rhytids are short, small aliquots of botulinum toxin A (for example, 1–2 U of Botox® or Xeomin®) are placed in four locations along the vermillion border. Dividing the lips into quadrants, the product

is injected one-quarter and three-quarters laterally in each quadrant and repeated on the contralateral side. Care should be taken to avoid the corners of the mouth, where chemodenervation can cause mouthdrooping and drooling. If the vertical lines of the lip are longer, injections can be made with 1–2 U of Botox® or Xeomin® (Dysport® requires slightly more), up to a maximum of 4 U for each lip. We dilute 1–2 U of Botox® or Xeomin® to a volume of 0.1 cm^3 and inject it along the vermillion border on each side, starting just lateral to the cupid's bow. The product is injected into the superficial orbicularis oris, as opposed to deep placement, to maintain adequate sphincter tone of the mouth. The technique can be repeated if desired for the lower lips.

Facial Contouring

Masseter muscle hypertrophy typically presents between the ages of 20 and 40 years [36] and can lead to a prominent mandibular angle that can make the face appear wider. This is primarily a concern among Asians, in which it known as square-jaw. Masseter hypertrophy is commonly considered undesirable, since Asian women prefer an oval or almond-shaped face [37]. Injections of botulinum toxin A into the masseter muscle in the treatment of masseteric hypertrophy was first reported in 1994 [38], and can be effective in reshaping and narrowing the face. Reduction in masseter hypertrophy is effective and relatively long lasting.

In an early study by Park *et al.*, 25–30 U of Botox® yielded results out to 10 months, with an average 18–20% reduction in mass demonstrated through ultrasonic and computed tomography imaging. Another group reported an average 31% reduction in masseter hypertrophy in 383 patients injected with 100–140 U of Dysport® [39]. The duration of efficacy and quantitative reduction in mass appeared to be doserelated. Effective treatment doses were evaluated using ultrasonic measurements of the masseter. Improved results were seen with 20–30 U of Botox®, as compared with

10 U [40]. In general, suggested doses include 25–30 U of Botox® and 50–70 U of Dysport® per side [41]. Adequate treatment shows a dose-dependent effect for 6–9 months. Side effects may include initial awkwardness upon smiling, fatigue with vigorous chewing, speech disturbance, and localized pain at injection sites. These side effects are transient and last approximately 1–4 weeks after injection.

Botulinum injections are distributed among five to six sites along the mandibular angle. Multiple injection sites allow for a more uniform reduction in masseter thickness without compensatory muscle bulging at other areas along the jawline. The product is placed from the level of the earlobe to the lower posterior portion of the masseter at the angle of the jaw. Injection sites are kept low on the jawline to prevent damage to the parotid duct and paralysis of the risorius and zygomaticus muscles. This textbook also contains a separate chapter with a comprehensive discussion of mandibular contouring and description of technique.

Other Cosmetic Applications

More recently, recontouring of enlarged gastrocnemius muscles has been achieved with botulinum toxin A [42,43]. The technique has been mainly described among Asians, and particularly Korean and Chinese, in whom slimmer calves are culturally desirable.

Both the appearance of the muscle prominence and actual leg circumference can be reduced. There are few studies on optimal dosing; however, as little as 30 U and as much as 70 U of Botox® and from 150 to 180 U of Dysport® per side have been used safely, with results lasting up to 8 months. Injections are placed into the medial head, since it is the most prominent muscle of the calf and is functionally redundant. No functional disabilities have been reported with these doses. This is also discussed further in a separate chapter in this textbook.

Conclusion

The unique properties and differences in skin and facial structure in skin of color affect aging. Although there are many treatment options to improve aging, specific variations are needed when treating ethnic skin. Actinic damage and superficial wrinkling can be minimal or absent, and dynamic wrinkling predominates. Changes in the brow and eye complex as well as laxity leading to mental crease and mouth frown are commonly seen. These changes in darker skinned patients can be addressed with botulinum toxin A. Early intervention of these rhytids becomes important in skin of color as treatment procedures such as resurfacing can be problematic. We advocate for prevention and early treatment, before rhytids become persistent. Botulinum toxin A is an effective and integral part of cosmetic enhancement in darker skin types. The key to a successful cosmetic outcome in people of color is having a clear understanding of their facial structure, basic histopathological differences and skin properties, as well as knowledge about specific ethnic backgrounds so that diverse and distinct traits are preserved.

References

1 American Society of Aesthetic Plastic Surgery. 2015 Statistics. Available at http://http://www.surgery.org/media/statistics. Accessed February 8, 2017.

2 Szabo G. Pigment cell biology. In: Gordon M, ed. *Mitochondria and Other Cytoplasmic Inclusions*. New York, NY: Academic Press; 1959.

3 Szabo G, Gerald AB, Patnak MA, Fitzpatrick TB. Racial differences in the fate of melanosomes in human epidermis. Nature 1969;222:1081–1082.

4 Toda K, Pathak MA, Parrish JA, *et al*. Alteration of racial differences in melanosome distribution in human epidermis after exposure to ultraviolet

light. Nat New Biol 1972;236(66):143–145.

5 Olson RL, Gaylor J, Everett MA. Skin color, melanin, and erythema. Arch Dermatol 1973;108:541–544.

6 Kaidbey KH, Agin PP, Sayre RM, Kligman AM. Photoprotection by melanin – a comparison of black and Caucasian skin. J Am Acad Dermatol 1979;1(3):249–260.

7 Montagna W, Kirchner S, Carlisle K. Histology of sun-damaged skin. J Am Acad Dermatol 1989;21(5):907–918.

8 Morizot F, Guehenneux S, Dheurle S, et al. Do features of aging differ between Asian and Caucasian women? J Invest Dermatol 2004;123:A67.

9 Nouveau-Richard S, Yang Z, Mac-Mary S, et al. Skin again: A comparison between Chinese and European populations: A pilot study. J Dermatol Sci 2005;40(3):187–193.

10 Griffiths CE, Goldfarb MT, Finkel LJ, et al. Topical tretinoin treatment of hyperpigmented lesions associated with photoaging in Chinese and Japanese patients: a vehicle-controlled trial. J Am Acad Dermatol 1994;30:76–84.

11 Goh SH. The treatment of visible signs of senescence: the Asian experience. Br J Dermatol 1990;122(Suppl 35):105–109.

12 Grimes PE. Beauty: A historical and societal perspective. In: Grimes PE, Kim J, Hexsel D, et al., eds. Aesthetic and Cosmetic Surgery for Darker Skin Types. Philadelphia, PA: Lippincott Williams & Wilkins; 2007:10.

13 Montagna W, Prota G, Kenney JA, eds. The structure of black skin. In: Black Skin Structure and Function. San Diego, CA: Academic Press; 1993:37–49.

14 Anh KY, Park MY, Park DH, Han DG. Botulinum toxin A for the treatment of facial hyperkinetic wrinkle lines in Koreans. Plast Reconstr Surg 2000;105(2):778–784.

15 Berardesca E, de Rigal J, Leveque JL, Maibach HI. In vivo biophysical differences in races. Dermatologica 1991;182:89–93.

16 Richards G, Oresajo C, Halder R. Structure and function of ethnic skin and hair. Dermatol Clin 2003;21:595–600.

17 Talakoub L, Wesley N. Differences in perceptions of beauty and cosmetic procedures performed in ethnic patients. Semin Cutan Med Surg 2009;28:115–129.

18 Shirakabe Y. A new paradigm for the aging Asian face. Aesthetic Plastic Surg 2003;27:397–402.

19 To EW, Ahuja AT, Ho WS, et al. A prospective study of the effect of botulinum toxin A on masseteric muscle hypertrophy with ultrasonographic and electromyographic measurement. Br J Plast Surg 2001;54(3):197–200.

20 Ortiz-Monasterio F, Olmedo A. Rhinoplasty on the mestizo nose. Clin Plast Surg 1977;4:89–102.

21 Sanchez AE. Rhinoplasty in the "Chata" nose of the Caribbean. Aesth Plast Surg 1980;4:169–177.

22 McCurdy JA. Cosmetic Surgery of the Asian Face. New York, NY: Thieme Medical Publishers; 1990.

23 Grimes PE. Beauty: A historical and societal perspective. In: Grimes PE, Kim J, Hexsel D, et al., eds. Aesthetic and Cosmetic Surgery for Darker Skin Types. Philadelphia, Pa: Lippincott Williams & Wilkins; 2007:9.

24 Kunjur J, Sabesan T, Ilankovan V. Anthropometric analysis of eyebows and eyelids: an inter-racial study. Br J Oral Maxillofac Surg 2006;44(2):89–93.

25 Lam SM, Kim YK. The partial-incision technique for the creation of the double eyelid. Aesthetic Surg 2003;23:170–176.

26 Odunze M, Rosenberg D, Few J. Periorbital aging and ethnic considerations: a focus on the lateral canthal complex. Plast Reconstr Surg 2008;121:1002–1008.

27 Hexsel D, Hexsel C, Brunetto L. Botulinum Toxin. In: Grimes PE, Kim J, Hexsel D, et al., eds. Aesthetic and Cosmetic Surgery for Darker Skin Types. Philadelphia, Pa: Lippincott Williams & Wilkins; 2007:214.

28 Lew H, Yun SY, Lee SY, Kim SJ. Effect of botulinum toxin A on facial wrinkle lines in Koreans. Ophthalmologica 2002;216:50–54.

29 Grimes PE, Shabazz D. A four-month randomized, double-blind evaluation of the efficacy of botulinum toxin type A for the treatment of glabellar lines in women with skin types V and VI. Dermatol Surg 2009; 35(3):429–435.

30 Wu Y, Zhao G, Li H, *et al*. Botulinum toxin type A for the treatment of glabellar lines in Chinese: a double blind, randomized, placebo-controlled study. Dermatol Surg 2010;36:102–108.

31 Kane M, Brandt F, Rohrich R, Narins R, *et al*., Reloxin Investigational Group. Evaluation of variable-dose treatment with a new US botulinum toxin type A (Dysport) for correction of moderate to severe glabellar lines: results from a phase II, randomized, double-blind, placebo-controlled study. Plas Reconstr Surg 2009;124(5):1619–1629.

32 Taylor SC, Callender VD, Albright CD, *et al*. Abobotulinumtoxin A for reduction of glabellar lines in patients with skin of color: post hoc analysis of pooled clinical trial data. Dermatol Surg 2012;38(11): 1804–1811.

33 Biller J, Kim D. A contemporary assessment of facial aesthetic preferences. Arch Facial Plast Surg 2009;11(2):91–97.

34 Huilgol SC, Carruthers A, Carruthers JDA. Raising eyebrows with botulinum toxin. Dermatol Surg 1999;25(5):373–376.

35 Flynn TC, Carruthers A, Carruthers JDA. Botulinum-A toxin treatment of the lower eyelid improves infraorbital rhytids and widens the eye. Dermatol Surg 2001;27(8): 703–708.

36 Von Lidern JJ, Niederhagen B, Appel T, *et al*. Type A botulinum toxin for the treatment of hypertophy of the masseter and temporal muscles; an alternative treatment. Plast Reconstr Surg 2001;107: 327–332.

37 Park MY, Ahn KY, Jung DS. Botulinum toxin type A treatment for contouring of the lower face. Dermatol Surg 2003;29(5): 477–483.

38 Moore AP, Wood GD. The medical management of masseteric hypertrophy with botulinum toxin type A. Br J Oral Maxillofac Surg 1994;32(1):26–28.

39 Kim NH, Chung JH, Park RH, Park JB. The use of botulinum toxin type A in aesthetic mandubular countouring. Plast Recontr Surg 2005;115(3):919–930.

40 Choe SW, Cho WI, Lee CK, Seo SJ. Effects of botulinum toxin type A on contouring of the lower face. Dermatol Surg 2005;31(5): 502–507.

41 Ahn J, Horn C, Blitzer A. Botulinum toxin for masseter reduction in Asian patients. Arch Facial Plast Surg 2004;6(3):188–191.

42 Lee HJ, Lee DW, Park YH, *et al*. Botulinum toxin A for aesthetic contouring of enlarged medial gastrocnemius muscle. Dermatol Surg 2004;30(6):867–871.

43 Han KH, Joo YH, Moon SE, Kim KH. Botulinum toxin A treatment for contouring of the lower leg. 2006;17(4): 250–254.

22

Axillary Hyperhidrosis

Ada Regina Trindade de Almeida, MD,[1] Joel L. Cohen, MD (FAAD, FACMS),[2,3,4] and Chinobu Chisaki, MD[1]

[1] Medical Assistant, Dermatology Clinic, Hospital do Servidor Público Municipal de São Paulo, São Paulo, Brazil
[2] Director, AboutSkin Dermatology and DermSurgery, Greenwood Village and Lone Tree, Colorado, USA
[3] Associate Clinical Professor, University of Colorado Department of Dermatology, Denver, USA
[4] Assistant Clinical Professor, University of California Irvine Department of Dermatology, Irvine, USA

Introduction

Sweat is the fluid excreted by eccrine glands. Its production occurs as a normal physiologic process and is the most effective way for humans to regulate their body temperature [1, 2].

Hyperhidrosis is the term used when sweating occurs in excess, beyond the body's thermoregulatory needs. It can be categorized into *focal* or *generalized* – depending on the extent of the affected area – and considered as *secondary* to some underlying cause, or when the etiology is unknown, as *primary or idiopathic*.

Focal hyperhidrosis affects localized areas such as the axillae, palms, soles, face, or other specific sites. *Generalized hyperhidrosis* usually affects the entire body surface area and can often be attributed to one of a variety of causes (including endocrine, infectious, menopause/physiologic, neurologic, oncologic, or adverse effects of medications such as antidepressants) [3].

The term "focal hyperhidrosis" usually refers to the primary or idiopathic form of hyperhidrosis, and its diagnostic criteria were described in 2004 [4] as focal, visible, excessive sweating for at least 6 months without secondary cause, and showing at least two of the following characteristics:

- Bilateral and relatively symmetric sweating
- Frequency of at least one episode per week
- Impairment of activities of daily living
- Age at onset < 25 years
- Positive family history
- Cessation of sweating during sleep.

A study assessing the prevalence of hyperhidrosis in the American population estimates that it may affect 2.8% of the population [5]. Of these, 50.8% have the axillary region affected either alone or in association with other areas. This disorder affects men and women equally, with the onset age being during adolescence, and it is more frequent in 25- to 64-year-old people [5].

Walling, in a retrospective chart review, found that 93% of patients with hyperhidrosis had primary disease, with isolated axillary distribution occurring in 29% of cases [6]. In all types of focal hyperhidrosis, emotional, thermal, and vasodilatory stimuli further accentuate the baseline problem. Hyperhidrosis impairs daily functions, social interactions, and work activities, and it can dramatically reduce patients' quality of life

Botulinum Toxins: Cosmetic and Clinical Applications, First Edition. Edited by Joel L. Cohen and David M. Ozog.
© 2017 John Wiley & Sons Ltd. Published 2017 by John Wiley & Sons Ltd.
Companion Website: www.wiley.com/go/cohen/botulinum

(QoL) [7–10]. When validated QoL scales are used to measure the burden of the disease, the effects of hyperhidrosis are comparable to severe psoriasis, end-stage renal disease, rheumatoid arthritis, and multiple sclerosis [7, 11].

Anatomy and Physiology

Sweat glands are distributed throughout the skin. Distinct anatomic areas have varying numbers of the three types of sweat glands: eccrine, apocrine, and apoeccrine.

At birth, 2–4 million eccrine glands are distributed over almost the entire body surface [12] and are most numerous on the palms, soles, forehead, axillae, and cheeks. Its clear cells contain the pump, co-transporter, and aquaporin channels required for fluid secretion [13]. In humans, sweat secreted in response to exercise or thermal stimulation is produced by these glands in the dermis that open directly onto the skin surface [14]. They are innervated by cholinergic postganglionic sympathetic nerve fibers [15].

Apocrine glands are far less numerous and open into the infundibular region of the hair follicle [14]. They are specifically located in the urogenital regions and the axillae, and they are stimulated by epinephrine and norepinephrine [16]. They produce a viscid secretion that can become malodorous due to bacterial breakdown [17].

According to previous studies, apoeccrine glands have morphological characteristics from both eccrine and apocrine types, develop during puberty, and may correspond to 10–45% of all axillary glands [12, 18]. They respond to cholinergic stimuli and intensely to epinephrine and isoproterenol infusion [12]; however, recent histologic studies have failed to show evidence of apoeccrine glands in the investigated axillary tissue samples [13, 19]. The existence of these glands presently remains controversial [19–21].

Hyperhidrosis is defined as excessive sweating that is produced by eccrine glands; however, histological studies comparing excessive sweating patients with normal controls have not shown any morphologic changes or increase in their number or size [13, 21].

The pathophysiology of primary focal hyperhidrosis is not currently well-understood [21]. Findings of several studies suggest that secretory clear cell of the eccrine gland has a key role in fluid transport and is probably the source of excessive sweating in the axillary type of hyperhidrosis [13, 19]. On the other hand, other studies suggest that the primary form of hyperhidrosis is possibly due to abnormal central control of emotional sweating because it affects the same body areas as those affected in emotional sweating (hands, feet, and axillae) [22, 23].

Diagnosis and Severity Documentation

In general, axillary hyperhidrosis diagnosis is clinical. It is based on the history, which should include the onset, duration, frequency, intensity, and distribution, as well as impact on daily living and family history. Physical examination and a review of systems will help rule out a secondary cause or associated conditions, such as pregnancy [24].

During evaluation of hyperhidrosis patients, it is important to determine their volume of sweat production, the affected area distribution, and the impact on their quality of life.

Gravimetric testing measures the volume of sweat produced over a fixed time under controlled conditions. The best way to perform the test is the following: the affected area is dried using absorbable tissue; then, a previously weighted filter paper is applied and left in place for a certain time. The weight difference between before and after the contact quantifies the sweat volume produced within that time interval. The evaluation period varies among authors [21]. One group prefers contact with the affected area for 1 minute [25], whereas other investigators prefer 5 [26, 27], 10 [28] or 15 minutes [29].

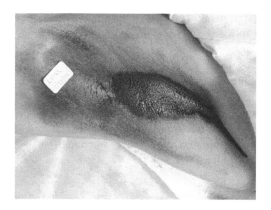

Figure 22.1 Minor starch test showing true sweaty (deep purple) area and regions of false positive test.

In a study comparing normal controls with excessive axillary sweating patients, Hund *et al.* considered axillary hyperhidrosis when the gravimetric tests showed values over 100 mg of sweating for 5 minutes for men and 50 mg for women [27]. While this method is useful in research trials, it is not practical for routine clinical practice.

The Minor starch-iodine test provides assessment of sweat production volume and extent of distribution [1] as well as identification of posttreatment residual sweating. Iodine in contact with starch turns the sweat dark purple making it easily identifiable (Figure 22.1). The test must be carried out before any topical or regional anesthesia and it is easy and cheap to perform [21, 30]. For a better performance, first dry the test area by touching it with absorbable paper. Then, apply a 3–5% iodine solution and allow it to dry for a little while. In some patients with constant sweating, the area has to be dried again with absorbable paper just before the starch application to prevent false positives. For patients with a history of sensitivity to iodine, Ponceau's red tincture may be used, which will turn sweat in contact with starch from red to pink [31]. The distribution and maximal perspiration sites can be recorded in photographs for future comparison.

Another important detail to observe is that, very often, the axillary hyperhidrotic area does not coincide with the hairy underarm region. In some cases, it assumes a bizarre shape and may be located outside the hairy area, while in others, by contrast, it is confined to smaller regions inside the hairy location. For this reason, we consider the Minor's test as mandatory to identify the affected area precisely, so that the toxin injection can be optimized and an effective treatment can be ensured. The association of the two previous methods – gravimetry and Minor test – with point counting using a transparent square-lattice grid was proposed by Bahmer *et al.* as the Hyperhidrosis Area and Severity Index (HASI). Each 1 centimeter (cm) represents 1 point. After estimating the sweating area, the volume of secretion weighted by gravimetry after 10 minutes is divided by the number of points in the affected area. The HASI score is given in mg of sweat by cm^2 per minute. Hyperhidrosis is assumed present with HASI values above $1 \, mg/cm^2$ per minute [28].

The QoL of patients affected by focal idiopathic hyperhidrosis can be measured with several tests, such as the Dermatology Life Quality Index (DLQI), the Hyperhidrosis Impact Questionnaire (HHIQ) [9, 10], the Hyperhidrosis Disease Severity Scale (HDSS) [5], and measures of psychiatric morbidity [32]. In routine clinical practice, they are not required.

Treatment of Axillary Hyperhidrosis

Topical

The treatment of focal hyperhidrosis generally begins with the use of topical antiperspirants that will locally reduce the sweat production. Today, aluminum chloride (AlCl) salts are the most common active ingredient. They reduce sweat by mechanical obstruction of eccrine sweat ducts [33, 34] and its long-term use may cause atrophy of the secretory cells [35]. The hexahydrate compound is more effective; this is seen in prescription formulations containing 10–35% absolute alcohol or salicylic acid gel [36, 37]. It should be applied every night on dry skin, and washed off after 6–8 hours. When sweating is reduced to a tolerable level, the frequency of application may be reduced accordingly, commonly decreasing to once every 1–3 weeks. If irritation occurs, especially with higher concentrations, the application of a 1% hydrocortisone cream the following morning would be useful [4, 37]. Currently, several companies are developing new vehicles, such as microemulsions and liquid crystals, to allow higher concentrations of antiperspirant with lower irritation and higher compliance [38].

Other topical agents, such as aldehydes, have also shown to effectively reduce hyperhidrosis; however, they are rarely used due to irritating, allergic contact dermatitis and/or yellow-brown skin staining [39].

Topical anticholinergic agents have been tried as a therapeutic option for hyperhidrosis. There were reports of patients successfully treated with topical glycopyrrolate for craniofacial and compensatory hyperhidrosis [40–42]. Unfortunately, cutaneous absorption is often insufficient and, when an additional volume is used to compensate the problem or to treat large areas, unpleasant systemic effects emerge [43–45].

Iontophoresis Therapy

Iontophoresis consists of introducing an ionized substance into intact skin through the application of a direct current [46, 47]. Its exact mechanism of action is still unclear. The most generally accepted explanation is poral plugging, as the effect is reversed by cellophane tape stripping of the skin overlying eccrine sweat gland [46]. Other possible explanations are rapid temporary interference with ion pumps and/or innervation of eccrine sweat glands [48] and a complex mechanism involving changes in reabsorption of ductal Na$^+$ [49].

Tap water is most frequently used, but anticholinergic agents are sometimes added to improve efficacy [46]. Irritation may occur, causing dry, peeling and cracked skin, which may be relieved with the use of moisturizers and/or by reducing the frequency of treatments.

Iontophoresis is considered as a second-line therapy for palmar or plantar hyperhidrosis when topical antiperspirants have failed, and it is not used for other affected areas, such as underarms and forehead due to practical problems [37, 50].

Systemic Agents

Oral anticholinergic agents have been used in the therapy of hyperhidrosis. Glycopyrrolate, amitriptyline, methantheline bromide, and oxybutynin have been described, especially when large or multiple areas are affected. They can be added to other topical therapies such as iontophoresis and botulinum toxin to enhance improvements. They act as competitive inhibitors of acetylcholine at muscarinic receptors, which are present throughout the central and autonomic nervous system [51]. However, the treatment is limited by side effects due to secondary blockage of physiologic cholinergic processes resulting in dry mouth, palpitations, blurred vision, constipation, and urinary retention that will be worsened depending on the chosen drug and dosage, the cumulative time of use, and individual susceptibility [1, 37, 50].

There are a few isolated case reports with some level of efficacy (mostly in generalized hyperhidrosis patients) with several other systemic drugs, including diazepam, propranolol, belladonna, indomethacin, clonidine, phentolamine, phenoxybenzamine, diltiazem, and Gabapentin [1].

Local Procedures

Local Excision

Removal of eccrine glands from the axilla can be achieved by curettage, liposuction, or even direct skin excision [1, 52]. There are several different treatment techniques, which differ in their type and size of incisions, type of cannula and curette used, and the aggressiveness of the procedure. The experience of the surgeon is also an important factor [53].

In a literature review, Wollina *et al.* counted 1,270 individuals who underwent suction curettage and 693 patients who underwent minor skin excisions [52]. Both surgical methods were considered effective and safe with only minor, temporary complications and no reports of compensatory sweating.

Refractory cases are described for all methods. Bechara *et al.* [54], when analyzing some of these cases, found three residual sweating patterns after local surgery. These are the *circular* one, in which surgeons mainly focus the central axillary area, leaving a circular region of residual sweat; *crescent*, which is related to the interference of a cupped depression between the pectoralis muscle and the axilla, making careful curettage difficult; and *spot-like* surrounding entry points of previous surgery that makes it difficult to reach by curettage regularly performed in a fan-like fashion.

Minimal skin resection – with or without the association of subcutaneous sweat gland curettage – is more effective in permanently reducing hyperhidrosis than suction curettage [52, 55]. However, they are both associated with higher rates of infection, bleeding, delayed healing, prolonged downtime, and significant scarring [1, 37, 56].

A combination of surgical resection and carbon dioxide laser vaporization was reported as effective for axillary hyperhidrosis with few complications [57, 58]. Because liposuction is less invasive and results in minimal residual scars in axillary hyperhidrosis, it is considered as the surgical treatment of choice by many authors [52, 59, 60].

Emerging Therapies

Devices that deliver heat targeting eccrine glands or the surrounding tissue may be able to injure those glands, thereby reducing sweat production. Various technologies such as lasers, radiofrequency, and ultrasound applied externally or inserted into the soft tissue, are used for this purpose, with limited available data so far, in treating hyperhidrosis [61].

A device recently approved by FDA – called MiraDry – uses microwave energy to destroy eccrine sweat glands. This energy is preferably absorbed by tissue with a high water content, such as the sweat glands, leading to rapid molecular rotation, generation of frictional heat, and cellular thermolysis [61].

After identification of the affected area by a starch-iodine test, the axillary vault is measured with the grid supplied and then injected with an anesthetic tumescent solution containing saline, lidocaine, and epinephrine. A hand piece with a single-use bioTip delivers focused microwave energy on to the dermal-adipose interface, regardless of the skin thickness [62, 63]. The skin temperature is simultaneously cooled and monitored during the energy cycle to prevent thermal transfer of heat into the epidermis.

The device was effective in reducing excessive sweating. Based on gravimetric assessments, 90% of patients experienced a 50% or greater reduction in axillary sweating, with an average reduction of 81.7%.

At 12 months after treatment, 85.5% of patients were satisfied with their treatment outcome [64]. Patients also noticed improvement of axillary odor [65].

Common, minor side effects include edema, axillary tenderness/pain for several days, and numbness and tingling in the upper arm or axilla for several weeks [66].

Endoscopic Thoracic Sympathectomy

Endoscopic (thoracoscopic or video-assisted) sympathectomy (ETS or VATS) is the most invasive of the therapeutic options. This is recommended for those with moderate-to-severe hyperhidrosis who have not responded to any other treatments [67]. The goal of any sympathectomy for hyperhidrosis is to disconnect the eccrine sweat glands from the sympathetic signals that trigger them to initiate sweating [68].

In this surgery, the sympathetic ganglia are interrupted by excision, ablation, or clipping [69]. ETS has been most frequently indicated for focal palmar hyperhidrosis, for which the success rates have been high [67–69]; however, there are still questions about its efficacy in treating axillary hyperhidrosis.

The appropriate level of division of the sympathetic chain is chosen according to the location of the primary symptoms. The recent consensus recommendations by the Society of Thoracic Surgeons include sympathetic chain interruption above the third rib for palmar hyperhidrosis, above the fourth and fifth rib for axillary hyperhidrosis, and above the third rib for craniofacial hyperhidrosis [68].

Milder reflex sweating – also known as compensatory sweating or compensatory hyperhidrosis – is the main problem when performing sympathectomies for focal hyperhidrosis, with very high incidence (more than 50%) occurring in most patients, as reported in most of the studies [67–69]. It affects other anatomical areas, such as the back, anterior chest, abdomen, buttocks, and less frequently, legs. Often mild in severity, it may remain stable or be reduced over time, although it can also be severe in some individuals. It typically begins 2–8 weeks after sympathectomy [1]. Due to the significance of this side effect, up to one third of patients treated with ETS are moderately dissatisfied with their treatment [69].

Other less commonly reported complications include chest wall paresthesia, Horner's syndrome, pneumothorax and hemothorax, and rarely, cardiac arrest or arrhythmias [1,67].

In a recent review of ETS publications, Krasna [70] found that "studies by ETS surgeons have claimed satisfaction rates around 85–95% with only 2% regretting the surgery, generally because of compensatory sweating". He concluded, however, that the exact results of ETS are unpredictable due to anatomic variations in the sympathetic nerve distribution and the surgical techniques chosen [70].

Botulinum Toxin

The use of botulinum toxin A (BoNTA) for axillary hyperhidrosis was first reported by Bushara et al. in 1996 [71], and since then, this therapeutic indication has emerged. Many open-label and controlled studies [25, 72–82] have supported the safety and efficacy of intradermal or subcutaneous botulinum toxin injections for axillary hyperhidrosis.

To date, **onabotulinumtoxinA** (Botox/Botox Cosmetic® in the US, Latin America, Allergan, Inc., Westport, Ireland) [83] is the only FDA-approved formulation for hyperhidrosis. It is also the most studied type for this indication, followed by abobotulinumtoxinA (Dysport® in the United States, Europe and Latin America, Ipsen Biopharm Ltd., Wrexham, UK [84] and rimabotulinumtoxinB (Myobloc®/Neurobloc® in the United States and Neurobloc® in Europe; Solstice Neurosciences Inc./Eisai Co., Ltd.) [85]. To date, there is only one study of incobotulinumtoxinA for axillary hyperhidrosis (Xeomin® in North and Latin Americas and in Europe; Merz Pharma, Frankfurt) [86,87].

After BoNTA injection, the anhidrotic effect usually begins within 7 to 10 days and lasts 6 to 10 months, with a mean duration of 7 to 9 months [1,2,25,76,80]. For axillary hyperhidrosis, reported average doses range from 50–100U of onabotulinumtoxinA or 100–250U of abobotulinumtoxinA, injected intradermally. [25, 88, 89]. Although two reports using high doses of onabotulinumtoxinA (200 units) per axilla described prolonged efficacy – for as long as 29 months [90, 91], other studies comparing different dosages found little advantages with doses higher than 50 onabotulinumtoxinA U [76] or 100 abobotulinumtoxinA U per axilla [92].

With regard to rimabotulinumtoxinB, studies suggested doses varying from 2,500 to 5,000 U/axilla and described quicker onset of anhidrotic effect – within 3–5 days, lasting around 9–16 weeks. Higher dosages were associated with systemic side effects such as dry mouth, accommodation difficulties, and corneal irritation, leading researchers to recommend 2000 U/axilla as the optimal effective dose [93–95].

There is no standardized dilution for botulinum toxin treatment of focal hyperhidrosis. Reported dilutions range from 1 to 10 ml of saline [2, 11] for onabotulinumtoxinA, with most clinicians using between 2–5 ml. As for abobotulinumtoxinA, dilution volumes vary from 1.25 to 10 ml, [2, 11, 92, 96] with the use of 2.5–5 ml being the most frequent. In the study of incobotulinumtoxinA compared with onabotulinumtoxinA for hyperhidrosis, the authors considered that both had similar efficacy; the dilution used was 10 U/ml for both products [87].

Some substances had been added to the toxin solution with no harm to the toxin, such as hyaluronidase, lidocaine, and epinephrine. Among these substances, the most interesting for axillary treatment is lidocaine, which showed similar efficacy and reduced pain, turning the procedure more comfortable [97–99] when compared to the saline alone.

No downtime is required for the axillary injection procedure and patients' quality of life has shown to dramatically improve after treatment [7–10, 79]. Although some studies found no reduction in the duration of symptom relief after repeated BoNTA injections [9, 26, 77, 89], others noticed increased efficacy after multiple treatments [21, 100].

The use of ice or a topical anesthetic cream can further minimize discomfort. Subcutaneous injections may also be less painful than dermal injections, while maintaining a similar level of efficacy [101].

No significant side effects were found with BoNTA injections into underarms. Pruritus in the treated region [76] and mild local urticaria lasting for 2 days were described [89]. Discrete compensatory sweating was observed in 5% of patients treated with onabotulinumtoxinA [26] and in 2 of 52 individuals of another study with abobotulinumtoxinA [89].

Studies suggest that body odor can be improved in healthy volunteers with the use of intradermal injections of onabotulinumtoxinA into the axillae. The underlying mechanisms may include interference with axillary bacterial growth by decrease of moist environment as well as denervation of apoeccrine sweat glands [102, 103]. Also, a complete [104] or partial [105] remission of moist and eroded axillary plaques of Hailey-Hailey disease have been anecdotally reported.

Botulinum Toxin Injection

After the iodine starch test, when the affected area is identified and photographed, it has to be delineated with a marker pen or gentian violet. Although some authors prefer to inject directly through the purple-colored residues, we like to remove them and make the interior of the highlighted region clear.

The soft, thin axillary skin is easily trespassed by 30G needles. In general, pain is not a big issue in this area; however, to make the procedure more comfortable, topical anesthetic creams can be applied at this moment and ice cubes or packs may be helpful just before the injections or following the procedure.

Cheshire self-injected 1 U of onabotulinumtoxinA into his forearm and observed an anhidrotic halo of $1.5\,cm^2$ [106], while Braune et al. found that 2.5 U of abobotulinumtoxinA was needed to obtain $1\,cm^2$ of anhidrotic skin [107]. The toxin concentration would be higher at the injection site and the concentration gradient rapidly decreases with distance from this site [108].

For hyperhidrosis, the goal is to place injections in such a pattern that creates confluent overlapping anhidrotic halos in order to achieve maximum outcome and minimize the risk of affecting underlying musculature [109].

Injections are administered by using small, delicate syringes with sharp short fixed 30G needles or luer lock syringes with 32G needles. The former is preferable because no toxin is lost in the idle space inside a removable needle (0.3 or 0.5-ml syringes

[Ultrafine II 30-U or 50-U insulin syringes; Becton-Dickinson Co, New Jersey, USA]). To avoid dulling the needles when trespassing the rubber stopper, BoNT vials should be opened with a bottle opener after saline reconstitution and syringes should be directly filled from the opened vial.

Our technique is to distribute intradermal injections across the previously identified hyperhidrotic regions, spaced 1–1.5 cm apart. The number of injections and the total dose should depend on the involved surface area. According to the surface area involved, we use approximately 10–20 intradermal injections in 0.1–0.2 ml aliquots, totaling 50–100 U onabotulinumtoxinA for each axilla. Injections into the axillae may also be performed in the superficial fat without adverse events or significant reduction in efficacy. In our practices, the treatment of the axillae results in successful improvement of hyperhidrosis in nearly all patients. The effects last approximately 6–9 months; however, in some cases, they may last more than 1 year, as shown in Figure 22.2, Figure 22.3, Figure 22.4, Figure 22.5 Figure 22.6 and Figure 22.7.

Transcutaneous Botulinum Toxin

Alternative methods of toxin delivery through the skin without the use of needles or punctures have been recently tried with promising results. However, botulinum

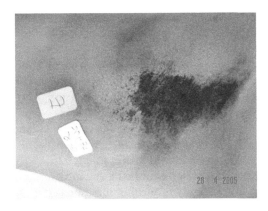

Figure 22.3 Left axilla of the same patient as shown in Figure 22.2 before treatment.

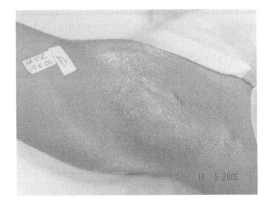

Figure 22.4 Right axilla 21 days after injection of 50 U of onabotulinumtoxinA.

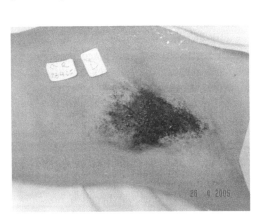

Figure 22.2 Right axilla of a 28-year-old woman before treatment.

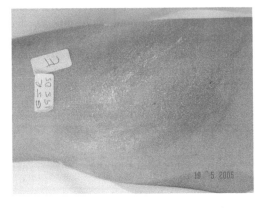

Figure 22.5 Left axilla 21 days after injection of 50 U of onabotulinumtoxinA.

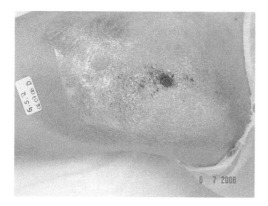

Figure 22.6 Right axilla 15 months after injection of 50 U of onabotulinumtoxinA.

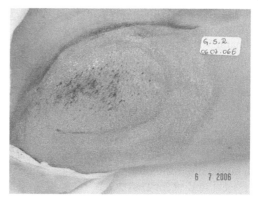

Figure 22.7 Left axilla 15 months after injection of 50 U of onabotulinumtoxinA.

toxin directly injected into the skin is not absorbed due to its large molecular size [110]. Some other driving force may be necessary to allow transcutaneous absorption [110]. Iontophoresis units to deliver onabotulinumtoxinA via electric current were reported in patients with palmar hyperhidrosis [111–113].

A small controlled clinical trial investigated a novel proprietary transport peptide to deliver botulinum toxin A through the skin. By using 200 U of onabotulinumtoxinA reconstituted with saline admixed with the transport peptide, the author found statistically significant reduction of sweat production in 12 cases of axillary hyperhidrosis. The duration of effect was not reported in that paper [114].

This innovative method is likely to open a window of opportunity to treat other hyperhidrosis-affected areas and may be useful in the future for other indications as well.

References

1 Cohen JL, Cohen G, Solish N, *et al.* Diagnosis, impact, and management of focal hyperhidrosis: treatment review including botulinum toxin therapy. Facial Plast Surg Clin North Am 2007;15:17–30, v–vi.

2 Grunfeld A, Murray CA, Solish N. Botulinum toxin for hyperhidrosis – A review. Am J Clin Dermatol 2009;10(2): 87–102.

3 Moraites E, Vaughn O, Hill S. Incidence and prevalence of hyperhidrosis. Dermatol Clin 2014;32:457–465.

4 Hornberger J, Grimes K, Naumann M, *et al.* Multi-Specialty Working Group on the Recognition, Diagnosis, and Treatment of Primary Focal Hyperhidrosis: Recognition, diagnosis, and treatment of primary focal hyperhidrosis. J Am Acad Dermatol 2004;51:274–286.

5 Strutton DR, Kowalski JW, Glaser DA, Stang PE. US prevalence of hyperhidrosis and impact on individuals with axillary hyperhidrosis: results from a national survey. J Am Acad Dermatol 2004;51: 241–248.

6 Walling H. Clinical differentiation of primary from secondary hyperhidrosis. J Am Acad Dermatol 2011;64(4):690–695.

7 Swartling C, Naver H, Lindberg M. Botulinum A toxin improves life quality in severe primary focal hyperhidrosis. Eur J Neurol 2001;8:247–252.

8 Tan SR, Solish N. Long-term efficacy and quality of life in the treatment of focal

hyperhidrosis with botulinum toxin A. Dermatol Surg 2002;28:495–499.

9 Naumann M, Hamm H, Lowe N. Effect of botulinum toxin A on quality of life measures in patients with excessive axillary sweating: a randomized controlled trial. Br J Dermatol 2002;147:1218–1226.

10 Campanati A, Penna L, Guzzo T, et al. A quality-of-life assessment in patients with hyperhidrosis before and after treatment with botulinum toxin: results of an open-label study. Clin Ther 2003 Jan;25(1):298–308.

11 Hamm H. Impact of hyperhidrosis on quality of life and its assessment. Dermatol Clin 2014;32:467–476.

12 Sato K, Kang WH, Saga KT. Biology of sweat glands and their disorders I. Normal sweat gland function. J Am Acad Dermatol 1989;20:537–563.

13 Bovell DL, MacDonald A, Meyer B, et al. The secretory clear cell of the eccrine sweat gland as the probable source of excess sweat production in hyperhidrosis. Exp Dermatol 2011;20(12):1017–1020.

14 Mota Juang J, Sotto MN. Anatomy and histology of sweat glands. In: Almeida ART, Hexsel DM. eds. Hyperhidrosis and Botulinum Toxin. Edition of authors. São Paulo, 2004;1:3–6.

15 Kreyden O, Scheidegger E. Anatomy of the sweat glands, pharmacology of botulinum toxin, and distinctive syndromes associated with hyperhidrosis. Clin Derm 2004;22:40–44.

16 Lindsay SL, Holmes S, Corbett AD, et al. Innervation and receptor profiles of the human apocrine (epitrichial) sweat gland: routes for intervention in bromhidrosis. Br J Dermatol 2008:159:653–660.

17 Atkins JL, Butler PEM. Hyperhidrosis: a review of current management. Plast Reconstr Surg 2002;110:222–228.

18 Sato K, Kang WT, Saga KT. Biology of sweat glands and their disorders II. Disorders of sweat gland function. J Am Acad Dermatol 1989;20:713–726.

19 Bovell D, Corbett A, Holmes S, et al. The absence of apoecrine glands in the human axilla has disease pathogenic implications, including axillary hyperhidrosis. Br J Dermatol 2007;156:1278–1286.

20 Bechara F. Do we have appocrine sweat glands? Int J Cosmetic Sci 2008;30:67–68.

21 Almeida ART, Montagner S. Botulinum toxin for axillary hyperhidrosis. Dermatol Clin 2014;32:495–504.

22 Lakraj A, Moghimi N, Jabbari B. Hyperhidrosis: anatomy, pathophysiology and treatment with emphasis on the role of botulinum toxins. Toxins (Basel) 2013;5:821–840.

23 Hamm H, Naumann MK, Kowalski JW, et al. Primary focal hyperhidrosis: disease characteristics and functional impairment. Dermatology 2006;212: 343–353.

24 Kreyden OP. Rare forms of hyperhidrosis. Curr Probl Dermatol 2002;30:178–187.

25 Heckmann M, Ceballos-Baumann AO, Plewig G. Botulinum toxin A for axillary hyperhidrosis (excessive sweating). N Engl J Med 2001;344(7):488–493.

26 Naumann M, Lowe N. Botulinum toxin type A in the treatment of bilateral primary axillary hyperhidrosis: randomized, parallel group, double-blind, placebo controlled trial. Br Med J 2001; 323:596–570.

27 Hund M, Kinkelin I, Naumann M, et al. Definition of axillary hyperhidrosis by gravimetric assessment. Arch Dermatol 2002;138:539–541.

28 Bahmer F, Sachse M. Hyperhidrosis area and severity index [letter]. Dermatol Surg 2008;34:1744–1745.

29 Odderson IR. Long-term quantitative benefits of botulinum toxin A in the treatment of axillary hyperhidrosis. Dermtol Surg 2002;28:480–483.

30 Glogau R. Hyperhidrosis and botulinum toxin A: patient selection and techniques. Clin Dermatol 2004;22:45–52.

31 Bushara KO, Park DM. Botulinum toxin and sweating [letter]. J Neurol Neurosurg Psychiat 1994;54(11):1437.

32 Weber A, Heger R, Sinkgraven M, et al. Psychosocial aspects of patients with focal

hyperhidrosis. Marked reduction of social phobia, anxiety and depression and increased quality of life after treatment with botulinum toxin A. Br J Dermatol 2005;114:343–345.

33 Shelley W, Hurley H Jr. Studies on topical and perspirant control of axillary hyperhydrosis. Acta Derm Venereal 1975;55(4):241–260.

34 Qualtrale RP, Coble DW, Stoner KL, *et al.* The mechanism of antiperspirant action by aluminum salts II. Histologic observations of human eccrine sweat glands inhibited by aluminum chlorohydrate. J Soc Cosmet Chem 1981;32:107–136.

35 Holzle E, Braun-Falco O. Structural alterations of axillary eccrine glands in hyperhidrosis following long-term treatment with aluminum chloride hexahydrate. Br J Dermatol 1984;110: 399–403.

36 Benohanian A, Dansereau A, Bolduc C, *et al.* Localized hyperhidrosis treated with aluminum chloride in a salicylic acid gel base. Int J Dermatol 1998;37:701–703.

37 Gelbard C, Epstein H, Hebert A. Primary pediatric hyperhidrosis: a review of current treatment options. Pediatr Dermatol 2008;25(6):591–598.

38 Boonme P, Songkro S. Antiperspirants and deodorants: active ingredients and novel formulations. J Clin Dermatol 2010;1(2):67–72.

39 Holzle E. Topical pharmacologic treatment. Curr Probl Dermatol 2002;30: 30–43.

40 Luh JY, Blackwell TA. Craniofacial hyperhidrosis successfully treated with topical glycopyrrolate. South Med J 2002;95:756–758.

41 Kim WO, Kil HK, Yoon DM, Cho MJ. Treatment of compensatory gustatory hyperhidrosis with topical glycopyrrolate. Yonsei Med J 2003:44:579–582.

42 Cladellas E, Callejas M, Grimalt R. A medical alternative to the treatment of compensatory sweating. Dermatol Ther 2008;21:406–408.

43 Kavanagh GM, Burns C, Aldridge RD. Topical glycopyrrolate should not be overlooked in treatment of focal hyperhidrosis. Br J Dermatol 2006;155: 487.

44 Madan V, Beck MH. Urinary retention caused by topical glycopyrrolate for hyperhidrosis. Br J Dermatol 2006:155: 634–635.

45 Panting KJ, Alkali AS, Newman WD, Sharpe GR. Dilated pupils caused by topical glycopyrrolate for hyperhidrosis. Br J Dermatol 2007: 158: 187–188.

46 Stolman L. Iontophoresis with the Fischer galvanic unit. In: Almeida ART, Hexsel DM, eds. *Hyperhidrosis and Botulinum Toxin.* Edition of authors. São Paulo. 2004;17:97–100.

47 Pariser D, Balard A. Iontophoresis for palmar and plantar hyperhidrosis. Dermatol Clin 2014;32:491–494.

48 Shams K, Kavanagh GM. Immediate reduction in sweat secretion with electric current application in primary palmar hyperhidrosis. Arch Dermatol 2011 Feb;147:241–242.

49 Ohshima Y, Shimizu H, Yanagishita T, *et al.* Changes in Na+, K+ concentrations in perspiration and perspiration volume with alternating current iontophoresis in palmoplantar hyperhidrosis patients. Arch Dermatol Res 2008;300:595–600.

50 Wang R, Solish N, Murray C. Primary focal hyperhidrosis: diagnosis and management. Dermatol Nurs 2008;20(6): 467–470.

51 Glaser D. Oral medications. Dermatol Clin 2014;32:527–532.

52 Wollina U, Kostler E, Schonlebe J, Haroske G. Tumescent suction curettage versus minimal skin resection with subcutaneous curettage of sweat glands in axillary hyperhidrosis. Dermatol Surg 2008;34:709–716.

53 Glaser DA, Galperin T. Local Procedural approaches for axillary hyperhidrosis. Dermatol Clin 2014;32:533–540.

54 Bechara FG, Sand EM, Altmeyer EP. Characteristics of refractory sweating

areas following minimally invasive surgery for axillary hyperhidrosis. Aesth Plast Surg 2009;33:308–311.

55 Lawrence CM, Lonsdale Eccles AA. Selective sweat gland removal with minimal skin excision in the treatment of axillary hyperhidrosis: a retrospective clinical and histological review of 15 patients. Br J Dermatol 2006;155:115–118.

56 Commons G, Lim A. Treatment of axillary hyperhidrosis/bromidrosis using VASER ultrasound. Aesth Plast Surg 2009;33: 312–323.

57 Klopper M, Fischer G, Blugerman G. Laser-assisted suction of axillary sweat glands and axillary epilation. In: Shiffman MA, Di Giuseppe A, eds. *Liposuction: Principles and Practice.* Berlin: Springer-Verlag Berlin; 2006:505–515.

58 Park JH, Cha SH, Park SD. Carbon dioxide laser treatment vs subcutaneous resection of axillary osmidrosis. Dermatol Surg 1997;23:247–251.

59 Bechara FG, Sand EM, Tomi NS, *et al.* Repeat liposuction-curettage treatment of axillary hyperhidrosis is safe and effective. Br J Dermatol 2007;157:739–743.

60 Kim WO, Song Y, Kil HK, *et al.* Suction–curettage with combination of two different cannulae in the treatment of axillary osmidrosis and hyperhidrosis. J Eur Acad Dermatol Venereol 2008;22: 1083–1088.

61 Glaser DA, Galperin T. Local procedural approaches for axillary hyperhidrosis. Dermatol Clin 2014;32:549–553.

62 Jacob C. Treatment of hyperhidrosis with microwave technology. Semin Cutan Med Surg 2013;32(1):2–8.

63 Johnson JE, O'Shaughnessy KF, Kim S. Microwave thermolysis of sweat glands. Lasers Surg Med 2012; 44(1):20–5.

64 Chih-Ho Hong H, Lupin M, O'Shaughnessy KF. Clinical evaluation of a microwave device for treating axillary hyperhidrosis. Dermatol Surg 2012;38(5): 728–735.

65 Lee SJ, Chang KY, Suh DH, *et al.* The efficacy of a microwave device for treating axillary hyperhidrosis and osmidrosis in Asians: a preliminary study. J Cosmet Laser Ther 2013;15(5):255–259.

66 Glaser DA, Coleman WP, Fan LK, *et al.* A randomized, blinded clinical evaluation of a novel microwave device for treating axillary hyperhidrosis: the dermatologic reduction in underarm perspiration study. Dermatol Surg 2012;38(2): 185–191

67 Vorkamp T, Foo JF, Khan S, *et al.* Hyperhidrosis: evolving concepts and a comprehensive review. Surgeon 2010;8: 287–292.

68 Moraites E, Vaughn O, Hill S. Endoscopic thoracic sympathectomy. Dermatol Clin 2014;32:541–548.

69 Callejas MA, Grimalt R, Cladellas E. Actualización em hiperhidrosis. Actas Dermosifiliogr 2010;101(2):110–118.

70 Krasna MJ. Thorascoscopic dympathectomy. Thorac Surg Clin 2010;20(2):323–330.

71 Bushara KO, DM Park, Jones JC. Botulinum toxin – a possible new treatment for axillary hyperhidrosis. Clin Exper Dermatol 1996;21:276–278.

72 Rompel R, Scholz S. Subcutaneous curettage vs. injection of botulinum toxin A for treatment of axillary hyperhidrosis. J Eur Acad Dermatol Venereol 2001;15: 207–211.

73 Schnider P, Moraru E, Kittler H, *et al.* Treatment of focal hyperhidrosis with botulinum toxin type A: long-term follow-up in 61 patients. Br J Dermatol 2001;145:289–293.

74 Salmanpoor R, Rahmanian MJ. Treatment of axillary hyperhidrosis with botulinum-A toxin. Int J Dermatol 2002;41:428–430.

75 Tan SR, Solish N. Long-term efficacy and quality of life in the treatment of focal hyperhidrosis with botulinum toxin A. Dermatol Surg 2002;28:495–499.

76 Lowe PL, Cerdan-Sanz S, lowe NJ. Botulinum toxin type A in the treatment of bilateral primary axillary hyperhidrosis: efficacy and duration with repeated

treatments. Dermatol Surg 2003;29(5): 545–548.

77 Glaser DA, Coleman WP, Daggett S, *et al.* Type A treatment for primary axillary hyperhidrosis: 12-month interim analysis of a multicenter, open-label trial. Scientific Poster presented at the American Academy of Dermatology Meeting, 2005.

78 James R, Phillips D, Collin J. Durability of botulinum toxin injection for axillary hyperhidrosis. Br J Dermatol 2005;92: 834–835.

79 Solish N, Benohanian A, Kowalski JW. Prospective open-label study of botulinum toxin type A in patients with axillary hyperhidrosis: effects on functional impairment and quality of life. Dermatol Surg 2005;31(4): 405–413.

80 Schnider P, Binder M, Kittler H, *et al.* A randomized, double-blinded, placebo-controlled trial of botulinum A toxin for severe axillary hyperhidrosis. Br J Dermatol 1999;140:677–680.

81 Odderson IR. Long-term quantitative benefits of botulinum toxin type A in the treatment of axillary hyperhidrosis. Dermatol Surg 2002;28:480–483.

82 Naumann M, Lowe NJ, Kumar CR, Hamm H. Botulinum toxin type A is a safe and effective treatment for axillary hyperhidrosis over 16 months: a prospective study. Arch Dermatol 2003; 139:731–736.

83 Package insert on Botox. Westport, Ireland: Allergan, Inc; August 2013.

84 Package insert on Dysport. Wrexham, UK: Ipsen Biopharm Ltd; April 2013.

85 Package insert on Myobloc. San Diego, CA: Elan Pharmaceuticals; September 2009.

86 Package insert on Xeomin. Germany: Merz Pharma GmbH & Co.; November 2013.

87 Dressler D. Comparing Botox® and Xeomin® for axillar hyperhidrosis. J Neural Transm 2010;117:317–319.

88 Lowe NJ, Glaser DA, Eadie N, *et al.* Botulinum toxin type A in the treatment

of primary hyperhidrosis: a 52-week multicenter double-blind, randomized, placebo-controlled study of efficacy and safety. J Am Acad Dermatol 2007;56(4): 604–611.

89 Absar MS, Onwudike M. Efficacy of botulinum toxin type A in the treatment of focal axillary hyperhidrosis. Dermatol Surg 2008;34:751–755.

90 Karamfilov T, Konrad H, Karte K, Wollina U. Lower relapse rate of botulinum toxin A therapy for axillary hyperhidrosis by dose increase. Arch Dermatol 2000;136: 487–490.

91 Wollina U, Karanfilov T, Konrad H. High dose botulinum toxin type A therapy for axillary hyperhidrosis markedly prolongs the relapse-free interval. J Am Acad Dermatol 2002;46:536–540.

92 Heckmann M, Plewig G. Low-dose efficacy of botulinum toxin A for axillary hyperhidrosis. Arch Dermatol 2005;141: 1255–1259.

93 Dressler D, Saberi FA, Benecke R. Botulinum toxin type B for treatment of axillar hyperhidrosis. J Neurol 2002;249: 1729–1732.

94 Baumann LS, Halem ML. Botulinum toxin-B and the management of hyperhidrosis. Clin Dermatol 2004;22: 60–65.

95 Nelson L, Bachoo P, Holmes J. Botulinum toxin type B: a new therapy for axillary hyperhidrosis. Br J Plast Surg 2005;58: 228–232.

96 Talarico-Filho S, Nascimento MM, Macedo FS, Pecora CS. A double-blind, randomized, comparative study of two type A botulinum toxins in the treatment of primary axillary hyperhidrosis. Dermatol Surg 2007;33:S44–S50.

97 Trindade De Almeida AR, Secco LC, Carruthers A. Handling botulinum toxins: an updated literature review. Dermatol Surg 2011;37(11):1553–1565.

98 Vadoud-Seyedi J, Simonart T. Treatment of axillary hyperhidrosis with botulinum toxin type A reconstituted in lidocaine or in normal saline: a randomized,

side-by-side, double-blind study. Br J Dermatol 2007;156:986–989.

99 Gullec AT. Dilution of botulinum toxin A in lidocaine vs. in normal saline for the treatment of primary axillary hyperhidrosis: a double-blind, randomized, comparative preliminary study. J Eur Acad Dermatol Venereol 2012;26:314–318.

100 Lecouflet M, Leux C, Fenot M, *et al.* Duration of efficacy increases with the repetition of botulinum toxin A injections in primary axillary hyperhidrosis: a study in 83 patients. J Am Acad Dermatol 2013;69(6):960–964.

101 Pearson IC, Cliff S. Botulinum toxin type A treatment for axillary hyperhidrosis: a comparison of intradermal and subcutaneous injection techniques. Br J Dermatol 2004;151(Suppl 68):95.

102 Heckmann M, Teichmann B, Pause BM, Plewig G. Amelioration of body odor after intracutaneous axillary injection of botulinum toxin A. Arch Dermatol 2003;139:57–59.

103 Heckmann M. Effect of Botulinum toxin type A on body odor. In: Almeida ART, Hexsel DM, eds. *Hyperhidrosis and Botulinum Toxin*. São Paulo: Edition of authors, 2004;239–246.

104 Lapiere JC, Hirsh A, Gordon KB, *et al.* Botulinum toxin type A for the treatment of axillary Hailey–Hailey disease. Dermatol Surg 2000;26:371–374.

105 Kang NG, Yoon TJ, Kim TH. Botulinum toxin type A as an effective adjuvant therapy for Hailey–Hayley disease. Dermatol Surg 2002;28:543.

106 Cheshire WP. Subcutaneous botulinum toxin type A inhibits regional sweating in an individual observation. Clin Auton Res 1996;6:123–124.

107 Braune C, Erbguth F, Birklein F. Dose thresholds and duration of the local anhidrotic effect of botulinum toxin injections: measured by sudometry. Br J Dermatol 2001;144:111–117.

108 Klein A.W. Complication, adverse reaction, and insights with the use of botulinum toxin. Dermatol Surg 2003;29:549–556.

109 Glogau R. Hyperhidrosis and botulinum toxin A: patient selection and technique. Clin Dermatol 2004;22:45–52.

110 Chow A, Wilder-Smith EP. Effect of transdermal botulinum toxin on sweat secretion in subjects with idiopathic palmar hyperhidrosis. Br J Dermatol 2009;160(3):721–723.

111 Kavanagh GM, Oh C, Shams K. Botox delivery by iontophoresis. Br J Dermatol 2004;15:1093–1095.

112 Kavanagh GM, Shams K. Botulinum toxin type A by iontophoresis for primary palmar hyperhidrosis. J Am Acad Dermatol 2006;55(5):S115–S117.

113 Davarian S, Kalantari KK, Rezasoltani A, Rahimi A. Effect and persistency of botulinum toxin iontophoresis in the treatment of palmar hyperhidrosis. Aus J Dermatol 2008;49:75–79.

114 Glogau RG. Topically applied botulinum toxin type A for the treatment of primary axillary hyperhidrosis: results of a randomized, blinded, vehicle-controlled study. Dermatol Surg 2007;33(1):S76–S80.

23

Primary Focal Palm, Sole, Craniofacial, and Compensatory Hyperhidrosis

Dee Anna Glaser, MD[1] and Adam R. Mattox, DO (MS)[2]

[1]*Professor and Interim Chairman, Department of Dermatology, Saint Louis University School of Medicine, Saint Louis, USA*
[2]*Micrographic Surgery & Dermatologic Oncology Fellow, Department of Dermatology, Saint Louis University School of Medicine, Saint Louis, USA*

Botulinum toxin can be safely and effectively used to treat a multitude of cutaneous secretory problems such as hyperhidrosis, chromhidrosis, and Frey's syndrome. The focus of this chapter is the rationale for and the practical application of using botulinum toxins in this clinical setting.

Sweating

Sweating is controlled by the sympathetic nervous system [1]. The postganglionic sympathetic nervous system predominantly utilizes the neurotransmitter norepinephrine to activate adrenergic receptors on peripheral tissues. Sweating is one exception. Muscarinic receptors on clear cells of eccrine glands are activated by acetylcholine.

Eccrine glands are unequally distributed in the skin. High concentrations occur in the palms, soles, and forehead (Table 23.1). Eccrine glands are stimulated by heat, exercise, anxiety, and stress [2, 3].

Sympathetic innervation also regulates apocrine sweat glands; however, they respond to adrenergic stimuli, from the neurotransmitter epinephrine. The highest concentration of apocrine sweat glands occurs in the nipples, axillae, and perineum. Apocrine glands produce a sterile, thick, milky, odorless fluid containing protein, lipids, fatty acids, and carbohydrates. An odor is only produced when the secretions are decomposed by bacteria at the skin surface [1, 2].

Hyperhidrosis

Hyperhidrosis describes excess sweating beyond that necessary for thermoregulation. The amount necessary to be considered "excessive" is not well defined and varies between individuals. Problems can occur within any portion of the system, from the hypothalamus to the sweat gland or duct [4]. The eccrine glands in patients with primary focal hyperhidrosis do not demonstrate any histopathologic changes or glandular hyperplasia.

A detailed history, comprehensive review of symptoms, and thorough physical examination are the first steps in identifying the type (bilateral or unilateral, symmetric or asymmetric, and primary or secondary origin) and cause of hyperhidrosis. Further workup is guided by the findings.

Furthermore, hyperhidrosis is classified as generalized or focal. Generalized hyperhidrosis affects the entire body whereas focal hyperhidrosis occurs in discrete anatomic sections [5]. Generalized hyperhidrosis

Botulinum Toxins: Cosmetic and Clinical Applications, First Edition. Edited by Joel L. Cohen and David M. Ozog.
© 2017 John Wiley & Sons Ltd. Published 2017 by John Wiley & Sons Ltd.
Companion Website: www.wiley.com/go/cohen/botulinum

Table 23.1 Eccrine sweat gland concentration.

Anatomic Area	Quantity/cm^2
Sole of foot	620
Forehead	360
Palms	300
Axillae	300
Thigh	120
Scrotum	80
Back	65
Lips	None
Nipple	None
Labia majora	None

typically occurs as the result of an under-lying cause (secondary). Focal or localized hyperhidrosis may have a secondary origin; for example, lesions of the peripheral nervous system [6, 7]. More commonly, focal hyperhidrosis is idiopathic (primary) and referred to simply as "hyperhidrosis." It is characterized by excessive sweating of small areas, usually the axillae, palms, soles, face, or groin (Figure 23.1) [8]. The onset is usually during adolescence to early adulthood but can begin in early childhood, especially the palmar-plantar variants [9].

Primary focal hyperhidrosis tends to have an age of onset before 25 years, and presents as bilateral, symmetric, and focal sweating. It does not occur during sleep. In cases of secondary hyperhidrosis, an extensive differential diagnosis exists for the underlying cause; commonly an endocrine or neurologic disease (Table 23.2).

This chapter will focus on primary focal hyperhidrosis henceforth identified simply as hyperhidrosis (HH). Diagnostic criteria for primary hyperhidrosis have been suggested by a consensus panel and described statistically in the literature (Table 23.3) [10, 11].

Quality of Life

The greatest impact of HH is the significant reduction in the quality of life and alteration of daily function [12]. Several questionnaire tools to assess disease severity and quality of life are described in the literature. The most common of which is the Hyperhidrosis Disease Severity Scale (HDSS), which is based

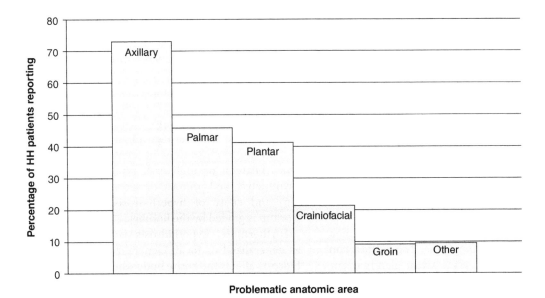

Figure 23.1 Sites of hyperhidrosis reported to be problematic.

Table 23.2 Hyperhidrosis classification.

Focal/localized	Generalized
Primary focal hyperhidrosis	Fever
Intrathoracic tumors	Infection
Rheumatoid arthritis	Malignancy
Spinal cord disease or injury	Tumors
Stroke	Thyrotoxicosis
Syringomelia	Pheochromocytoma
Ross syndrome	Diabetes mellitus
Atrioventricular fistula	Diabetes insipidus
Gustatory sweating	Hypoglycemia
Frey's syndrome	Hypopituitarism
Localized unilateral hyperhidrosis[a]	Endocarditis
Cold-induced hyperhidrosis	Gout
Eccrine nevus	Medications
Social anxiety disorder	Menopause
Granulosis rubra nasi	Anxiety
	Drug withdrawal

[a] Also referred to as unilateral circumscribed idiopathic hyperhidrosis.

Table 23.3 Criteria to diagnose primary focal hyperhidrosis.

Focal, visible excessive sweating of at least 6 months' duration

And

No apparent secondary cause

And

At least two of the following characteristics:

Impairs daily activities

Bilateral and relatively symmetric

Frequency of episodes at least once a week

Age of onset <25 years

Positive family history

Cessation of focal sweating during sleep

Table 23.4 Hyperhidrosis Disease Severity Scale (27). Question: Which best describes the impact of sweating on your daily activity?

Score	Answer
1	My (underarm) sweating is never noticeable and never interferes with my daily activity.
2	My (underarm) sweating is tolerable but sometimes interferes with my daily activity.
3	My (underarm) sweating is barely tolerable and frequently interferes with my daily activity.
4	My (underarm) sweating is intolerable and always interferes with my daily activity.

on one question the patient can answer in the office, "Which best describes the impact of sweating on your daily activity?" Answer choices are assigned integer values 1–4 with 3–4 corresponding to severe uncontrolled HH (Table 23.4).

Measuring Hyperhidrosis

It is essential to objectively assess hyperhidrosis before prescribing treatment. The Minor's Starch-Iodine test is a simple way to detect the presence of sweat and localize the area involved. The skin to be tested is dried thoroughly and an iodine solution is painted over the field. When the solution is thoroughly dry, a starch powder is sprinkled on the surface. A modified starch-iodine test can use Betadine^{TM} solution, which is available in most offices (Figure 23.2). Plain cooking corn starch is effective and inexpensive. Starch is applied with a brush, cotton ball, sifter or loose gauze (Figure 23.3). Accurate colorimetric results are achieved when the amount of powder is minimized. Moisture from sweat dissolves the iodine and starch followed by a chemical reaction producing polyiodide chains which are purple to black.

Gravimetric testing is quantitative and determines the rate of sweat production. It is typically reserved for research purposes. It

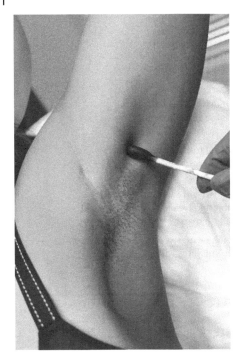

Figure 23.2 Iodine is applied to a clean dry surface.

is performed by thoroughly drying the skin and placing preweighed filter paper on the affected skin. Conventionally, paper is left in place for 5 minutes (accurately timed) and reweighed. Results are operator dependent as care must be taken to prevent paper saturation and evaporation before reweighing. No standard or validated quantity has been established to separate hyperhidrosis from euhidrosis. HH can exceed 30 times that of nonhyperhidrotic individuals. The mean

palmar HH gravimetric measurement was ~300 mg/5 min [13].

The HDSS has been statistically analyzed and is used in clinic to measure disease severity and quality of life. A score from 1 to 4 is generated and correlates with treatment response. A 1-point HDSS improvement corresponds to an approximate 50% reduction in sweat. This validated scale can aid in selecting patients appropriate for therapy and assessing the effectiveness of treatment [14].

Therapy

Many treatments are available for primary focal HH. Therapy should be tailored to the needs of the individual based on skin region, severity, age, and occupation (Table 23.5). Consensus groups have established indication guidelines for each modality [10]. Prior to treatment, one must be sure there is no treatable underlying etiology. If discovered, it must be treated before proceeding with the guidelines.

Antiperspirants are first-line therapy and decrease sweat by blockage of the distal eccrine ducts. Over-the-counter products rarely control HH in patients with severe disease (HDSS 3 or 4) [8, 9, 15, 16]. Prescription strength products containing high concentrations of metal salts, most commonly aluminum chloride, can be more effective [17]. Nonetheless, efficacy remains limited, and

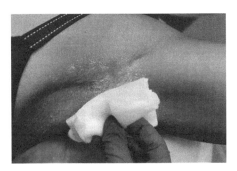

Figure 23.3 Cornstarch is applied sparingly after iodine has dried.

Table 23.5 Therapies most commonly used for hyperhydrosis.

Anitperspirants, over the counter

Antiperspirants, prescription strength

Iontophoresis

Systemic oral medication

Botulinum toxin type A

Local excision of eccrine glands

Liposuction and/or curettage

Endoscopic transthoracic sympathectomy

irritation, erythema, dryness, and pruritus are frequent.

Systemic anticholinergic drugs such as glycopyrrolate, atropine, or oxbutynin provide a generalized acetylcholine blockade [15, 18–20]. Dry eyes, dry mouth, and urinary retention may be encountered at the doses required to achieve symptom relief. Additionally, generalized sweat reduction can increase the risk of hyperthermia.

Iontophoresis is an electrical device most suited to treat palmar-plantar HH. It uses direct current connected to trays of tap water and treatment can be performed at home. The mechanism of action is unknown but may reduce gland secretion, or physically block sweat ducts via ions carried into the ducts. For increased efficacy, anticholinergic agents (crushed glycopyrrolate) can be added to the tap water [21]. Side effects are relatively minimal but cost and time-commitment limit its use for many patients [22].

Local surgical excision, liposuction, curettage, and microwave ablation techniques can be used to remove and destroy eccrine units [23]. Though technology is improving, efficacy is technique dependent and is usually limited to the axillae.

Endoscopic thoracic sympathectomy (ETS) can offer long-term improvement for axillary and palmar symptoms but is not universally accepted. During the procedure, the sympathetic chain is interrupted by destruction or clipping at the appropriate level [24, 25]. The most significant potential adverse effect of ETS surgery is the development of compensatory HH [26]. The incidence varies, but it affects approximately 60–70% of patients. Severity is unpredictable, having the potential to affect large portions of body surface area [24, 27, 28].

Botulinum Toxin Therapy

OnabotulinumtoxinA, abobotulinumtoxinA and incobotulinumtoxinA are derived from botulinum toxin type A (BoNTA). OnabotulinumtoxinA and abobotulinumtoxinA have been the most extensively studied in HH. Botulinum toxin type B has been studied and found to be effective. Despite its efficacy, the side effect profile is quite different from BoNTA [29, 30]. Given the effectiveness and safety profile of onabotulinumtoxinA, it has emerged as the clinically preferred treatment.

As with other treatment modalities, prior to treating excessive sweating with BoNTs, one must objectively identify the area of excessive sweating using a colorimetric test such as a starch-iodine test (Figure 23.2 and Figure 23.3). For optimal BoNT interaction at the neuron–eccrine interface (typically at the junction of the dermis and subcutaneous fat), it should be delivered as a deep intradermal injection. Injections are generally placed 1–2 cm apart. Avoid injecting deeper structures to prevent unwanted denervation.

Different philosophies exist for choosing a toxin dilution volume. The prevailing sentiment is that high dilution volume (lower concentration) will diffuse and treat more area. One location where high volume is appropriate is inguinal HH. However, treating the forehead requires precision to avoid adverse effects and higher concentration is preferred [31].

Compensatory hyperhidrosis is a common side effect of ETS. The phenomenon is considered rare in BoNT injection therapy. Occasionally patients report the perception of increased sweating in untreated anatomic locations after therapy. Literature supporting and refuting this phenomenon can be found [32, 33].

Axillary Hyperhidrosis

No area has been as extensively studied as the axillae. Numerous studies show the benefit and safety of BoNTA, including large, multicenter, randomized, placebo-controlled trials in Europe and the United States. Techniques are reviewed in Chapter 22.

Palmar Hyperhidrosis

BoNT injections are useful in the treatment of palmar HH. Multiple small studies have demonstrated the ability of BoNT to establish clinical improvement in symptoms [13, 34, 35]. Several challenges exist when treating hands such as choosing optimal doses, control of pain during injection, and the side effects which include muscle weakness [13, 36–40].

The optimum dose of BoNTA to control palmar HH is unknown and the issue is complicated by large variations in hand size (Figure 23.4). AbobotulinumtoxinA doses have ranged from 120–500 U per hand [34, 41, 42]. Published studies report onabotulinumtoxinA doses of 50–200 U per hand [35, 43]. OnabotulinumtoxinA is most commonly used. Some authors have suggested a defined dose per unit area, with Swartling's group using 0.8 U/cm^2. Naumann's group used 2 U every 1.5 cm on the palm but three injections per fingertip and two injections into each of the middle and proximal phalanx using 1–2 U per injection [35, 44]. The Canadian advisory committee recommends 1.5–2 U/cm^2 with a mean dose of 100 U onabotulinumtoxinA per palm [9]. It is unclear whether larger doses add to the duration of symptom relief or increase the risk of developing muscle weakness. When Wollina used 200 U of onabotulinumtoxinA per hand in 10 patients, his relapse time varied from 3–22 months [43]. Saadia studied 24 patients: 11 received 50 U onabotulinumtoxinA per hand and 13 received 100 U/hand. Despite more hand and finger weakness, higher patient satisfaction was reported in the high-dose group. There was no difference in duration of efficacy [35]. Until larger studies are available, 75–100 U onabotulinumtoxinA per hand is a good starting point. Adjustments should be made for the size of the hand and efficacy of past treatment doses [16].

Another challenge with palmar BoNT therapy is an apparent shorter duration of efficacy compared to axillary injections [36]. Responses range from 3 to 12 months [45]. Aghaei found that anhidrosis lasted up to 5 months for patients treated with 500 U abobotulinumtoxinA per hand; however, hypohidrosis lasted an average of 10 months [42]. The reason for this shorter duration is unknown but may be related to a smaller diffusion radius in the thicker palm skin and compartmentalized areas of the phalanges [45]. Another possibility is a higher number of cholinergic nerve endings or a faster recovery rate in nerves of the hands.

Injection of the hand is painful due to the high density of nerve receptors and large number of injections required. Using a visual analogue scale (1–100), the pain during injection of the palm has been rated an average 68.1 ± 31.8 compared to 29.9 ± 24.5 for axillary treatment [46]. Several methods of pain control have been tried (Table 23.6). Topical anesthetic containing lidocaine and cold packs is often inadequate. More intense cold exposure is more effective; for example, dichlorotetrafluoroethane, submersion of the hand in an ice bath, and direct exposure of an ice cube [47, 48]. Kreyden describes a technique of iontophoresis with 2% lidocaine for 30 minutes, followed by a light spray of liquid nitrogen just prior to injecting BoNTA [49]. The use of a needleless pressure unit to inject BoNTA was found to be less painful than

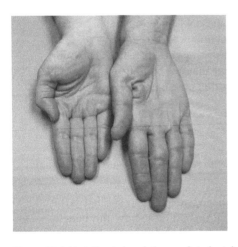

Figure 23.4 Variation in hand size needs to be taken into consideration when dosing botulinum toxin for treatment of palmar hyperhidrosis.

Table 23.6 Anesthesia techniques used for palmar injections.

Class	Specific
Topical	
Nerve blocks	
Cryoanalgesia	Dichlorotetrafluoroethane
	Liquid nitrogen spray
	Ice cubes, ice pack, or ice bath
	Cold packs
	Machine-assisted cold air
Vibration	
Intravenous regional anesthesia (Bier's Block)	
Conscious sedation or general anesthesia	

standard needle injections, but was much less effective. As a result, needleless injection of BoNTA cannot be recommended [50]. Benohanian has described the use of a needleless pressure unit to inject lidocaine into the palms and soles before conventional injections of BoNTA [51]. The Med-JetMBX II (MIT Canada) [52] is approved by Health Canada and the European Union. Once anesthetic wheals appear, BoNT can be administered with a standard needle.

Nerve blocks are effective [40, 44, 53, 54] The palm is innervated by the median, ulnar and radial nerves. All three can be anesthetized at the level of the wrist (Figure 23.5). Risks include nerve injury and vascular puncture. Furthermore, temporary hand weakness limits the patient's activities for several hours. This effect does not permit the treatment of both hands in one session. A 30G 0.5 inch needle should be used to minimize any nerve trauma. Approximately 2 mL of 1–2% lidocaine is injected around each of the nerves. If the patient feels any unusual tingling or sensation during the injection, the needle should be withdrawn slightly. Twenty minutes or more may be necessary for the full effect to develop. Intravenous regional anesthesia (IVRA), also known as a Bier's block is effective [55, 56] but requires additional time, equipment, and cardiovascular monitoring.

Vibratory anesthesia is gaining popularity [57]. Theoretically, the nervous system is unable to perceive fully two different sensory inputs simultaneously. Handheld vibrators can be applied to the volar and dorsal surface of the hand near the site of injection (Figure 23.6). This requires an assistant and

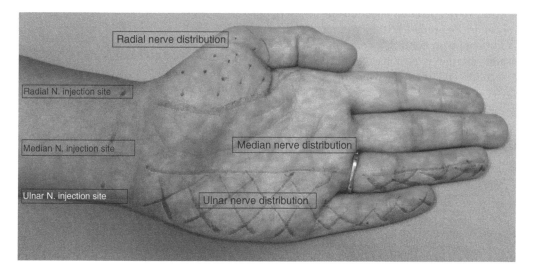

Figure 23.5 The palm is innervated by the ulnar, median, and radial nerves. Nerve blocks may be performed at the level of the wrist.

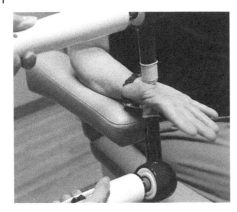

Figure 23.6 Use of a two-vibrator technique for pain control.

creates movement of the patient's hand, making injections more challenging. Despite being easier to maneuver, the use of one vibrator on the volar aspect is not as effective as the use of two (personal experience). Neither technique results in a pain-free injection, but rather diminished perceived pain. A study by Scherer found that the pain threshold is significantly higher during vibration compared to pre- or postvibration, and vibration applied distal to the site of pain was superior to proximal [58].

The author most commonly uses ice with pressure for palmar injections. An ice cube is applied firmly to the planned injection site for 7–10 seconds (Figure 23.7). If the patient requires additional pain control, a combination of ice and vibration is used. Ice is applied for 7–10 seconds and then the vibrator is

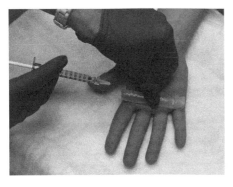

Figure 23.7 Ice and pressure should be applied for 7–10 seconds.

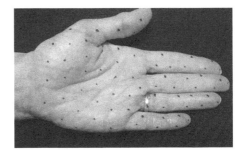

Figure 23.8 Typical injection pattern for palmar hyperhidrosis.

applied immediately adjacent to the site for no more than 1–2 seconds prior to the injection. The injection is delivered during vibration. This technique requires an assistant and time coordinated movement. A 30G 0.5-inch needle with a leur lock syringe or insulin type syringe is especially helpful for the thick skin and higher pressure needed to inject the palm. Injections should be placed every 1–1.5 cm but the digits will usually need two to three injection sites per phalangeal unit (Figure 23.8).

Bruising is common but temporary with palmar injections. Subepidermal injections may increase the incidence of hematoma [37]. Injections of BoNTA should be in the dermal layer, to limit the chance that the drug will come into contact with the deeper muscle tissue. Weakness can result, with the incidence varying in published series from 0 to 77% [13, 35–37, 59]. The most commonly affected area is in the thenar eminence. Strength can be measured in the thumb-index finger pinch, whereas gross and grip strength are usually unaffected [35, 38]. There is one report of atrophy of the intrinsic musculature of the hands with "debilitating" weakness associated with BoNTA injections. This effect occurred after the fifth session using 500 U abobotulinumtoxinA per palm every 9 months [60]. Recent case reports have noted transient dexterity limitations while text messaging [61]. Patients should be adequately counseled on the risks of weakness, which is usually mild and transient.

Zaiac found the average depth of the eccrine glands in ten consecutive palmar biopsies to be 2.6 mm. In an attempt to control the depth of needle insertion and prevent muscle weakness, he advocates the use of the ADG® needle, a device designed for collagen injection [62]. By adjusting the needle to a length of 2.6 mm and using a total of 60–70 U onabotulinmtoxinA per palm, he had no weakness in a series of ten patients. Likewise, cut needle caps can function as an adapter to shorten 7 mm 30G needles to measure 2.5–3.0 mm [40, 63]. Other physicians find these techniques insufficient as ADG® needles can be difficult to obtain and adaptors obstruct the physician's view of the needle. One group has advocated the use of a sterile clamp to make a right-angle bend in the needle 2.6 mm from the tip. The 2.6 mm length can be inserted with full visualization and depth control. They report, but do not quantify reduced complications and improved patient satisfaction [64].

Children with palmar hyperhidrosis can be treated with BoNTs but pain control remains the biggest challenge. Less is known about the dosing, duration, and adverse events associated with pediatric use. Coutinho dos Santos published a series of nine children aged 6.5–15 years with palmar HH successfully treated with onabotulinumtoxinA. Nerve block anesthesia and doses of 75–150 U per palm were used [65].

Plantar Hyperhidrosis

Little has been published on BoNT therapy for plantar HH. Like the palms, there is no consensus on the optimal dose, the duration is variable and the injections are painful. Naumann used 42 and 48 U of onabotulinumtoxinA to treat two soles by injecting 3 U onabotulinumtoxinA (0.15 ml) into each 2 × 2 cm squares [66]. Blaheta's and Campanati's groups report success using 100 U onabotulinumtoxinA per sole (100 U/5 ml saline) [60]. All patients had an improvement in symptoms and a "significant decrease of Minor's test" for 12 weeks without significant side effects [67].

Minor's Starch-Iodine test delineates the hyperhidrotic area, which can extend up the sides and onto the dorsum of the foot. BoNTA should be evenly distributed every 1–2 cm using small gauge needles and injecting into the deep dermis. Injections of the plantar surface can be technically more challenging due to the thickness of the stratum corneum, especially if calloused. The physician has to adjust for the variation in depth to accurately place BoNTA.

As for palmar injections, pain control must be addressed. IVRA can provide sufficient anesthesia for the sole. In a small series of eight patients, IVRA was found to be more effective than nerve blocks [68]. Nerve blocks used are generally performed at the level of the ankle. For sole anesthesia, the tibial and sural nerves are blocked. If the dorsum of the foot must be injected, the superficial peroneal nerve can be included [63].

Vadoud-Seyedi reported on using the Dermojet to inject BoNTA for plantar HH. Ten patients were treated with 50 U BoNTA/5 ml saline per foot; 15–20 points were injected per foot and no analgesia was used. The injections were tolerated well by all patients, although one developed a localized hematoma. The duration of benefit lasted 3–6 months; however, 20% of patients reported the treatment had no effect [69].

At this time, the author's preferred method of pain control is ice combined with vibration as described earlier (Figure 23.9). Doses of 100–200 U onabotulinumtoxinA per foot are

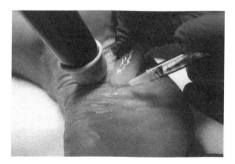

Figure 23.9 When using a combination of ice and vibration, ice is applied for 7–10 seconds and vibration is applied in the treatment area immediately before injection.

typically required. Bruising and pain with injection are the most common side effects. In the published literature, one patient reported weakness of plantar flexor muscles in both feet following BoNTA injections, with resolution in 10 days [70].

Facial Hyperhidrosis

Primary facial HH has several patterns with involvement of the forehead, scalp perimeter, entire scalp, cheeks, nose, upper lip, chin, or a combination of the areas (Figure 23.10). The most common pattern affects the forehead with or without the scalp. All forms of facial HH tend to respond to BoNTA, with the duration of gustatory response being exceptionally long.

There is a paucity of literature published on BoNTA therapy for craniofacial hyperhidrosis. Kinkelin's group injected a mean of 86 U onabotulinumtoxinA (3 U per injection site)

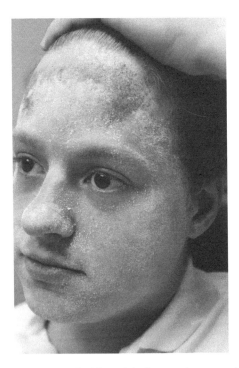

Figure 23.10 Facial starch-iodine test demonstrating excessive sweating of the forehead and to lesser extent the upper lip.

over the forehead at equidistant locations (1–1.5 .5) in 10 men with frontal hyperhidrosis [71]. Intracutaneous injections were placed ≥1 cm superior to the eyebrow to prevent eyelid ptosis. Five of ten patients had partial disability in frowning, but was limited to ≤8 weeks. No ptosis was noted and satisfaction was good or excellent in 90% of subjects. Effects were maintained ≥5 months in 90% of patients. Similarly, Tan and Solish report that symptoms return on average 4.5 months after treatment of the forehead [46].

Boger treated 12 men suffering from bilateral craniofacial hyperhidrosis with abobotulinumtoxinA 0.1 ng per injection [72]. Half of the forehead was treated using a total of 2.5–4 ng injected equidistantly with a total of 25–40 injections. Decreased sweating lasted ≥3 months (up to 27 months). Side effects were limited to temporary weakness of the frontalis (100%), and brow asymmetry lasting 1–12 months (17%).

It is the observation of the author that patients typically present with forehead sweating that may be combined with scalp sweating in a diffuse pattern or an ophiasis pattern. OnabotulinumtoxinA injections are performed with 2–3 U every 1–2 cm avoiding the inferior 1–2 cm of the forehead to reduce the risk of brow ptosis [73]. The forehead can be treated more inferiorly if the response is not sufficient and the patient is willing to accept temporary brow ptosis. Typical doses of onabotulinumtoxinA used by the author are 50–100 U to treat the forehead and frontal hairline, 200 U to treat the forehead and the perimeter of the scalp, and 300 U when treating the forehead and entire scalp [73].

Gustatory Sweating (Frey's Syndrome)

Gustatory sweating is a relatively common complication after surgery or injury in the region of the parotid gland. It may result from misdirection of autonomic nerve fibers after surgery and is frequently observed in diseases

Table 23.7 Selected studies on BoNTA treatment of gustatory sweating.

Author	Year	Design	n	Dose (mean)	Duration (months)
Naumann et al. [101]	1997	Open	45	21 mu OnabotulinumtoxinA	6
Bjerkhoel and Trobbe [102]	1997	Open	15	37 mu OnabotulinumtoxinA	13
Laskawi et al. [103]	1998	Open	19	31 mu OnabotulinumtoxinA	11–27
Laccourreye et al. [104]	1999	Open	33	86 mu AbobotulinumtoxinA	12–36

of the parotid gland and diabetes. Sweating occurs on the cheek in response to salivation or anticipation of food.

BoNTA is a highly effective treatment option for gustatory sweating as shown by several uncontrolled studies (Table 23.7) [74–78]. In a large open study of 45 patients, there was a significant reduction of local facial sweating after injection of onabotulinumtoxinA using a mean dose of 21 U (range 5–72 U) and no recurrence of sweating was observed during the follow-up period of six months. A marked long-lasting benefit of 11–36 months was also observed in three other open studies [76–78]. The reason for BoNTA's long-lasting effect on gustatory sweating is unknown.

It is important to perform a starch-iodine test before injection to visualize the affected area. After the iodine and starch have been applied, it is helpful for the patient to chew candy or food to stimulate facial sweating. Injections with 2–3 U onabotulinumtoxinA or 8 U abobotulinumtoxinA are given intradermally at sites 2–2.5.5 apart and evenly distributed over the affected area. Specific side effects include pain on injection, local hematomas, and transient local muscle weakness with facial asymmetry. Care must be taken to avoid affecting the zygomatic muscles.

Other Sweating Disorders

Inguinal sweating affects 2–10% of individuals with HH [8]. It usually develops in adolescence and can be associated with HH in other body sites. Intradermal injections of BoNTA can control symptoms for

≥ 6 months. As with other body sites, a starch-iodine test is valuable in identifying the areas producing sweat, but often is technically challenging. Treatment is with 2–3 U onabotulinumtoxinA injected every 1–2 cm within the affected field; typical doses range 60–100 U per side [79].

Compensatory sweating is the most common complication of endoscopic transthoracic sympathectomy (ETS), ranging from 44 to 91% [80]. Often affecting large areas, treatment is particularly difficult but success has been reported using BoNTA. Belin and Polo reported good results treating the upper abdomen with onabotulinumtoxinA. Unfortunately this patient's total area affected was too large to be treated in one sitting (involved his nipple line to knees) [26]. Huh used 300 U abobotulinumtoxinA to treat the chest and abdomen after identifying the area with an starch-iodine test [80]. Each 100 U of onabotulinumtoxinA was diluted in 10 ml saline and 0.1 ml/cm^2 was injected. Efficacy gradually diminished, but was maintained for 8 months. Kim and colleagues reported 17 patients treated with 100–500 U of onabotulinumtoxinA, administering 2 U every 1.5 cm. The injections were well-tolerated, but they noted incomplete resolution due to insufficient dosing, and limited duration of only 4 months [81].

Chromhidrosis is a rare disorder characterized by the excretion of colored or pigmented sweat. It is most commonly confined to the face or axilla. Matarasso used 15 U onabotulinumtoxinA to treat the affected area of each cheek which measured 3 cm in diameter. Within 48 hours, the patient had a marked reduction in the amount of discharged black sweat [82].

Ross Syndrome

First described by the neurologist Alexander T. Ross in 1958, it is characterized by the triad of unilateral tonic pupils, generalized areflexia (Holmes-Adie syndrome), and progressive segmental anhidrosis with a compensatory band of excessive perspiration. Patients usually do not perceive the anhidrosis. Instead, the compensatory segmental hyperhidrosis is bothersome [83]. The pathogenesis of Ross syndrome is unknown. There is no histologic evidence of nerve fiber destruction. Therefore, Ross postulated a defect in acetylcholine cholinesterase activity, rather than the degeneration of sweat glands. Although there is no therapy for the progressive segmental anhidrosis, the compensatory hyperhidrosis can be improved with systemic antimuscarinic drugs or BoNTA injections to the affected areas.

Localized Unilateral Hyperhidrosis

Localized unilateral hyperhidrosis (LUH) is idiopathic and rare. It is a confined area of hyperhidrosis of less than 10×10 cm, mainly found on the forehead or forearm. Not only is LUH unusual in localization, but also has no trigger and occurs while patients sleep. The etiology may be due to a misdirected reconnection of the sympathetic nerves after injury, similar to the Frey syndrome [1]. Excellent results are achieved following injection the affected area with 30 U of onabotulinumtoxinA.

Use of Botulinum Toxin Type B for Hyperhidrosis

Botulinum toxin type B (BoNTB) use has been limited to treatment of cervical dystonia, but there are reports of its use for HH. Injection of BoNTB can induce focal anhidrosis in a dose-dependent fashion. Birklein reported durations up to 6 months using 125 U [84].

Despite its efficacy, the use of BoNTB is limited by the occurrence of systemic adverse events [85]. A patient treated with 2500 U BoNTB to each palm for HH developed bilateral blurred vision, indigestion, dry sore throat, and dysphagia [86]. Another palmar HH study of 20 subjects used 5000 U BoNTB per palm [87]. Adverse events were common: dry mouth or throat (90%), indigestion (60%), excessively dry hands (60%), muscle weakness (60%), and decreased grip strength (50%).

Lower dosing may be the key to reducing the high incidence of side effects [88]. However, the incidence of systemic side effects using BoNTB and the high safety profile using BoNTA to treat focal hyperhidrosis, to date, BoNTA remains the neurotoxin of choice.

Future Directions

The use of botulinum toxins has revolutionized the treatment of HH and other secretory disorders. Compared with other treatments, it is unmatched in its efficacy, ease of administration, and patient satisfaction. Development of quick, safe, and effective pain control is needed for the treatment of more tender areas. New delivery devices are being researched to provide the most comfortable and efficient therapy. Kavanagh and colleagues have successfully used a small iontophoresis machine to deliver BoNTA to two patients, sparing them the injections [89]. Glogau demonstrated that onabotulinumtoxinA can be successfully delivered into the axillary skin when combined with a proprietary transport peptide molecule [90]. Research is ongoing for different BoNT serotypes. For the present, BoNT therapy is a valuable, well-tolerated therapy and can provide meaningful improvement in the quality of life of patients with HH and other secretory disorders.

References

1 Goldsmith L. Biology of ecrine and apocrine sweat glands. In: Freedberg IM, Fitzpatrick TB, eds. *Fitzpatrick's Dermatology in General Medicine*. 5th edn. New York: McGraw-Hill, Health Professions Division; 1999:157–164.

2 Stenn K, Bhawan J. The normal histology of the skin. In: Farmer ER, Hood AF, eds. *Pathology of the Skin*. New York: McGraw-Hill; 2000.

3 Glogau RG. Botulinum A neurotoxin for axillary hyperhidrosis. No sweat Botox. Dermatol Surg Aug 1998;24(8):817–819.

4 Goldsmith L. Disorders of the eccrine sweat gland. In: Freedberg IM, Fitzpatrick TB, eds. *Fitzpatrick's Dermatology in General Medicine*. 5th edn. New York: McGraw-Hill, Health Professions Division; 1999:800–809.

5 Kreyden OP, Scheidegger EP. Anatomy of the sweat glands, pharmacology of botulinum toxin, and distinctive syndromes associated with hyperhidrosis. Clin Dermatol Jan-Feb 2004;22(1):40–44.

6 Cheshire WP, Freeman R. Disorders of sweating. Semin Neurol Dec 2003;23(4): 399–406.

7 Grazziotin TC, Buffon RB, da Silva Manzoni AP, Libis AS, Weber MB. Treatment of granulosis rubra nasi with botulinum toxin type A. Dermatol Surg Aug 2009;35(8):1298–1299.

8 Lear W, Kessler E, Solish N, Glaser DA. An epidemiological study of hyperhidrosis. Dermatol Surg Jan 2007;33(1 Spec No.): S69–75.

9 Solish N, Bertucci V, Dansereau A, *et al.* A comprehensive approach to the recognition, diagnosis, and severity-based treatment of focal hyperhidrosis: recommendations of the Canadian Hyperhidrosis Advisory Committee. Dermatol Surg Aug 2007;33(8):908–923.

10 Hornberger J, Grimes K, Naumann M, *et al.* Recognition, diagnosis, and treatment of primary focal hyperhidrosis. J Am Acad Dermatol Aug 2004;51(2):274–286.

11 Walling HW. Clinical differentiation of primary from secondary hyperhidrosis. J Am Acad Dermatol Apr 2011;64(4): 690–695.

12 Hamm H, Naumann MK, Kowalski JW, Kutt S, Kozma C, Teale C. Primary focal hyperhidrosis: disease characteristics and functional impairment. Dermatology 2006; 212(4):343–353.

13 Lowe NJ, Yamauchi PS, Lask GP, Patnaik R, Iyer S. Efficacy and safety of botulinum toxin type a in the treatment of palmar hyperhidrosis: a double-blind, randomized, placebo-controlled study. Dermatol Surg 2002 Sep;28(9):822–827.

14 Hyperhidrosis disease severity scale (HDSS): Validity and reliability results from three studies. Glaser, D., Kowalski, J., Eadie, N. *et al.* Washington, D.C.: American Academy of Dermatology:P198.

15 Stolman LP. Treatment of hyperhidrosis. Dermatol Clin Oct 1998;16(4):863–869.

16 Glaser DA, Hebert AA, Pariser DM, Solish N. Palmar and plantar hyperhidrosis: best practice recommendations and special considerations. Cutis 2007 May; 79(5 Suppl):18–28.

17 Benohanian A, Dansereau A, Bolduc C, Bloom E. Localized hyperhidrosis treated with aluminum chloride in a salicylic acid gel base. Int J Dermatol 1998 Sep;37(9): 701–703.

18 Praharaj SK, Arora M. Paroxetine useful for palmar-plantar hyperhidrosis. Ann Pharmacother 2006 Oct;40(10):1884–1886.

19 Bajaj V, Langtry JA. Use of oral glycopyrronium bromide in hyperhidrosis. Br J Dermatol 2007 Jul;157(1):118–121.

20 Klaber M, Catterall M. Treating hyperhidrosis. Anticholinergic drugs were not mentioned. BMJ 2000 Sep 16; 321(7262):703.

21 Naumann M, Davidson J, Glaser DA. Hyperhidrosis: Current Understanding, Current Therapy CME. 2002.

22 Stolman LP. Treatment of excess sweating of the palms by iontophoresis. Arch Dermatol 1987 Jul;123(7):893–896.

23 Swinehart JM. Treatment of axillary hyperhidrosis: combination of the starch-iodine test with the tumescent liposuction technique. Dermatol Surg 2000 Apr;26(4):392–396.

24 Gossot D, Galetta D, Pascal A, *et al*. Long-term results of endoscopic thoracic sympathectomy for upper limb hyperhidrosis. Ann Thorac Surg 2003 Apr; 75(4):1075–1079.

25 Kim BY, Oh BS, Park YK, *et al*. Microinvasive video-assisted thoracoscopic sympathicotomy for primary palmar hyperhidrosis. Am J Surg 2001 Jun;181(6): 540–542.

26 Belin EE, Polo J. Treatment of compensatory hyperhidrosis with botulinum toxin type A. Cutis 2003 Jan; 71(1):68–70.

27 Andrews BT, Rennie JA. Predicting changes in the distribution of sweating following thoracoscopic sympathectomy. Br J Surg 1997 Dec;84(12):1702–1704.

28 Kao MC, Chen YL, Lin JY, *et al*. Endoscopic sympathectomy treatment for craniofacial hyperhidrosis. Arch Surg 1996 Oct;131(10):1091–1094.

29 Dressler D, Adib Saberi F, Benecke R. Botulinum toxin type B for treatment of axillar hyperhidrosis. J Neurol 2002 Dec; 249(12):1729–1732.

30 Frasson E, Brigo F, Acler M, *et al*. Botulinum toxin type A vs type B for axillary hyperhidrosis in a case series of patients observed for 6 months. Arch Dermatol 2011 Jan;147(1):122–123.

31 Hexsel DM, Soirefmann M, Rodrigues TC, do Prado DZ. Increasing the field effects of similar doses of Clostridium botulinum type A toxin-hemagglutinin complex in the treatment of compensatory hyperhidrosis. Arch Dermatol 2009 Jul;145(7):837–840.

32 Krogstad AL, Skymne A, Pegenius G, *et al*. No compensatory sweating after botulinum toxin treatment of palmar hyperhidrosis. Br J Dermatol 2005 Feb;152(2):329–333.

33 Gregoriou S, Rigopoulos D, Makris M, *et al*. Effects of botulinum toxin-a therapy for palmar hyperhidrosis in plantar sweat production. Dermatol Surg 2010 Apr; 36(4):496–498.

34 Simonetta Moreau M, Cauhepe C, Magues JP, Senard JM. A double-blind, randomized, comparative study of Dysport vs. Botox in primary palmar hyperhidrosis. Br J Dermatol 2003 Nov;149(5):1041–1045.

35 Saadia D, Voustianiouk A, Wang AK, Kaufmann H. Botulinum toxin type A in primary palmar hyperhidrosis: randomized, single-blind, two-dose study. Neurology 11 2001 Dec;57(11):2095–2099.

36 Naver H, Swartling C, Aquilonius SM. Palmar and axillary hyperhidrosis treated with botulinum toxin: one-year clinical follow-up. Eur J Neurol 2000 Jan;7(1): 55–62.

37 Vadoud-Seyedi J, Heenen M, Simonart T. Treatment of idiopathic palmar hyperhidrosis with botulinum toxin. Report of 23 cases and review of the literature. Dermatology 2001;203(4):318–321.

38 Glaser DA, Kokoska M, Kardesch C. Botulinum toxin type A in the treatment of palmar hyperhidrosis: the effect of dilution and number of injection sites. American Academy of Dermatology Annual Meeting; 2001.

39 Baumann L, Frankel S, Welsh E, Halem M. Cryoanalgesia with dichlorotetrafluoroethane lessens the pain of botulinum toxin injections for the treatment of palmar hyperhidrosis. Dermatol Surg 2003 Oct; 29(10):1057–1059; discussion 1060.

40 de Almeida AR, Kadunc BV, de Oliveira EM. Improving botulinum toxin therapy for palmar hyperhidrosis: wrist block and technical considerations. Dermatol Surg 2001 Jan;27(1):34–36.

41 Schnider P, Binder M, Auff E, Kittler H, Berger T, Wolff K. Double-blind trial of botulinum A toxin for the treatment of focal hyperhidrosis of the palms. Br J Dermatol 1997 Apr;136(4):548–552.

42 Aghaei S. Botulinum toxin therapy for palmar hyperhidrosis: experience in an Iranian population. Int J Dermatol 2007 Feb;46(2):212–214.

43 Wollina U, Karamfilov T. Botulinum toxin A for palmar hyperhidrosis. J Eur Acad Dermatol Venereol 2001 Nov;15(6): 555–558.

44 Hund M, Rickert S, Kinkelin I, *et al*. Does wrist nerve block influence the result of botulinum toxin A treatment in palmar hyperhidrosis? J Am Acad Dermatol 2004 Jan;50(1):61–62.

45 Perez-Bernal AM, Avalos-Peralta P, Moreno-Ramirez D, Camacho F. Treatment of palmar hyperhidrosis with botulinum toxin type A: 44 months of experience. J Cosmet Dermatol 2005 Sep; 4(3):163–166.

46 Tan SR, Solish N. Long-term efficacy and quality of life in the treatment of focal hyperhidrosis with botulinum toxin A. Dermatol Surg 2002 Jun;28(6):495–499.

47 Kontochristopoulos G, Gregoriou S, Zakopoulou N, Rigopoulos D. Cryoanalgesia with dichlorotetrafluoroethane spray versus ice packs in patients treated with botulinum toxin-a for palmar hyperhidrosis: Self-controlled study. Dermatol Surg 2006 Jun;32(6):873–874.

48 Smith KC, Comite SL, Storwick GS. Ice minimizes discomfort associated with injection of botulinum toxin type A for the treatment of palmar and plantar hyperhidrosis. Dermatol Surg 2007 Jan; 33(1 Spec No.):S88–S91.

49 Kreyden O. Botulinum Toxin in the Management of Focal Hyperhidrosis. In: Benedetto AV, ed. *Botulinum Toxin in Clinical Dermatology*: Taylor & Francis; 2006:281–285.

50 Naumann M, Bergmann I, Hofmann U, Hamm H, Reiners K. Botulinum toxin for focal hyperhidrosis: technical considerations and improvements in application. Br J Dermatol 1998 Dec;139(6): 1123–1124.

51 Benohanian A. Needle-free anaesthesia prior to botulinum toxin type A injection treatment of palmar and plantar hyperhidrosis. Br J Dermatol 2007 Mar; 156(3):593–596.

52 Benohanian A. What stands in the way of treating palmar hyperhidrosis as effectively as axillary hyperhidrosis with botulinum toxin type A. Dermatol Online J 2009; 15(4):12.

53 Hayton MJ, Stanley JK, Lowe NJ. A review of peripheral nerve blockade as local anaesthesia in the treatment of palmar hyperhidrosis. Br J Dermatol 2003 Sep; 149(3):447–451.

54 Campanati A, Lagalla G, Penna L, *et al*. Local neural block at the wrist for treatment of palmar hyperhidrosis with botulinum toxin: technical improvements. J Am Acad Dermatol 2004 Sep;51(3): 345–348.

55 Vollert B, Blaheta HJ, Moehrle E, *et al*. Intravenous regional anaesthesia for treatment of palmar hyperhidrosis with botulinum toxin type A. Br J Dermatol 2001 Mar;144(3):632–633.

56 Ponce-Olivera RM, Tirado-Sanchez A, Arellano-Mendoza MI, *et al*. Palmar hyperhidrosis. Safety efficacy of two anaesthetic techniques for botulinum toxin therapy. Dermatol Online J 2006; 12(2):9.

57 Reed ML. Surgical pearl: mechanoanesthesia to reduce the pain of local injections. J Am Acad Dermatol 2001 Apr;44(4):671–672.

58 Sherer CL, Clelland JA, O'Sullivan P, *et al*. The effect of two sites of high frequency vibration on cutaneous pain threshold. Pain 1986 Apr;25(1):133–138.

59 Solomon BA, Hayman R. Botulinum toxin type A therapy for palmar and digital hyperhidrosis. J Am Acad Dermatol 2000 Jun;42(6):1026–1029.

60 Glass GE, Hussain M, Fleming AN, Powell BW. Atrophy of the intrinsic musculature of the hands associated with the use of botulinum toxin-A injections for hyperhidrosis: a case report and review of

the literature. J Plast Reconstr Aesthet Surg 2009 Aug;62(8):e274–e276.

61 Lehman JS. Writer's Block: "Texting" Impairment as a complication of botulinum toxin type a therapy for palmar hyperhidrosis. Arch Dermatol 2011 Jun; 147(6):752.

62 Zaiac M, Weiss E, Elgart G. Botulinum toxin therapy for palmar hyperhidrosis with ADG needle. Dermatol Surg 2000 Mar; 26(3):230.

63 de Almeida AR, Boraso R. Palmar Hyperhidrosis. In: de Almeida AR, Hexsel DM, eds. *Hyperhidrosis and Botulinum Toxin*. Sao Paulo: Know-How Editorial Ltd.; 2004:155–162.

64 Blugerman G, Schavelzon D, Labaronnie H, *et al.* Our trick to control the depth of injection of the botulinum toxin in the treatment of hyperhidrosis. Plast Reconstr Surg 2011 Jun;127(6):165e–166e.

65 Coutinho dos Santos LH, Gomes AM, Giraldi S, *et al.* Palmar hyperhidrosis: long-term follow-up of nine children and adolescents treated with botulinum toxin type A. Pediatr Dermatol 2009 Jul–Aug; 26(4):439–444.

66 Naumann M, Hofmann U, Bergmann I, *et al.* Focal hyperhidrosis: effective treatment with intracutaneous botulinum toxin. Arch Dermatol 1998 Mar;134(3): 301–304.

67 Campanati A, Bernardini ML, Gesuita R, Offidani A. Plantar focal idiopathic hyperhidrosis and botulinum toxin: a pilot study. Eur J Dermatol 2007 Jan–Feb;17(1): 52–54.

68 Blaheta HJ, Deusch H, Rassner G, Vollert B. Intravenous regional anesthesia (Bier's block) is superior to a peripheral nerve block for painless treatment of plantar hyperhidrosis with botulinum toxin. J Am Acad Dermatol 2003 Feb;48(2):302–304.

69 Vadoud-Seyedi J. Treatment of plantar hyperhidrosis with botulinum toxin type A. Int J Dermatol 2004 Dec;43(12):969–971.

70 Sevim S, Dogu O, Kaleagasi H. Botulinum toxin-A therapy for palmar and plantar

hyperhidrosis. Acta Neurol Belg 2002 Dec;102(4):167–170.

71 Kinkelin I, Hund M, Naumann M, Hamm H. Effective treatment of frontal hyperhidrosis with botulinum toxin A. Br J Dermatol 2000 Oct;143(4):824–827.

72 Boger A, Herath H, Rompel R, Ferbert A. Botulinum toxin for treatment of craniofacial hyperhidrosis. J Neurol Nov 2000;247(11):857–861.

73 Glaser DA, Hebert AA, Pariser DM, Solish N. Facial hyperhidrosis: best practice recommendations and special considerations. Cutis 2007 May; 79(5 Suppl):29–32.

74 Drobik C, Laskawi R. Frey's syndrome: treatment with botulinum toxin. Acta Otolaryngol 1995 May;115(3):459–461.

75 Naumann M, Zellner M, Toyka KV, Reiners K. Treatment of gustatory sweating with botulinum toxin. Ann Neurol 1997 Dec; 42(6):973–975.

76 Bjerkhoel A, Trobbe O. Frey's syndrome: treatment with botulinum toxin. J Laryngol Otol 1997 Sep;111(9):839–844.

77 Laskawi R, Drobik C, Schonebeck C. Up-to-date report of botulinum toxin type A treatment in patients with gustatory sweating (Frey's syndrome). Laryngoscope 1998 Mar;108(3):381–384.

78 Laccourreye O, Akl E, Gutierrez-Fonseca R, *et al.* Recurrent gustatory sweating (Frey syndrome) after intracutaneous injection of botulinum toxin type A: incidence, management, and outcome. Arch Otolaryngol Head Neck Surg 1999 Mar; 125(3):283–286.

79 Hexsel DM, Dal'forno T, Hexsel CL. Inguinal, or Hexsel's hyperhidrosis. Clin Dermatol 2004 Jan–Feb;22(1):53–59.

80 Huh CH, Han KH, Seo KI, Eun HC. Botulinum toxin treatment for a compensatory hyperhidrosis subsequent to an upper thoracic sympathectomy. J Dermatolog Treat 2002 Jun;13(2):91–93.

81 Kim WO, Kil HK, Yoon KB, Noh KU. Botulinum toxin: a treatment for compensatory hyperhidrosis in the trunk.

Dermatol Surg 2009 May;35(5):833–838; discussion 838.

82 Matarasso SL. Treatment of facial chromhidrosis with botulinum toxin type A. J Am Acad Dermatol 2005 Jan;52(1): 89–91.

83 Naumann M, Lowe NJ. Botulinum toxin type A in treatment of bilateral primary axillary hyperhidrosis: randomised, parallel group, double blind, placebo controlled trial. BMJ 2001 Sep 15;323(7313):596–599.

84 Birklein F, Eisenbarth G, Erbguth F, Winterholler M. Botulinum toxin type B blocks sudomotor function effectively: a 6 month follow up. J Invest Dermatol 2003 Dec;121(6):1312–1316.

85 Schlereth T, Mouka I, Eisenbarth G, *et al.* Botulinum toxin A (Botox) and sweating-dose efficacy and comparison to other BoNT preparations. Auton Neurosci 2005 Feb 7;117(2):120–126.

86 Baumann LS, Halem ML. Systemic adverse effects after botulinum toxin type B (myobloc) injections for the treatment of palmar hyperhidrosis. Arch Dermatol 2003 Feb;139(2):226–227.

87 Baumann L, Slezinger A, Vujevich J, *et al.* A double-blinded, randomized, placebo-controlled pilot study of the safety and efficacy of Myobloc (botulinum toxin type B)-purified neurotoxin complex for the treatment of crow's feet: a double-blinded, placebo-controlled trial. Dermatol Surg 2003 May;29(5):508–515.

88 Hecht MJ, Birklein F, Winterholler M. Successful treatment of axillary hyperhidrosis with very low doses of botulinum toxin B: a pilot study. Arch Dermatol Res 2004 Feb;295(8–9):318–319.

89 Kavanagh GM, Oh C, Shams K. BOTOX delivery by iontophoresis. Br J Dermatol 2004 Nov;151(5):1093–1095.

90 Glogau RG. Topically applied botulinum toxin type A for the treatment of primary axillary hyperhidrosis: results of a randomized, blinded, vehicle-controlled study. Dermatol Surg 2007 Jan; 33(1 Spec No.):S76–S80.

24

Topical Botulinum Toxin

Richard G. Glogau, MD[1] and Eileen Axibal, MD[2]

[1]*Clinical Professor of Dermatology, University of California San Francisco, USA*
[2]*Department of Dermatology, University of Colorado, Aurora, USA*

Introduction

Ten years after initial publication by the Carruthers of the use of botulinum toxin type A (BoNTA) for the treatment of glabellar lines [1], the Food and Drug Administration (FDA) approved the drug in 2002 for "temporary improvement in the appearance of moderate to severe glabellar lines associated with corrugator and/or procerus muscle activity in adult patients 65 or younger" [2]. This was the first elective cosmetic indication for a commercially available botulinum toxin in the United States market. Prior to this time, FDA approved therapeutic uses included the treatment of strabismus, blepharospasm, and cervical dystonia. In 2013, the FDA expanded its approval for BoNTA to include a new use for the temporary improvement in the appearance of moderate to severe lateral canthal lines, known as "crow's feet," in adults [3]. Widespread off-label use of the drug for cosmetic purposes has targeted other facial muscles including the frontalis muscle for horizontal lines, depressor anguli oris for the downturned corners of the mouth, and orbicularis oris for lip rhytides.

BoNTA is currently available in three commercial forms in the United States: Allergan's Botox® Cosmetic (onabotulinumtoxinA) [4], Ipsen & Galderma's Dysport® (abobotulinumtoxinA) [5], and Merz' Xeomin® (incobotulinumtoxinA) [6]. Two other forms are manufactured in Korea and China and these are marketed under the names Meditoxin®/Neuronox® and Hengli®/Prosigne®, respectively. All of these forms of BoNTA are prepared in dilute form for injection and, as such, they all share the potential problems of pain, erythema, bruising, tenderness, and potential risk of infection from needle penetration [7–9]. Because of the disadvantage of requiring injection as the route of administration, alternative methods of drug delivery have been developed that can address some of these concerns.

Current Transepidermal Delivery Mechanisms

Current transepidermal approaches in drug delivery systems can only deliver small molecules. Some examples of smaller molecules that can be delivered through the skin topically include progesterone, certain antibiotics, and nicotine. These are readily delivered in topical preparations, creams, ointments, adhesive patches, etc. These vehicles, however, are very inefficient in delivering biologically active proteins and other macromolecules across the skin barrier. The stratum corneum and upper layers of the epidermis are lipid-rich barriers to entry for most of the larger molecules;

Botulinum Toxins: Cosmetic and Clinical Applications, First Edition. Edited by Joel L. Cohen and David M. Ozog.
© 2017 John Wiley & Sons Ltd. Published 2017 by John Wiley & Sons Ltd.
Companion Website: www.wiley.com/go/cohen/botulinum

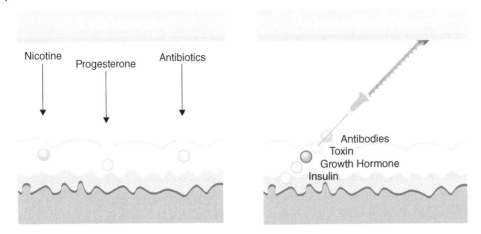

Figure 24.1 Small molecules can penetrate skin directly (left), while larger molecules have traditionally required direct injection to penetrate the skin (right). Reproduced with permission of Revance Therapeutics.

the exclusion of assaults on the inner host by biologically active macromolecules is, after all, the skin's primary function. For this reason, the flux of most proteins across the skin barrier is essentially zero.

Attempts to increase penetration by manipulation of drug structure have been rudimentary to date. For example, conjugation of a drug to a carrier can compromise drug activity. Permeation enhancers may disrupt protein linkages and tertiary structures vital to biological activity of the protein. At present, delivery of most macromolecules across the skin barrier requires direct injection; for example, insulin, antibodies, toxins, growth hormone (Figure 24.1).

The stratum corneum and upper layers of the epidermis are essentially a multilayered arrangement of the mature and differentiated horny cells of the epidermis that are interwoven in a lipid matrix with a lamellar structure (Figure 24.2). This lipid matrix provides a potential route for the passage of molecules into the skin by a process called "lipid rafting." This process is energy independent and involves the passive movement of the molecules along the pathways of the lipid matrix, in the spaces between the horny cells of the stratum corneum (Figure 24.3). This process is highly time dependent, concentration dependent, and obviously becomes much less efficient as the size of the molecule

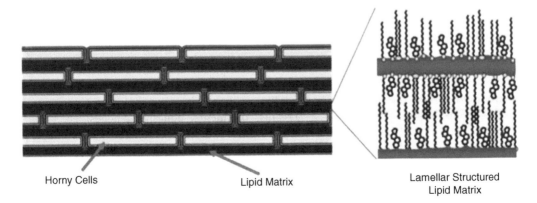

Figure 24.2 The epidermis consists of cells interspersed in a lipid matrix (left) which demonstrates a lamellar structure on further examination (right). Reproduced with permission of Revance Therapeutics.

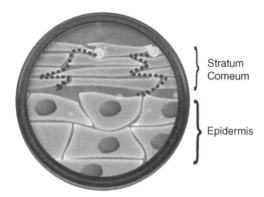

Stratum
Corneum

Epidermis

Figure 24.3 The lipid matrix provides a route between skin cells which permits passive, non-energy dependent, "lipid rafting" of molecules through the skin, a very slow and concentration dependent process. Reproduced with permission of Revance Therapeutics.

in question increases. Highly ionic and/or aqueous entities are also less likely to penetrate the lipid matrix.

There are several ongoing investigational studies that aim to determine if various excipients may be able to promote the passive diffusion of topical botulinum toxin without barrier disruption, as well as if barrier disruption techniques may be effective in promoting pure toxin delivery.

Investigational Transepidermal Delivery Systems

Botulinum toxin type A topical formulations that are currently under investigation include RT-001 (Revance Therapeutics, Inc., Newark, CA) and ANT-1207 (Allergan Plc., Parsippany-Troy Hills, NJ – acquired from Anterios, Inc. in 2016). RT-001 topical gel contains an albumin-free 150-kDa BoNTA and a novel cell-penetrating peptide (CPP) that enables transcutaneous delivery of the BoNTA. ANT-1207 utilizes a proprietary NDS^{TM} (Nanodermal Society) platform delivery technology focused on the local, targeted delivery of macromolecules across the skin; the specifics of the NDS^{TM} platform are not yet elucidated but the manufacturers

describe long-term stability of BoNTA in their preparation which does not require reconstitution of a lyophilized toxin at the time of use. RT-001 and ANT-1207 are currently under phase III and phase IIb investigation, respectively, for the treatment of moderate to severe lateral canthal lines (LCLs). This novel approach to BoNTA administration may eliminate the local pain and ecchymoses associated with injections in the lateral canthus and orbicularis oculi regions.

The development of the Revance proprietary peptide that is the transport molecule joined to the cargo molecule, in this case botulinum toxin A, was a serendipitous discovery that grew out of study of one of the human immunodeficiency virus (HIV) genes called "TAT", for "trans-activator of transcription." TAT was originally characterized in 1988 by two research teams: Frankel & Pabo [10] and Green & Loewenstein [11]. TAT causes accelerated production of the HIV double-stranded RNA by binding to cellular factors, controlling their phosphorylation, resulting in increased transcription of all the HIV genes. TAT has, within it, a protein transduction domain (PTD) that is capable of penetrating cell membranes and it functionally responsible for the propagation of the virus genomes.

The novelty of the Revance peptide is that it represents a *reverse* sequence of basic residues of the TAT gene. The backbone peptide consists of approximately 35 L-amino acids in a reverse sequence of TAT. Despite the reversal of the sequence, the protein transduction domains continue to function in the same way. The peptide backbone is bound through noncovalent (electrostatic) bonds, with the positive charge of the peptide attracted to the relatively negatively charged 150 kDa botulinum toxin (Figure 24.5 (a)–(c)) [12]. The toxin is surrounded by peptides with the PTDs directed outward where they are free to attach to the cell surfaces. The cells then absorb the peptide-covered toxin into the cytoplasm of the cell where it crosses to the cell membrane on the other side and passes out and into the next cell. This is an

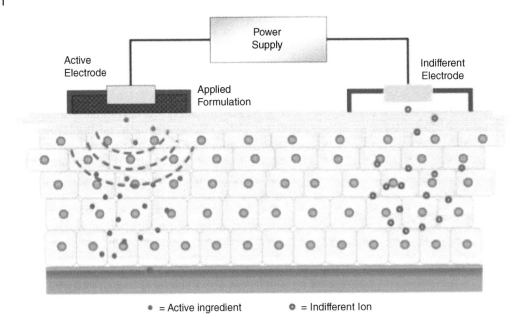

= Active ingredient   **= Indifferent Ion**

Figure 24.4 Iontophoresis uses an electric current to drive molecules below the active electrode into the skin, a process that is dependent on current and concentration. The method has been used for hyperhidrosis but is cumbersome at best. Reproduced with permission of Revance Therapeutics.

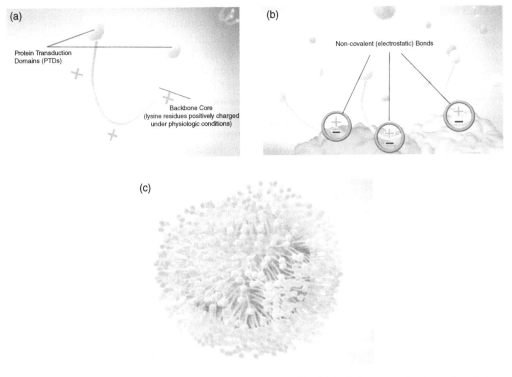

Figure 24.5 The TAT gene has a protein transduction domain (PTD) which binds noncovalently to the relatively negatively charged botulinum toxin. The toxin becomes surrounded by the peptides with the PTDs binding to cell surfaces and permitting active energy transport of the toxin into the cell, then out the cell and into the next cell. Reproduced with permission of Revance Therapeutics.

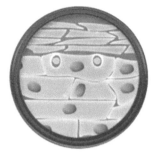 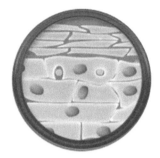 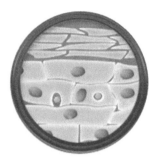

Figure 24.6 Now instead of depending on passive movement through the intracellular spaces, the peptide-covered toxin is actively transported through cells into the neighboring cell, repeating the process until the toxin exits the epidermis on the dermal side. Reproduced with permission of Revance Therapeutics.

active energy transport system and is not specific to botulinum toxin. It is a variant of induced macropinocytosis where the cell takes a "drink" of the surrounding media and conveys it out the other side without harming the cell or the cell membranes (Figure 24.6). The peptide can be joined to other types of molecules and may provide an alternative delivery system for other molecules and indications.

Once the complex has traversed the cell, it moves through the next cell, and the next, until it exits the epidermis on the dermal side. At this point the toxin is released from the carrier peptide and is free to exert its usual action on the SNAP-25 protein, producing the cholinergic blockade that is characteristic of BoNTA. This action appears identical to the action of the injected toxin in every way except, of course, that the total dose delivered varies depending on the concentration of the toxin, concentration of the peptide, and length of time it is in contact with the skin.

Investigational Studies

The digital abduction score as reported by Aoki uses the startle reflex of the mouse to demonstrate the amount of botulinum-induced muscle weakness in the hind limb that, in turn, inhibits the splay or spread of the mouse's toes when lifted by the tail.[13] In a normal startle reflex, the toes on the mouse's foot spread far apart in a rapid reflex. If the hind limb is injected with botulinum toxin, the movement is inhibited. In 2011, Waugh and associates demonstrated that limbs treated with a topical peptide–botulinum complex resulted in statistically significant reflex inhibition compared with the application of toxin alone, highlighting the role of cell-penetrating peptides in transcutaneous drug delivery (Figure 24.7) [12]. They also demonstrated that application of a topical peptide–botulinum complex produced a nearly complete reflex inhibition that was comparable to the effect seen with injected toxin. The first study to directly compare the application of topical toxin, without a carrier, to local intramuscular injection in human subjects for the treatment of LCLs was published by Mahmoud and associates in 2016 [14]. Topical application of 50 units of Dysport® to one side of the face and injection of 50 units of Dysport® to the contralateral side was given to 10 individuals. When evaluated in a dynamic state at 1 week and 1 month, the topical side showed no statistically significant difference in facial rhytides and the difference between the two treatment types was statistically significant showing improved LCLs on the injected side. This confirmed the assumption upon which several prior studies have relied: topical application of BoNTA solution on the surface of the skin is ineffective and, for a topical application to be effective, the molecule should either be formulated in a way to penetrate the skin or the stratum corneum barrier should bypassed.

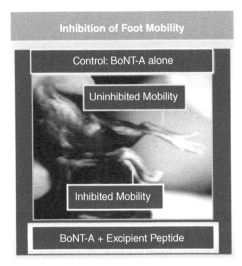
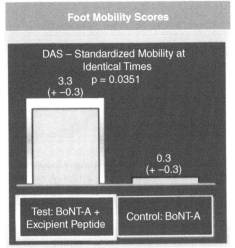

Figure 24.7 The combination of toxin plus peptide shows classic inhibition of muscular action of the mouse's hind foot, with inhibition significantly greater than that of topical botulinum toxin without the peptide. Reproduced with permission of Revance Therapeutics.

Several techniques have been developed to alter the stratum corneum barrier function, including the use of active energy sources (iontophoresis, electroporation, sonophoresis, and magnetophorsis) and stratum corneum abruption (microneedling, microdermabrasion, fractional CO_2 laser, tape-stripping, and suction) to facilitate transepidermal drug delivery [15]. Two of these techniques, ionotophoresis and fractional CO_2 laser, have been studied in association with topical BoNTA. Iontophoresis utilizes direct current of low amplitude to enhance drug transfer into the skin, but lacks targeting and delivery specificity and is very time dependent. With this technique, an active electrode is placed on the drug formulation that is to be driven into the skin by the electrons streaming from the active electrode. The ionic charge imparted to the target molecule allows the molecule to be driven into the skin as the indifferent ions are pulled from the skin by the indifferent electrode to complete the circuit (Figure 24.4). Iontophoresis has been reported to be successful with botulinum toxin [16, 17]. The disadvantages are that the technique is very

time and concentration dependent, requires that the patient can tolerate the sensation of the direct current, and is less effective with delivery of lipophilic molecules. In 2015, Mahmoud, Burnett, and Ozog demonstrated that the combination of CO_2 laser with concentrated topically applied BoNTA resulted in a statistically significant improvement in LCLs compared to CO_2 laser alone [18]. This result is plausibly the result of the fractional ablative laser removing the stratum corneum by creating microscopic columns in the epidermis and dermis, allowing the large molecules of BoNTA to reach the lower dermis and ultimately their target in the orbicularis oculi muscle. In 2016, these authors demonstrated that topical BoNTA without laser was ineffective for improving LCL. This is the only published clinical study on the inability of the large BoNTA molecule to cross an intact cutaneous surface. Another 2016 study by Zhu and colleagues demonstrated that topical application of BoNTA applied after fractional CO_2 laser could enhance the facial rejuvenation effect [19].

The first proof-of-concept study using a peptide–botulinum complex in humans

Minor Test: Patient L-RAC-RGG-022

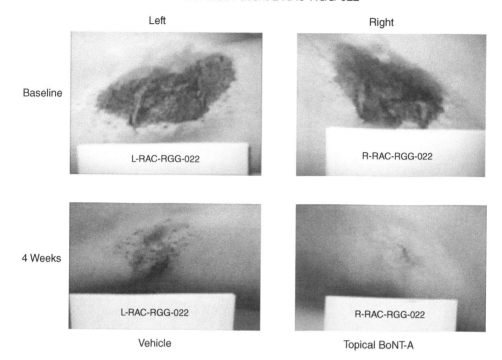

Figure 24.8 Toxin plus peptide topically demonstrated a qualitative inhibition of sweating as demonstrated by the Minor starch iodide test of axillary sweating compared to baseline. *Source:* Glogau 2007 [20]. Reproduced with permission of John Wiley & Sons.

with idiopathic axillary hyperhidrosis was reported by Glogau in 2007 in a randomized, blinded, vehicle-controlled study [20]. Application of the topical peptide–botulinum complex showed significant inhibition of sweating measured by the Minor starch-iodine test at 4 weeks after the initial application (Figure 24.8). Limitations of this pilot study included the aqueous vehicle, which was very unwieldy and difficult to keep in full skin contact for the required 30 minutes; day-to-day variability in sweating in both placebo and active patients, which made consistency in data capture difficult; and a recognized effect of the sweating inhibition produced by the topical toxin on one axillary vault producing a parallel drop in sweating on the non-treated side likely due to inhibition from higher cortical function. These factors limited the interpretation of magnitude of effect when comparing patient to patient.

Nevertheless, demonstration of the qualitative activity of the peptide–toxin moiety was firmly established.

Phase I studies examining sensitization and safety in 41 subjects in a single center with four repeat doses on the forearm showed minimal side effects [21]. This was followed by several phase II studies for treatment of LCLs with topical BoNTA, the first presented by Glogau in 2008 at the American Society for Dermatologic Surgery Annual meeting [22]. Enrolled subjects were aged 30–55 years with moderate to severe lateral canthal lines at maximal smile and no treatment in the head or neck with botulinum toxin in the preceding 9 months. There were 30 subjects in each of two participating centers that were randomly assigned to a range of doses in five cohorts. Three of five cohorts (concentrations of 11, 22, and 25 ng/mL) were considered treatment successes at 4 weeks

(a)

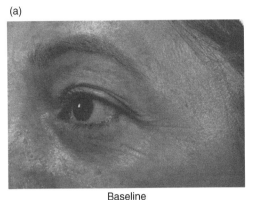

Baseline

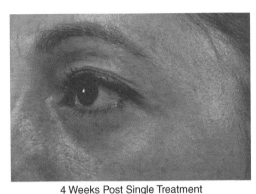

4 Weeks Post Single Treatment

Subject 014

Case 1L: Topically Delivered BoNT-A

(b)

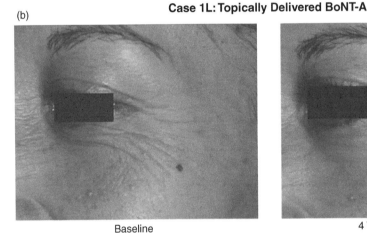

Baseline

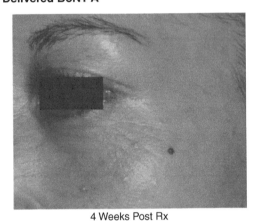

4 Weeks Post Rx

Single Topical Application of BoNT-A

Figure 24.9 Single application of toxin plus peptide demonstrated qualitative inhibition of muscular movement in the lateral canthal lines evaluated at smile and rest.

with no significant irritation or safety issues reported and a 1- or 2-point change in grade from the pretreatment assessment of the canthal lines (Figure 24.9). Patients in this study were evaluated at smile (primary endpoint) and at rest (secondary endpoint). Significant results from this study showed, in addition to the expected effects of increasing dose of toxin with peptide on the primary and secondary endpoints (Figure 24.10), that measurement of the canthal lines at rest was a more stable measurement endpoint with higher reliability and that all observed study side effects were nonsignificant and equally distributed between active and placebo groups (Figure 24.11). Of the subjects, 18% had mild to moderate treatment-related adverse events (AEs), with the most common AEs being application site erythema, burning sensation, and eye dryness. Notably, as efficacy increases were observed with escalating doses of RT001, there was no accompanying dose-dependent increase in AEs.

Brandt and associates reported another phase II double-blinded, placebo-controlled, repeat dosing study in 2010. Subjects underwent topical treatment at baseline and repeated again at 4 weeks. The primary

Overall Efficacy Results

• *Dose response seen with fixed peptide and escalating toxin*

% 1-Point Improvement at Smile 4 Weeks Post Treatment

% 2-Point Improvement at Rest 4 Weeks Post Treatment

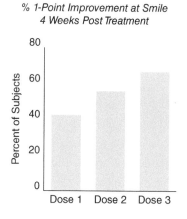
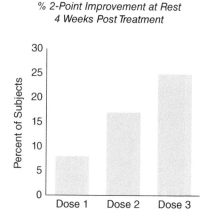

Figure 24.10 The toxin-peptide complex demonstrated an increasing effect with increasing doses, in some cases comparable to that seen with injected toxin.

endpoint was improvement in baseline LCL severity using the Investigator's Global Assessment of Lateral Canthal Lines (IGA-LCL) assesment [23, 24]. At 8 weeks, 50% of LCLs treated with RT001 showed a 2-point or greater improvement in baseline IGA-LCL severity compared to 0% of the placebo-treated subjects, and 94.7% of LCLs treated with RT001 showed a 1-point or more improvement compared to 14.7% of placebo-treated LCLs. There were no treatment-related adverse events. Clinical responses seen in this study were comparable to those seen in injectable BoNTA studies

At Rest

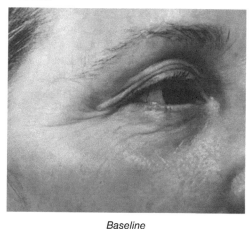
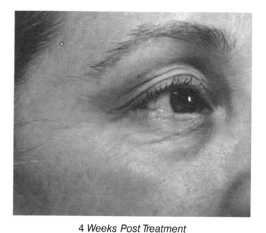

Baseline   *4 Weeks Post Treatment*

Subject 008–010; *Dose* 3

Figure 24.11 Measurement of canthal lines at rest was a more stable measurement endpoint with higher reliability.

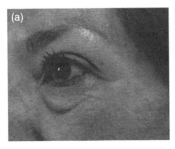 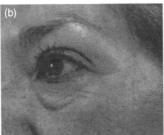 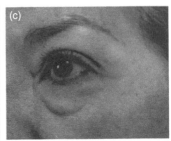

Figure 24.12 Representative subject photographs showing shorter and shallower LCLs. (a) Screening, (b) 4 weeks post first application of RT001, and (c) 8 weeks post first application of RT001 (4 weeks post second application of RT001). *Source:* Brandt 2010 [24]. Reproduced with permission of John Wiley & Sons.

[7, 25] as well as earlier phase 2 studies (Figure 24.12).

In 2012, Glogau and associates published results of another phase II, randomized, double-blinded, placebo-controlled study to evaluate the efficacy and safety of topical RT001 BoNTA for LCLs [26]. Of 90 patients who were enrolled, 45 underwent single treatment of RT001 to the lateral canthal area and 45 underwent placebo. The primary endpoint was a rigorous composite of 2-point or greater improvement on both the IGA-LCL and patient severity assessment (PSA) scales. At 4 weeks, 44.4% of subjects treated with RT001 achieved improvement as defined by the primary endpoint compared to 0% for the placebo group, and 88.9% of patients achieved clinically relevant improvement by investigator assessment alone. There were no clinically meaningful or significant differences in safety assessments between treatment and placebo group.

Future Directions

Given the success of topical botulinum toxin delivery demonstrated with iontophoresis and fractional CO_2 laser, further studies exploring active energy systems and temporary stratum corneum disruption to facilitate topical botulinum – and other drug – delivery to target areas should be considered. The ability to pair topical BoNTA application with elective cosmetic procedures such as laser treatments, microdermabrasion, and microneedling may be a desirable adjunct for patients wishing to avoid the adverse effects of BoNTA injection. These techniques are unlikely to supplant traditional injections given the additional cost and time, but may fill niche indications.

Now that previous trials have established stable outcome measures, established dose ranges, reproducible patient satisfaction, and optimized toxin/peptide gel formulations, further trials of transcutaneous delivery via botulinum–peptide complexes were completed. REALISE 1, a phase III clinical trial investigating the safety and efficacy study of the Revance topical RT001 gel in subjects with LCLs, were completed in 2016 but failed to achieve statistical significance on the primary endpoints. Revance has since moved their focus of clinical development to the use of the toxin-peptide complex in injected form. Early evidence suggests a longer duration of action than seen with other toxins. Allergan is also planning to pursue phase IIb studies evaluating the use of ANT-1207 to treat LCLs.

Transcutaneous topical botulinum toxin delivery may offer opportunities to treat anatomic sites that are difficult to manage with injection and patients who prefer to avoid injectables. There may also be useful roles for topical botulinum therapies as adjunctive or extender therapies for the injectable techniques currently in use. Clearly, molecules besides neurotoxin may be joined to the carrier peptide to deliver payloads to the dermis. Potential areas of therapy may include melasma, hyperpigmentation, acne, hirsutism, and vitiligo. The utility of topical botulinum toxin will likely extend the novelty of this peptide carrier drug delivery system to other areas, both in dermatology and general medicine.

References

1 Carruthers JD, Carruthers JA. Treatment of glabellar frown lines with C. botulinum-A exotoxin. J Dermatol Surg Oncol 1992; 18(1):17–21.

2 FDA. BOTOX Cosmetic Approval Letter. 2002. https://www.accessdata.fda.gov/ drugsatfda_docs/appletter/2002/ botuall041202L.htm.

3 FDA. FDA approves Botox Cosmetic to improve the appearance of crow's feet lines. September 2013; http://www.fda.gov/News Events/Newsroom/PressAnnouncements/ ucm367662.htm. Accessed 4 February 2017.

4 BOTOX® Cosmetic (onabotulinumtoxinA) for injection, for intramuscular use. Prescribing information. Irvine, CA: Allergan; 2016.

5 DYSPORT® for injection (abobotulinumtoxinA). Prescribing information. Slough, UK: Ipsen, Galderma, 2012.

6 XEOMIN® (incobotulinumtoxinA) for injection, for intramuscular use. Prescribing information. Germany: Merz Pharmaceuticals GmbH, 2014.

7 Lowe NJ, Lask G, Yamauchi P, Moore D. Bilateral, double-blind, randomized comparison of 3 doses of botulinum toxin type A and placebo in patients with crow's feet. J Am Acad Dermatol 2002;47(6): 834–840.

8 Lowe NJ, Ascher B, Heckmann M, *et al.* Double-blind, randomized, placebo-controlled, dose-response study of the safety and efficacy of botulinum toxin type A in subjects with crow's feet. Dermatol Surg 2005;31(3):257–262.

9 Coté TR, Mohan AK, Polder JA, *et al.* Botulinum toxin type A injections: adverse events reported to the US Food and Drug Administration in therapeutic and cosmetic cases. J Am Acad Dermatol 2005;53(3):407–415.

10 Frankel AD, Pabo CO. Cellular uptake of the tat protein from human immunodeficiency virus. Cell 1988;55(6): 1189–1193.

11 Green M, Loewenstein PM. Autonomous functional domains of chemically synthesized human immunodeficiency virus tat trans-activator protein. Cell 1988;55(6):1179–1188.

12 Waugh JM, Lee J, Dake MD, Browne D. Nonclinical and clinical experiences with CPP-based self-assembling peptide systems in topical drug development. Methods Mol Biol 2011;683:553–572.

13 Aoki KR. A comparison of the safety margins of botulinum neurotoxin serotypes A, B, and F in mice. Toxicon 2001;39(12): 1815–1820.

14 Mahmoud BH, Ozog D, Burnett C, Cohen JL. Prospective randomized split-face comparative study between topical botulinum toxin a surface application and local injection for crow's feet. Dermatol Surg 2016;42(4):554–556.

15 Parhi R, Suresh P, Patnaik S. Physical means of stratum corneum barrier manipulation to enhance transdermal drug delivery. Curr Drug Deliv 2015;12(2):122–138.

16 Kavanagh GM, Oh C, Shams K. BOTOX delivery by iontophoresis. Br J Dermatol 2004;151(5):1093–1095.

17 Solomon P. Delivery of Botox by iontophoresis. Br J Dermatol 2005;153(5): 1075; author reply 1076.

18 Mahmoud BH, Burnett C, Ozog D. Prospective randomized controlled study to

determine the effect of topical application of botulinum toxin A for crow's feet after treatment with ablative fractional CO2 laser. Dermatol Surg 2015;41(Suppl 1): S75–S81.

19 Zhu J, Ji X, Li M, *et al.* The efficacy and safety of fractional CO_2 laser combined with topical type A botulinum toxin for facial rejuvenation: A randomized controlled split-face study. Biomed Res Int 2016;2016:3853754.

20 Glogau RG. Topically applied botulinum toxin type A for the treatment of primary axillary hyperhidrosis: results of a randomized, blinded, vehicle-controlled study. Dermatol Surg 2007;33(1 Spec No.): S76–S80.

21 Jones T, Scott J, Tranowski D, T. J. Safety and tolerability of topical botulinum toxin type A in healthy adults. Poster presentation at the 69th Annual Meeting of the Society for Investigative Dermatology, Montreal, Canada, May 2009.

22 Glogau R. Topical delivery systems and botulinum toxins. Poster presentation at the American Society for Dermatologic Surgery Annual Meeting, Orlando, Florida, November 2008.

23 Kane MA, Blitzer A, Brandt FS, *et al.* Development and validation of a new clinically-meaningful rating scale for measuring lateral canthal line severity. Aesthet Surg J 2012;32(3):275–285.

24 Brandt F, O'Connell C, Cazzaniga A, Waugh JM. Efficacy and safety evaluation of a novel botulinum toxin topical gel for the treatment of moderate to severe lateral canthal lines. Dermatol Surg 2010; 36(Suppl 4):2111–2118.

25 Ascher B, Rzany BJ, Grover R. Efficacy and safety of botulinum toxin type A in the treatment of lateral crow's feet: double-blind, placebo-controlled, dose-ranging study. Dermatol Surg 2009;35(10):1478–1486.

26 Glogau R, Blitzer A, Brandt F, Kane M, Monheit GD, Waugh JM. Results of a randomized, double-blind, placebo-controlled study to evaluate the efficacy and safety of a botulinum toxin type A topical gel for the treatment of moderate-to-severe lateral canthal lines. J Drugs Dermatol 2012;11(1):38–45.

25

Exciting New Uses of Botulinum Toxin Type A:
Dermatology/Dermatologic Surgery and Beyond

Donna Bilu Martin, MD (FAAD)[1,2] and Stephen Mandy, MD (FAAD)[2,3]

[1]Dermatologist, Premier Dermatology, Aventura, USA
[2]Volunteer Professor of Dermatology and Cutaneous Surgery, Miller School of Medicine University of Miami, Miami, USA
[3]Premier Dermatology, South Beach Dermatology, Miami Beach, USA

Introduction

Botulinum toxin type A (BoNTA) is currently approved by the Food and Drug Administration (FDA) in the United States for the treatment of glabellar rhytides, strabismus, primary axillary hyperhidrosis, blepharospasm, hemifacial spasm, cervical dystonia in adults, and, most recently, chronic migraine, overactive bladder, upper/lower limb spasticity, and crow's feet [1–5]. Small studies and case reports in the literature have demonstrated positive results using BoNTA for the treatment of challenging painful and pruritic conditions, dyshidrotic eczema, inverse psoriasis, Hailey–Hailey and Darier's disease, facial flushing, ischemic digits, parotid duct injury, and more. (Table 25.1). The treatments described in this chapter are all off-label (not approved by the FDA). While many show promise for new approaches for often difficult to treat disorders, large, well-designed, controlled clinical studies are needed to establish safety and efficacy.

Pain

Pain is an unfortunate and often difficult to manage symptom in many conditions. BoNTA may reduce both nociceptive and neurogenic pain. The activation and sensitization of A- and C-nociceptors by neuropeptides released in tissue damage, infections, inflammation, and other stressors results in nociceptive pain [6]. BoNTA is theorized to block the local release of these neuropeptides, such as glutamate [7], substance P [8, 9], vasopressin [10], and calcitonin gene-related peptides (CGRPs) [7, 11] (Figure 25.1). BoNTA also appears to increase the heat pain threshold, likely by affecting transient receptor potential vanilloid receptor 1 (TRPV1-receptors) located on sensory nerve endings [10]. Capsaicin is a ligand for the VR1 receptor [12]. TRPV1-receptors are expressed on the plasma membrane via soluble N-ethylmaleimide-sensitive factor attachment protein receptor (SNARE) proteins, the complex that BoNTA cleaves [2, 10]. TRPV1 expression has also been shown to be increased in keratinocytes in patients with prurigo nodularis [13], and is likely involved in the sensation of both pain and pruritus. Low pH levels, as seen in contracting muscles and ischemic muscle pain, can also activate VR1 receptors [12].

BoNTA may also alleviate neurogenic pain. In a recent study, BoNTA injected in the foreheads of healthy males was found to target C-fibers [10]. Patients demonstrated reduced capsaicin-induced trigeminal pain,

Table 25.1 Conditions reported to improve with botulinum toxin type A.

Dynamic rhytides	Hailey-hailey disease	Dyshidrotic eczema
Blepharospasm	Darier's disease	Inverse psoriasis
Strabismus	Epidermolysis bullosa simplex, Weber-Cockayne type	Severe knee pain
Hemifacial spasm	Persistent facial flushing	Tennis elbow
Cervical dystonia	Migraine headache	Breast reconstruction
Post herpetic neuralgia	Back pain	Notalgia paresthetica
Multiple cutaneous piloleiomyomas	Wound healing	Granulosis rubra nasi
Primary axillary hyperhidrosis	Anal sphincter spasm	Eccrine hidrocystomas
Frey's syndrome	Compensatory hyperhidrosis	Raynaud's syndrome
Parotid duct injury (post surgery)	Drooling	Depression
Benign prostatic hyperplasia	Penile retraction	Lichen simplex chronicus
Pachydermoperiostosis pachydermia rhytides	Hypertrophic scars	Arthritic joint pain

sensitization, and inflammation. Post-herpetic neuralgia (PHN) is a complication that can occur following herpes zoster and may cause chronic pain (Figure 25.2). Three patients suffering from PHN for 2.5 months were injected with 100 U onabotulinumtoxinA (Botox®, Allergan, Inc., Irvine, CA). A dilution of 4 ml per 100 U was used [14]. The patients reported pain relief within 72 hours. The mean visual analogue scale (VAS) score decreased from a baseline of 8.3 to 2 in week 2, although by week 12 it had increased to 4. A larger randomized, double-blinded, placebo-controlled study

was then conducted with 30 patients. Of all patients in active treatment, 13 (87%) from the experimental arm achieved at least a 50% reduction in VAS pain score, compared with none of the placebo patients. Pain relief occurred as early as 1 week after BoNTA (BTX-A) administration, and it was maintained until the week 16 of the study. The therapeutic effect on pain was consistent with improvement on the secondary outcome of sleep disturbance by week 1, which was sustained throughout a 12-week period [15]. The inhibition of neuropeptides such as substance P and CGRP may reduce neurogenic

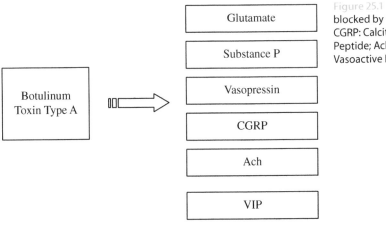

Figure 25.1 Neuropeptides likely blocked by botulinum toxin type A. CGRP: Calcitonin Gene Related Peptide; Ach: Acetylcholine; VIP: Vasoactive Intestinal Peptide.

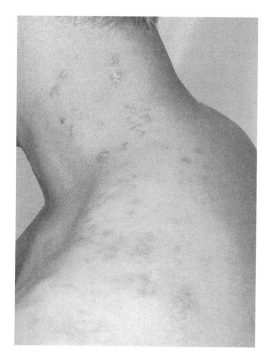

Figure 25.2 Herpes zoster, photo courtesy of Drs. Jason Emer and Gary Goldenberg.

inflammation and pain [16, 17]. Multiple painful cutaneous piloleimyomas in a patient were injected with 200 U of Botox®, resulting in a decrease in pain lasting for 3 months [18] (Figure 25.2).

Patients with painful disorders in areas of medicine outside of dermatology have been treated with BoNTA. Recent studies

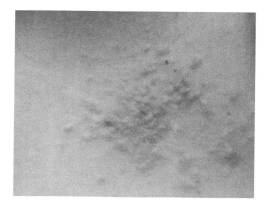

Figure 25.3 Piloleimyoma, photo courtesy of Dr. Michael Paltiel.

have shown promise for the treatment of arthritic joint pain. Synovial blood vessels and subsynovial nerve fibers are positive for substance P and CGRP [19]. In a study of 42 patients with moderate to severe knee pain, patients were randomized to receive 100 U of BoNTA plus lidocaine or placebo (saline) injections [19]. A statistically significant reduction in severe knee pain (48% at 1 month) was seen in the group treated with BoNTA.

Chronic lateral epicondylitis, or tennis elbow, is another painful condition. In a randomized, controlled study, 24 patients with the condition received an injection of BoNTA (60 U reconstituted in 1 ml normal saline) and 24 patients received a placebo saline injection at a point one-third the length of the forearm from the tip of the lateral epicondyle overlying the posterior interosseous nerve [20]. There was a statistically significant decrease in pain at rest in the group treated with BoNTA, but not during gripping. Adverse events included a decline in grip strength.

BoNTA has been used as a treatment for migraine headaches, low back pain, and headaches of musculoskeletal origin associated with strain and discomfort along the back, neck, and shoulders [2, 21]. The FDA has approved Botox® for the treatment of chronic migraines in adults (defined as headache for more than 14 days in a month) [5]. Multiple injections around the head and neck can be administered every 12 weeks to prevent future headache symptoms. In an open-label study, 18 patients with a history of imploding, exploding, and ocular type migraines received Botox® diluted with 5 ml of preserved 0.9% saline in the glabella, forehead, and periorbital areas for cosmetic purposes [22]. The mean dose injected was 45.7 T per treatment. Three months after the initial treatment, patients were interviewed to evaluate the response of their migraine symptoms. Of the patients, 13 with imploding or ocular headaches and 3 with exploding headaches reported a decrease in migraine frequency. Of note, 10 patients also received injections in sites of muscle tenderness (temporalis, occipitalis, cervical paraspinal, and trapezius muscles), although the authors stated that these additional injections did not seem to determine response. Vasoactive intestinal peptide (VIP) and substance P released from parasympathetic neurons may play a role in vasodilation and pain in migraine [21]. The exact mechanism of action of BoNTA is unclear, but it may act on the aforementioned neuropeptides, as well as CRGP [23].

Women who have undergone mastectomy for breast cancer may elect reconstruction with breast implants. The procedure often involves subpectoral tissue expansion, which can be very painful due to spasm and contraction of the pectoralis muscle [24]. Of patients undergoing mastectomy with tissue expander placement, 22 received infiltration of Botox® (100 U, diluted with 40–60 ml of normal saline) into the pectoralis major, serratus anterior, and rectus abdominis insertion [25]; 26 patients had standard mastectomy with tissue expander placement and no BoNTA. The group treated with BoNTA had significantly less pain and less narcotic use during their initial and final expansions. The authors observed a noted improvement following 1 day of BoNTA injection, due to an onset of action of 6–36 hours [25].

Pruritus

Many of the aforementioned neuropeptides released in pain also play a role in pruritus. Histamine activates C-fibers in the skin and causes the release of neuropeptides (substance P, VIP, neuropeptide Y, acetylcholine, bradykinin, serotonin, and prostaglandin E) that results in the further release of histamine from mast cells [26]. Substance P sensitizes mast cells, increases blood vessel permeability, and induces the synthesis of bradykinin and prostaglandins [12,27]. In a double-blind, placebo-controlled study in 14 male patients, 5 U of BoNTA (dilution of 2.5 ml unpreserved saline per 100 U/vial) was injected into the forearm, with the same volume of sterile saline injected

into the contralateral forearm as a control [28]. Histamine prick tests were performed at the treatment sites before treatment with BoNTA, on days 1, 3, and 7 after treatment. BoNTA reduced histamine-induced itch and vasomotor responses for 1 week after application. Such findings may have future applications and benefits for many pruritic and recalcitrant diseases seen in dermatology, such as lichen simplex chronicus (LSC) (Figure 25.4). In a small open pilot study, four patients with LSC were injected with 20–80 U (20 U per 2 × 2 cm²) of abobotulinumtoxinA (Dysport®; Ipsen Ltd, Slough, United Kingdom) in the affected area [29]. All patients reported alleviation of itching after 1 week according to a VAS, with three patients free of symptoms at 12 weeks. After 4 weeks, five of six lesions had cleared. The inhibition of acetylcholine release by BoNTA may play a role in the alleviation of itch in LSC.

In addition to itch in inflamed skin, BoNTA may improve noninflammatory pruritus. In a small study, four patients with notalgia paresthetica, one with meralgia paresthetica, and one with neuropathic itch on the foot were injected with 18–100 U of BoNTA (dilution of 3 ml unpreserved saline per 100 U/vial) for a mean dose of 1 U/cm² [30]. All but one patient had previously failed topical capsaicin treatment. Five of six patients had some improvement of pruritus 1-week posttreatment, but had a mean improvement of only 28% at the 6-week evaluation

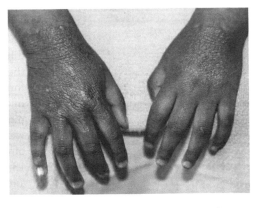

Figure 25.4 Lichen simplex chronicus (LSC), photo courtesy of Dr. Tor Shwayder.

(comparable to placebo). The one patient who had full improvement with BoNTA had not tried capsaicin previously. The authors postulated that as both capsaicin and BoNTA act through TRPV1, patients that fail capsaicin treatment may not respond to BoNTA for relief of pruritus.

A case report describes a 55-year-old woman with intractable pruritus on the right side of her forehead for 6 years [31]. She failed to respond to various treatments, including neurontin and novocaine injections. The uninflamed pruritic area was in close proximity to a surgical scar resulting from frontal sinus surgery 14 years earlier. The pruritic area was injected with 15 U of Botox® and – to maintain symmetry – 15 U were injected into the nonpruritic side. The patient reported a significant improvement in pruritus that lasted for 2 months.

Role of Hyperhidrosis in Dermatologic Conditions

BoNTA is approved to treat primary axillary hyperhidrosis. Hyperhidrosis has been shown to exacerbate several dermatologic conditions. There are several case reports and small studies in the literature reporting the benefit of BoNTA in the treatment of such disorders.

Dyshidrotic Eczema

Patients with dyshidrotic eczema present with recurrent or chronic pruritic, vesicular eruptions on the hands and feet. (Figure 25.5). Repeated exposure to moisture, heat, and occlusion may worsen the condition. Corticosteroids, immunosuppressive medications, and ultraviolet light are all possible treatment modalities. Hyperhidrosis often aggravates the condition. A small study of 10 patients with dyshidrotic eczema was conducted in which Botox® was injected intradermally to one palm and fingers with the untreated side as a control [32]. A dilution of 1.0 ml of unpreserved saline per 100 U of Botox® was

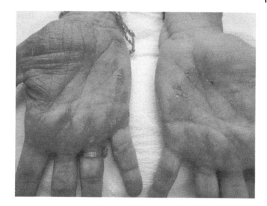

Figure 25.5 Dyshidrotic eczema.

prepared (10 w/0.1 ml); 2 U were injected intradermally every 15 mm, with a mean dose of 162 U injected. An improvement in their hand dermatitis within 5–6 weeks was experienced by 7 of 10 patients, including a decrease in pruritus, occurrence of vesicles, infiltration, erythema, and decrease in disease activity scores. Transient muscle weakness in the treated hand is a possible side effect.

In a study of eight patients with dyshidrotic eczema, patients were treated with either topical corticosteroids alone or corticosteroids plus 100 U of Botox® per palm [33]. The dilution of the toxin was not specified. Six of eight patients had significant improvement in hyperhidrosis, fewer episodes of eczema, and decreased pruritus in the hand treated with Botox®. In both studies, improvement was likely due to anhidrosis induced by the toxin through inhibition of acetylcholine release and the action on smooth muscle associated with sweat glands. Improvement in pruritus and pain were also likely due to inhibition of substance P. Botulinum toxin type A may be a useful addition to the current treatment options available for dyshidrotic eczema.

Inverse Psoriasis

Inverse psoriasis presents as erythematous, well-demarcated plaques in intertriginous areas (Figure 25.6). Botulinum toxin has been hypothesized to reduce local sweating in

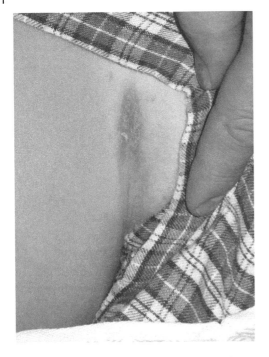

Figure 25.6 Inverse psoriasis, photo courtesy of Dr. Tor Shwayder.

the affected sites, thereby limiting irritation and possible infection, and well as having anti-inflammatory effects [34]. In a recent study, 15 patients received Botox® injections to the affected areas [35]; 87% of patients had improvement 12 weeks posttreatment. In addition to the reduction in sweat, improvement may have resulted from the blockage of the release of neuropeptides such as prostaglandins and nitric oxide that influence pain and itch [35, 36].

Granulosis Rubra Nasi

Children and young adults are more likely to have granulosis rubra nasi, a disorder of the eccrine glands of the nose and cheeks. Hyperhidrosis can occur first, followed by erythematous papules, pustules, and telangiectasias. The condition is difficult to treat. A 16-year-old male patient with granulosis rubra nasi was treated with 10 intradermal injections of 0.1 ml of Botox® to each side of his nose [37]. The dilution of the toxin was

not specified. His overall condition improved for 6 months, with hyperhidrosis recurring at 1 year.

Hailey–Hailey, Darier's Disease, Epidermolysis Bullosa Simplex

Hyperhidrosis is a known aggravating factor in autosomal dominant conditions such as Benign Familial Pemphigus (Hailey–Hailey disease), keratosis follicularis (Darier's Disease), and epidermolysis bullosa simplex (EBS)-Weber-Cockayne (WC) type [38–40]. A patient with Hailey–Hailey disease had Botox® 100 U (diluted with 5 ml of 0.9% sodium chloride) injected in the bilateral submammary areas. Her hyperhidrosis resolved within 3 days and lesions cleared within 2 weeks (Figure 25.7). No relapse was observed after 12 months [41]. A patient with Darier's disease was treated with 40 U of Botox® into each inguinal fold and 20 U into the anal fold [39] (Figure 25.8). She

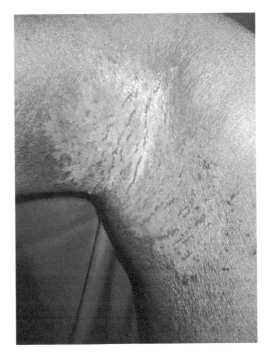

Figure 25.7 Hailey-Hailey, photo courtesy of Dr. Henry Lim.

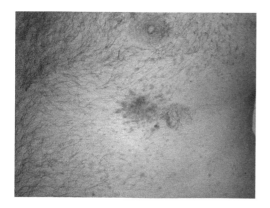

Figure 25.8 Darier's disease, photo courtesy of Dr. Tor Shwayder.

demonstrated improvement in both hyperhidrosis and Darier's for up to 2 months posttreatment. The dilution of the toxin was not specified. A patient with EBS-WC was treated with 100 U of Botox® to the right sole of the foot, with saline injected to the left sole as a control [40] (Figure 25.9). She experienced a therapeutic benefit 3 weeks after the treatment that persisted for 3 months.

Frey's Syndrome and Eccrine Hidrocystomas

Frey's syndrome, or gustatory sweating, is caused by inappropriately regenerated parasympathetic fibers of the auriculotemporal branch of the facial nerve, resulting in

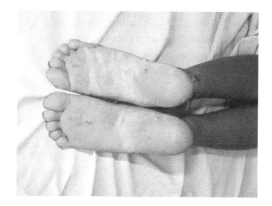

Figure 25.9 Epidermolysis bullosa simplex, photo courtesy of Dr. Tor Shwayder.

facial hyperhidrosis [2, 42]. It often results from parotid surgery, and as a rare complication of diabetes mellitus, where it can occur bilaterally. Intradermal injection of botulinum toxin over the parotid gland has been used to decrease sweat production, likely due to relaxation of the smooth muscle surrounding the glands [2,42]. Eccrine hidrocystomas are common cystic lesions that may be solitary or multiple. A patient with multiple periorbital eccrine hidrocystomas failed incision and drainage alone but had flattening of the lesions lasting for 4 months following concomitant Botox® injection (2 –3 U per cystic space) [43]. The successful results suggest that sweat production in eccrine hidrocystomas may be regulated by acetylcholine. Another study reported that BoNTA also reduces axillary odor in healthy patients [44].

Compensatory Hyperhidrosis

Sympathectomy is a permanent resolution for patients with palmar hyperhidrosis who fail conventional therapies; however, most of these patients often develop truncal compensatory hyperhidrosis, which is difficult to manage and irreversible. A retrospective analysis of 17 patients with severe truncal compensatory hyperhidrosis following sympathectomies was performed. Each patient received intradermal injections of Botox®, total dose 100–500 U. The vial of Botox® was diluted with 5 ml of 1% lidocaine (2 U/0.1 ml). Of 17 patients, 15 had resolution of hyperhidrosis within 5 days. The two remaining patients had improvement of hyperhidrosis. Resolution persisted for 2–8 months following treatment [45]. The side effects were minor and included skin irritation.

Persistent Facial Flushing

Facial flushing is a vasomotor condition commonly seen in Caucasians, causing erythema during exercise, anxiety, temperature changes, and strong emotion. A recent case report describes a patient treated with 10 U of Botox® (diluted with 5 ml of normal saline) resulting in a substantial improvement in his flushing after two weeks [3]. Small amounts of toxin placed subdermally are crucial to avoid facial paralysis. Although the mechanism of action of the treatment is currently unclear, BoNTA may improve the flushing through a reduction in local inflammatory mediators such as substance P, TRPV1, and CGRP [46]. In a larger case series, twenty-five subjects 35–70 years of age with skin types I–IV and facial erythema from erythematotelangiectatic rosacea were studied prospectively. Subjects received 15–45 U of intradermal injections of abobotulinumtoxinA to the nasal tip, nasal bridge, and nasal alae. Blinded observers reported statistically significant improvement in erythema grade at 1, 2, and 3 months after treatment when compared with baseline. Only 15 patients completed all visits and were included for data analysis. Larger, placebo controlled studies are necessary to confirm these interesting outcomes [47].

Raynaud's and Ischemic Digits

Raynaud's phenomenon is a circulatory disorder in which stress and cold exposure induces reversible intermittent constriction and ischemia of small digital arteries. Clinically, patients present with pain, fingertip ulceration, and livido reticularis. In a retrospective study of 19 patients with Raynaud's phenomenon, 50–100 U of Botox® (diluted with 20 ml of normal saline) was injected into the palm around neurovascular bundles at the level of the metacarpophalangeal joint [48]. Of 19 patients, 16 had resolution of their pain, with 12 patients pain free for 13–59 months. BoNTA has been shown to block the cholinergic autonomic innervation of smooth muscle (in addition to that of sweat glands, tear ducts, and salivary glands) [49]. Inhibition of neuromuscular smooth muscle cells by BoNTA may lead to vasodilation [50]. The authors postulated that reduction of pain-related neurotransmitters by BoNTA is likely play a role in clinical improvement. Three

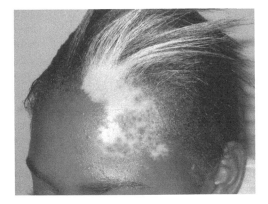

Figure 25.10 Vitiligo, photo courtesy of Dr. Tor Shwayder.

patients in the study experienced intrinsic muscle paralysis for 2 months.

Pigmentation Disorders

Vitiligo is an autoimmune disorder in which focal pigment loss is seen (Figure 25.10). Melanocytes express muscarinic acetylcholine (Ach) receptors on their membranes [51], and Ach is increased in the depigmentation of acute vitiligo [52]. A patient with periorbital vitiligo received BoNTA injections to treat rhytides in the glabella and crow's feet, and subsequently developed repigmentation in the vitiliginous area in the months after treatment [53]. To evaluate BoNTA as a possible treatment for vitiligo, 10 patients received Botox® injections (100 U vial diluted with 1 ml unpreserved saline) in one patch of vitiligo [53]. Another patch of vitiligo was left untreated as a control. None of the treated lesions showed evidence of repigmentation; however, the authors note that a longer follow-up duration for repigmentation or more BoNTA may be needed. More studies would need to be performed to prove the utility of BoNTA as an effective treatment for vitiligo.

Pachydermoperiostosis Pachydermia (PDP)

Patients with PDP, or primary hypertrophic osteoarthropathy, present with clubbing of the digits, periostosis, and pachydermia, or severe rhytides of the face [54]. The wrinkles are thought to be a result of thickening of the dermis, rather than repeated movement. Often cosmetic facial surgery treatment is the only option. In a small study, 3 patients with PDP were injected with BoNTA. A total of 70–80 U of BoNTA were injected in the procerus, corrugator muscles, tail of the eyebrow, and forehead (Neuronox, Medytox Inc, Kak-rl, Ochang-myeon, Cheongwongun, Korea). A dilution of 2.0 ml of preserved sterile saline was used, for a concentration of 5 o/0.1 ml. All patients demonstrated some degree of improvement of wrinkles that started 1-week posttreatment with some effect remaining 6 months posttreatment. The mechanism of action is unknown.

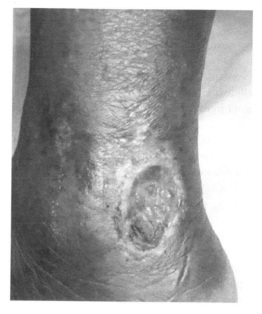

Figure 25.11 Ulceration.

Wound Healing and Hypertrophic Scars

Botulinum toxin administered 1-week preopererratively may improve wound healing and reduce scarring in areas such as the forehead, glabella, or upper lip by reducing tension and motion. BoNTA may inhibit myofibroblasts during primary and secondary intention healing, limiting contraction [46]. Similarly, temporary reduction of anal sphincter spasm with BoNTA allows anal fissures, or small cuts in anal skin, to heal [55]. A patient with paralysis secondary to a traumatic spinal cord injury developed recurrent muscular spasms and a chronic gluteal ulcer [56]. Dysport® was injected in the left gluteus maximus and the muscular area around the ulcer. The reduction in spasm and contraction allowed for easier wound care and facilitated healing of the ulcer. The authors state that BoNTA also improves blood microcirculation at the ulcer site. (Figure 25.11). In a recent study, five children less than 6 months old born with complete cleft lip and palate were injected with 10 U of BoNTA during surgical repair [57]; 3 U were injected in the orbicularis oris medially and 2 U in each lateral portion. The decrease in movement of the muscle decreased tension on the wound.

Hypertrophic scars can be difficult to treat and are often painful or pruritic. In a recent study, 19 patients with one hypertrophic scar for at least 2 years were treated monthly with intralesional BoNTA (Lanzou Biochemical Company, Lanzou City, P.R. China) for 3 months [58]. The dilution was adjusted to $2.5 \, U/cm^3$ and did not exceed 100 U per patient. Six months postinjection, all patients reported subjective improvement of their scar. A statistically significant reduction in erythema, itching sensation, and pliability was seen. While the exact mechanism of action is unknown, it may be similar to that seen in wound healing. BoNTA has been shown to affect the cell cycle distribution of fibroblasts seen in hypertrophic scars [59]. Additionally, fibroblasts isolated from hypertrophic scar tissue incubated with BoNTA (Lanzou Biochemical Company, Lanzou City, P.R. China) demonstrated slower growth than untreated fibroblasts as well as a decrease in transforming growth factor β1 (TGF-β1) protein expression [60].

Infiltrative skin cancers on the cheek may involve the parotid duct. Mohs micrographic surgery was utilized to treat a large squamous cell carcinoma on the cheek [61]. A parotid duct injury resulted in the formation of a sialocele 5 days after surgery; 23 U of Botox® (dilution of 50 U/ml) were injected directly into the parotid gland, with complete resolution of symptoms 2 weeks after injection that lasted 6 months. Salivary fistulas following parotidectomy may respond to botulinum toxin injections [62]. Similarly, sialorrhea (drooling) is seen in many neurological disorders. The resulting blockage of acetylcholine from the injection of BoNTA into the parotid, submaxillary, and salivary glands decreases the excess secretion of saliva [63]. Recently, 131 children with moderate to severe drooling from neurological disorders were treated with injections of BoNTA to the submandibular glands [64]. Clinical improvement in drooling was seen in 46.6% of children for a median of 22 weeks. Dysphagia and chewing difficulties are possible side effects of treatment.

Depression

Depression affects millions of Americans and is often treated with oral medications and psychotherapy. Such treatments can be costly and often have unwanted side effects. Recent studies have investigated the role BoNTA plays in emotion/mood. In one study, 20 healthy volunteers with no history of psychiatric or neurological disease received Dysport® (200 U/ml) injections in the corrugator supercilli muscles only [65]. Photos were taken of the volunteers contracting the remaining muscles of the face 1 week before and after treatment. Forty healthy volunteers (not injected) were shown the facial images and asked to rate the emotions on a five-point scale. Photos of faces treated with BoNTA were rated as expressing more happiness and less anger, fear, and sadness. The authors acknowledge that it

is unknown if the treated patients actually felt happier as well. However, the passive facial feedback hypothesis states that facial expression can affect mood, and therefore, it has been suggested that botulinum toxin may decrease negative emotions in those treated [66, 67]. Similarly, decreasing negative facial expressions and emotions may in turn stimulate positive emotional expressions, resulting in smiling and feeling positive emotions [67].

Exploring this concept further, 10 patients with moderate to severe depression (according to their self-reported Beck Depression Inventory II test scores; BDI-II and American Psychiatric Association's Diagnostic and Statistical Manual of Mental Disorders, fourth edition; DSM-IV) and no change to their medication or psychotherapy treatment during the prior 3 months, were injected with 29 U BoNTA into the procerus and corrugator supercilli muscles [68]. The patients were evaluated by a clinical psychologist 2 months posttreatment and given a repeat BDI-II test. All patients had improvement in mood, with, according to the authors, nine patients no longer meeting the clinical criteria for depression by their BDI-II test or DSM-IV scores. The tenth patient had bipolar disorder. Of note, this was not a controlled, randomized trial, and was not statistically significant, due to the small number of patients treated. Considering the high costs of treating depression in the United States, clinical trials to determine the utility and cost effectiveness of botulinum toxin in this disorder would be warranted [69].

Benign Prostatic Hyperplasia, resulting in enlargement of the prostate, is a common condition seen in older men. In a small study with no control group, 11 elderly males with BPE and no evidence of prostate cancer, received total of 200 U of Botox® (diluted with 8 ml of saline) under transrectal ultrasound guidance to two places in the prostate [70]. The mean prostate volume progressively decreased until month 6, with a return to baseline by month 18. BoNTA may induce prostate gland apoptosis in rats by blocking sympathetic innervation and decreasing adenergic stimulation to the gland [71].

Tinnitus

Tinnitus can result from multiple factors, such as infection, malignancy, medication, and repeated exposure to loud noises. In a patient with tinnitus due to stapedius myoclonus, gelfoam infused with BoNTA (25 U/ml, Lanzhou Institute of Biological Products, Lanzhou, China) was placed through a perforation in the left tempanic membrane close to the stapedius [72]; 2 days after treatment, the tinnitus resolved, and did not recur until 4 months posttreatment. At that time, the same treatment was performed, with resolution of the tinnitus again. The authors postulated that in patients with an intact tympanic membrane, the BoNTA could be administered by microinjection. The mechanism of action is unclear.

Atrial Fibrillation

Arrhythmias such as atrial fibrillation can occur after cardiac surgery, and are associated with patient morbidity [73]. Denervation may play a role in atrial fibrillation. In a small study, the right atrium-pulmonary vein and left atrium-inferior vena cava fat pads in six dogs were injected with BoNTA (50 U/ml) [74]. Atrial fibrillation was significantly reduced, and vagal stimulation effects on the sinus node were eliminated. Large, controlled, and long-term studies would need to be performed in humans to evaluate the efficacy and safety of botulinum toxin for short-term autonomic denervation of the atria.

Penile Retraction and Premature Ejaculation

Contraction of the bulbospongiosus and ischiocavernosus muscles contributes to the expulsion of semen during ejaculation [75]. Although no trials have been conducted, it has been hypothesized that the inhibition of the contraction of these muscles may play a role in the treatment of premature ejaculation [76]. A possible side effect could be anejaculation. Currently, there is a vast market for products and surgical procedures to correct penile retraction, or the appearance of a "short/small penis." Contraction of the dartos muscle results in retraction of the non-erect penis. In a recent study, the dartos muscle of 10 male patients with flaccid short penises (although average length when erect) was injected with 100 units of BoNTA [77]. Seven of ten patients had a subjective decrease in the frequency and amplitude of penis retraction, with an objective measurement of less retraction, and no side effects, for 6 months.

Linear Immunoglobulin A Bullous Dermatosis (LABD)

LABD is an immunobullous disease in which IgA auto-antibodies react to components of the hemidesmosome and basement membrane and cause a split in the dermo-epidermal junction. Clinically, bullae and blisters form, often in an annular or linear arrangement, although the eruption can be polymorphic in adults. It is the most common bullous disease in children. Recently, a single case report was published of a 17 year old female with LABD who developed a flare of blisters in the axillae bilaterally despite receiving treatment with dapsone [78]. 500 of BoNTA were injected in her left axillae only. Six weeks post treatment, only 1 lesion was seen in the left axillae, whereas the right axillae continued to develop lesions. The right axilla was subsequently treated as well, with a resulting decrease in blisters that persisted for 6 months, and then recurred. The authors postulated that the improvement from BoNTA was likely due to the decrease in sweating and inflammation in the axilla.

Summary

The uses of botulinum toxin type A have expanded since its FDA approval in 1989 to treat blepharospasm and strabismus [46]. Recent discoveries in the use of botulinum toxin for painful and pruritic conditions have applications in many fields of medicine. More applications are likely on the horizon. Currently, a phase 3 study is underway to investigate the safety and efficacy of Botox® in mild to moderate acne vulgaris [78]. A phase 1 study is investigating botulinum toxin for the treatment of seborrheic dermatitis in Parkinsonian patients [79]. Although large, controlled studies are needed for the treatments discussed in this chapter, the future looks promising.

References

1 Carruthers J, Carruthers A. The evolution of botulinum neurotoxin type A for cosmetic applications. Journal of Cosmetic and Laser Therapy 2007;9:186–192.

2 Zalvan C, Bentsianov B, Gonzalez-Yanes O, et al. Noncosmetic uses of botulinum toxin. Dermtol Clin 2004;22:187–195.

3 Yuraitis M, Jacob C. Botulinum Toxin for the Treatment of Facial Flushing. Dermatol Surg 2004;30:102–104.

4 Klein A. The Therapeutic Potential of Botulinum Toxin. Dermatol Surg 2004;30: 452–455.

5 FDA approves Botox to treat chronic migraine. www.fda.gov 2010.

6 Stucky C, Gold M, Zhang X. Mechanisms of pain. Proc Natl Acad Sci USA 2001; 98(21):11845–6.

7 Cui M, Khanijou S, Rubino J, et al. Subcutaneous administration of botulinum toxin A reduces formalin-induced pain. Pain 2004;107:125–133.

8 Prukiss J, Welch M, Droward S, et al. Capsaicin stimulates release of substance P from dorsal root ganglion neurons via two distinct mechanisms. Biochem Soc Trans 1997;25:542S.

9 Iskawa H, Mitsui Y, Yoshitomi T, et al. Presynaptic effects of botulinum toxin type A on the neuronally evoked response of albino and pigmented rabbit iris sphincter and dilator muscles. Jpn J Ophthalmol 2000;44:106–9.

10 Gazerani P, Pedersen N, Staahl C, et al. Subcutaneous Botulinum toxin type A reduces capsaicin-induced trigeminal pain and vasomotor reactions in human skin. Pain 2008;epub ahead of print.

11 Sala C, Andresose J, Fumagalli G, et al. Calcitonin gene-related peptide: possible role in formation and maintenance of neuromuscular junctions. J Neuroscience 1995;15:520–8.

12 Mense S. Neurobiological basis for the use of botulinum toxin in pain therapy. J Neurol 2004;251(Suppl 1):1/1–1/7.

13 Steinhoff M, Bienstock J, Schmelz M, et al. Neurophysiological, neuroimmunodermatological, and neuroendocrine basis of pruritis. J Invest Dermatol 2006;126:1705–18.

14 Sotiriou E, Apalla Z, Panagiotidou D, et al. Severe post-herpetic neuralgia sucessfully treated with botulinum toxin A: three case reports. Acta Derm Venerol 2009;89(2): 214–5.

15 Apalla Z, Sotiriou E, Lallas A, Lazaridou E, Ioannides D. Botulinum toxin A in postherpetic neuralgia: a parallel, randomized, double-blind, single-dose, placebo-controlled trial. The Clinical journal of pain 2013;29:857–64.

16 Purkiss J, Welch M, Doward S, et al. Capsaicin-stimulated release of substance P from cultured dorsal root ganglion neurons: involvement of two distinct mechanisms. Biochem Pharmacol 2000; 59(11):1403–6.

17 Meng J, Wang J, Lawrence G, et al. Synaptobrevin I mediates exocytosis of CGRP from sensory neurons and inhibition by botulinum toxins reflects their anti-nociceptive potential. J Cell Sci 2007; 120(Pt 16):2864–74.

18 Sifaki M, Krueger-Krasagakis S, Koutsopoulos A, et al. Botulinum Toxin

Type A—Treatment of a Patient with Multiple Cutaneous Piloleiomyomas. Dermatology 2008;218(1): 44–47.

19 Mahowald M, Krug H, Singh J, et al. Intra-articular Botulinum Toxin Type A: A new approach to treat arthritis joint pain. Toxicon 2009;54(5):658–67.

20 Espandar R, Heidari P, Rasouli M. Use of anatomic measurement to guide injection of botulinum toxin for the management of chronic lateral epicondylitis: a randomized controlled trial. CMAJ 2010;182(8): 768–73.

21 W, Brin M, Blitzer A, et al. Botulinum toxin type A (BOTOX) for treatment of migraine. Dis Mon 2002;48:323–35.

22 Kim C, Bogart M, Wee S. Predicting Migrain Responsiveness to Botulinum Toxin Type A Injections. Arch Dermatol 2010;146(2):159–163.

23 Durham P, Cady R, Cady R. Regulation of calcitonin gene-related peptide secretion from trigeminal nerve cells by botulinum toxin type A: implications for migraine therapy. Headache 2004;44(1):35–43.

24 Senior M. Botox and the management of pectoral spasm after subpectoral implant insertion. Plast Reconstr Surg 2000;106: 224.

25 Layeeque R, Hochberg J, Siegel E, et al. Botulinum Toxin Infiltration for Pain Control After Mastectomy and Expander Reconstruction. Annals of Surgery 2004; 240(4):608–614.

26 Wallengren J. Neuroanatomy and neurophysiology of itch. Dermatol Ther 2005;18:292–303.

27 Yosipovitch G, Greaves M, Schmelz M. Itch. Lancet 2003;361:690–694.

28 Gazerani P, Pedersen N, Drewes A. Botulinum toxin type A reduces histamine-induced itch and vasomotor responses in human skin. Br J Dermatol 2009(May).

29 Heckmann M, Heyer G, Brunner B, et al. Botulinum toxin type A injection in the treatment of lichen simplex: An open pilot study. J Am Acad Dermatol 2002;46:617–9.

30 Wallengren J, Bartosik J. Botulinum toxin type A for neuropathic itch. Br J Dermatol 2010;163:424–437.

31 Salardini A, Richardson D, Jabbari B. Relief of Intractable Pruritus After Administration of Botulinum Toxin A (Botox): A Case Report. Clin Neuropharmacol 2008;31:303–306.

32 Swartling C, Naver H, Lindberg M, et al. Treatment of dyshidrotic hand dermatitis with intradermal botulinum toxin. J Am Acad Dermatol 2002;47:667–71.

33 Wollina U, Karamfilov T. Adjuvant botulinum toxin A in dyshidrotic hand eczema: a controlled, prospective pilot study with left-right hand comparison. J Eur Acad Dermatol Venereol 2002;16: 40–2.

34 Eedy D, Johnston C, Shaw C, et al. Neuropeptides in psoriasis: an immunocytochemical and radioimmunoassay study. J Invest Dermatol 1991;96:434–438.

35 Zanchi M, Favot F, Bizzarini M, et al. Botulinum toxin type-A for the treatment of inverse psoriasis. European Acad Dermatol and Venereol 2007;22:431–436.

36 Bonifati C, Carducci M, Mussi A, et al. IL-1 alpha, IL-1 beta and psoriasis: conflicting results in the literature. Opposite behaviour of the two cytokines in lesional or no-lesional extracts of whole skin. J Biol Regul Homeost Agents 1997;11:133–136.

37 Grazziotin T, Buffin R, Manzoni A, et al. Treatment of Granulosis Rubra Nasi with Botulinum Toxin Type A. Dermatol Surg 2009;35:1298–1299.

38 Burge S. Hailey-Hailey disease: the clininical features, response to treatment and prognosis. British Journal of Dermatology 1992;126:275–82.

39 Santiago-Et-Sanchez-Mateos J, Bea S, Fernandez M, et al. Botulinum Toxin Type A for the Preventative Treatment of Intertrigo in a Patient with Darier's Disease and Inguinal Hyperhidrosis. Dermatol Surg 2008;34:1733–1737.

40 Abitbol R, Zhou L. Treatment of Epidermolysis Bullosa Simplex,

Weber-Cockayne Type, With Botulinum Toxin Type A. Arch Dermatol 2009;145(1): 13–15.

41 Konrad H, Karamfilov T, Wollina U. Intracutaneous botulinum toxin A versus ablative therapy of Hailey-Hailey disease- a case report. J Cosmetic & Laser Ther 2001; 3:181–184.

42 Arad-Cohen A, Blitzer A. Botulinum toxin treatment for symptomatic Frey's syndrome. Otolaryngology-Head Neck Surg 2000;122:237–40.

43 Woolery-Lloyd H, Rajpara V, Nijhawan R. Treatment for Multiple Periorbital Eccrine Hidrocystomas: Botulinum Toxin A. J Drugs Dermatol 2009;8(1):71–73.

44 Heckmann M, Kutt S, Dittmar S, et al. Making scents: Improvement of olfactory profile after botulinum toxin-A treatment in healthy individuals. Dermatol Surg 2007;33:S81–7.

45 Kim W, Kil H, Yoon K. Botulinum Toxin: A Treatment for Compensatory Hyperhidrosis in the Trunk. Dermatol Surg 2009;35(5):833–838.

46 Bansal C, Omlin K, Hayes C, et al. Novel cutaneous uses for botulinum toxin type A. J of Cosmetic Dermatology 2006;5: 278–272.

47 Bloom BS, Payongayong L, Mourin A, Goldberg DJ. Impact of intradermal abobotulinumtoxinA on facial erythema of rosacea. Dermatologic surgery : official publication for American Society for Dermatologic Surgery [et al] 2015;41 Suppl 1:S9–16

48 Neumeister M, Chambers C, Heron M, et al. Botox Therapy for Ischemic Digits. Plast Reconstr Surg 2009;124(1):191–201.

49 Emer J, Waldorf H. Neurotoxin Update and Review, Part 1: The Science. Cosmetic Dermatology 2010;23(9):413–418.

50 Van Beek A, Lim P, Gear A, et al. Management of vasospastic disorders with botulinum toxin. Plast Reconstr Surg 2007;119:217–226.

51 Buchli R, Ndoye A, Arredondo J. Identification and characterization of muscarinic acetylcholine receptor subtypes expressed in human skin melanocytes. Molec Cell Biochem 2001;228(1–2):57–72.

52 Schallreuter K, Elwary S, Gibbons N, et al. Activation/deactivation of acetylcholinesterase by H202: More evidence for oxidative stress in vitiligo. Biochem Biophys Res Commun 2004; 315(502–508).

53 BinSaif G, Al Samary A, Al Mohizea S. Failure of Botulinum Toxin Treatment for Localized Vitligo. J Drugs Dermatol 2010; 9(9):1092–1094.

54 Ghosn S, Uthman I, Dahdah M, et al. Treatment of pachydermoperiostosis pachydermia with botulinum toxin type A. J Am Acad Dermatol 2010.

55 Madalinski M, Chodorowski Z. Why the most potent toxin may heal anal fissure. Adv Ther 2006;23(4):627–34.

56 Intiso D, Basciani M. Botulinum Toxin Type A in the healing of a chronic buttock ulcer in a patient with spastic paraplegia after spinal cord injury. J Rehabil Med 2009;41:1100–1102.

57 Galarraga I. Use of botulinum toxin in cheiloplasty: A new method to decrease tension. Can J Plast Surg 2009;17(3):e1–2.

58 Xiao Z, Zhang F, Cui Z. Treatment of Hypertrophic Scars with Intralesional Botulinum Toxin Type A Injections: A preliminary Report. Aesth Plast Surg 2009;33:409–412.

59 Xiao Z, Zhang M. Botulinum toxin type A affects cell cycle distribution of fibroblasts derived from hypertrophic scar. Plast Reconstr Surg 2008;61:1128–1129.2.

60 Xiao Z, Zhang F, Lin W, et al. Effect of Botulinum Toxin Type A of Transforming Growth Factor B1 in Fibroblasts Derived from Hypertrophic Scar: A Preliminary Report. Aesth Plast Surg 2010;34:424–427.

61 Krishnan R, Clark D, Donnelly H. The Use of Botulinum Toxin in the Treatment of a Parotid Duct Injury During Mohs Surgery and Review of Management Options. Dermatol Surg 2009;35:941–947.

62 Ting-Yeung L, Tam-Lin C, Pro-Yin K. Management of salivary fistula with botulinum toxin Type A. Annals of the

College of Surgeons of Hong Kong 2001;5(4):156–157.

63 Bhogal P, Hutton A, Monaghan A. Review of the current uses of Botox for dentally-related procedures. Dental Update 2006;33(3):165–168.

64 Scheffer A, Erasmus C, Van Hulst K, et al. Efficacy and Duration of Botulinum Toxin Treatment for Drooling in 131 Children. Arch Otolaryngol Head Neck Surg 2010;136(9):873–877.

65 Heckmann M, Teichmann B, Schroder U. Pharmacologic denervation of frown muscles enhances baseline expression of happiness and decreases baseline expression of anger, sadness, and fear. J Am Acad Dermatol 2003;49:213–6.

66 Mori K, Mori H. Another test of the passive facial feedback hypothesis: when your face smiles, you feel happy. Percept Mot Skills 2009;109(1):76–8.

67 Alam M, Barrett K, Hodapp R, et al. Botulinum Toxin and the facial feedback hypothesis: Can looking better make you feel happier? J Am Acad Dermatol 2007; 58:1061–72.

68 Finzi E, Wasserman E. Treatment of Depression with Botulinum Toxin A: A Case Series. Dermatol Surg 2006;32: 645–650.

69 Beer K. Cost Effectiveness of Botulinum Toxin for the Treatment of Depression: Preliminary Observations. J Drugs Dermatol 2010;9(1):27–30.

70 Silva J, Pinto R, Carvalho T, et al. Intraprostatic Botulinum Toxin Type A injection in patients with benign prostatic enlargement: duration of the effect of a single treatment. BMC Urology 2009;9(9).

71 Silva J, Pinto R, Carvalho T, et al. Mechanisms of Prostate Atrophy after Glandular Botulinum Neurotoxin Type A Injections: An Experimental Study in the Rat. Eur Urol 2009;56:134–141.

72 Liu H, Fan J, Zhao S, et al. Botox transient treatment of tinnitus due to stapedius myoclonus: Case report. Clin Neurol Neurosurg 2010;epub ahead of print.

73 Nair S. Atrial fibrillation after cardiac surgery. Ann Card Anaesth 2010;13(3): 196–205.

74 Seil O, Choi E-K, Choi Y-S. Short-Term Autonomic Denervation of the Atria Using Botulinum Toxin. Korean Circ J 2010;40: 387–390.

75 McKenna C, Chung S, McVary K. A model for the study of sexual function in anesthetized male and female rats. Am J Physiol 1991;261:R1276–85.

76 Serefoglu E, Silay M. Botulinum Toxin- An injection may be beneficial in the treatment of life-long premature ejaculation. Medical Hypotheses 2009;74(1):83–4.

77 Shaeer O, Shaeer K, Shaeer A. Botulinum Toxin (Botox) for Relieving Penis Retraction. J Sex Med 2009.

78 Legendre L, Maza A, Almalki A, et al. Botulinum Toxin A: An Effective Treatment for Linear Immunoglobulin A Bullous Dermatosis Located in the Axillae. Acta Derm Venereol 2016; 96: 122–123.

79 Clinical Trial Review. J Drugs Dermatol 2009;8(2):195–197.

26

Modulating Affect and Mood with Botulinum Toxin Injections: Psychosocial Implications of Neuromodulators

James L. Griffith, MD (MSci),[1] Kevin C. Smith, MD (FRCPC (DERM)),[2] and Murad Alam, MD (MSCI, MBA)[3]

[1]Dermatology Resident, Department of Dermatology, Henry Ford Hospital, Detroit, USA
[2]Private Practice Dermatologist, Niagara Falls, Ontario, Canada
[3]Professor and Vice-Chair, Department of Dermatology, Section of Cutaneous and Aesthetic Surgery, Departments of Dermatology, Otolaryngology, and Surgery, Northwestern University, Chicago, USA

Introduction

"Can there be emotion without facial expression?"

Paul Ekman [1]

While the answer is yes, this seemingly simple question highlights the importance of facial expression in conveying emotion, and poses a subtler, second question: Does facial expression influence our emotional experience?

A growing body of observational, experimental, and radiologic evidence indicates that muscles of facial expression not only *are* influenced by an individual's emotional state, but also *have* an influence on one's emotional experience and his/her interpretation of another's emotions, experience and intentions. Interestingly, this influence does not appear to correspond with aesthetic-induced improvements, which by itself, could impart a positive emotional state through improved personal and social feedback. Thus, manipulating muscles of facial expression (MFE) may alter the neuronal firing at emotional epicenters of the cortex affecting an individual's emotional context (affect, mood, and interpretation of social interactions), and in turn, open up new therapeutic avenues to normalize dysregulated cerebral activity in those with psychiatric disease.

To evaluate the accuracy of this assertion, this chapter will first briefly discuss the displays of facial emotion and the relevant aesthetic targets on the upper face for botulinum toxin (BoNTA) injection before examining its recent clinical trials in major depressive disorder and the evidence for/against relevant psychologic theories that postulate a dynamic two-way relationship between one's MFE and emotional context. Lastly, the future direction of investigations on botulinum's use in neuropsychiatric disease and potential prognostic factors for identifying both good and poor responders to BoNTA therapy will be discussed.

For the purposes of this discussion, facial expressions of fear, anger, sadness, disgust, and contempt will be considered "negative" emotions, and happiness (laughing, smiling, and joy) will be considered "positive"; surprise will be considered "neutral."

Botulinum Toxins: Cosmetic and Clinical Applications, First Edition. Edited by Joel L. Cohen and David M. Ozog.
© 2017 John Wiley & Sons Ltd. Published 2017 by John Wiley & Sons Ltd.
Companion Website: www.wiley.com/go/cohen/botulinum

Indicators of Facial Emotion and their Aesthetic Targets for Neuromodulation

There are six, very clear facial indications of emotion — anger, sadness, fear, surprise, disgust, contempt and happiness (Figure 26.1) [2]. Often, each expressions requires multiple muscles to be recruited. In so doing, each facial muscle is involved (to varying degrees) in a range of facial expressions – positive, negative, and neutral (Figure 26.2). For example, anger is expressed through eight muscles of facial expression (Figure 26.3). However, anger is primarily conveyed through corrugator muscle activity, which also can express the neutral and positive emotions of surprise and happiness (when laughing), respectively.

Still, systematic investigations have demonstrated a strong association between negative emotions and activation of the corrugator, procerus, and frontalis muscles [3–6] while positive emotions primarily correlate with orbicularis oculi activity [7, 8].

Although the primary aesthetic targets for BoNTA injection on the upper face include the glabellar rhytides (corrugator supercilii and procerus), horizontal forehead lines (frontalis), and crow's feet (orbicularis oculi), it is important to remember that the effects of treatment cannot be limited to a single muscle as:

1. Mechanical approaches, such as holding a pen between the teeth [9] or lifting the cheeks with tape [10] to simulate a smile, will inevitably affect a variety of target and

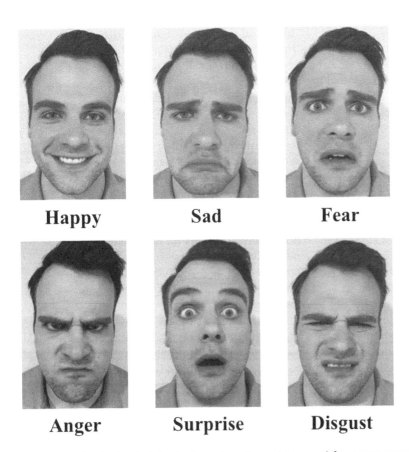

Happy   **Sad**   **Fear**

Anger   **Surprise**   **Disgust**

Figure 26.1 The six clear facial indications of emotion — happy, sad, fear, anger, surprise, and disgust.

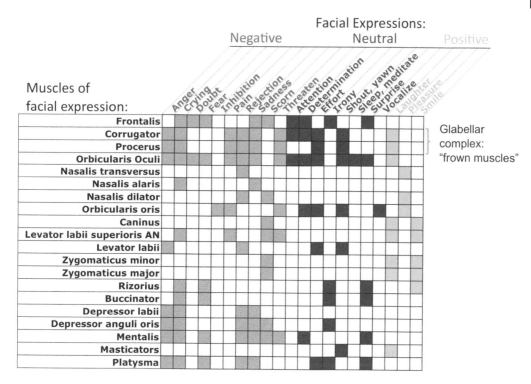

Figure 26.2 Muscles of facial expression and the expressions they participate in. *Source:* Victoria Contreras. Reproduced with permission of ARTNATOMYA.

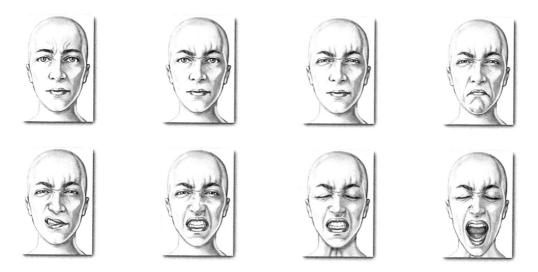

Figure 26.3 The muscles of facial expression that play roles in the facial expression of a single emotion: anger. *Source:* Alam 2008 [25]. Reproduced with permission of Elsevier.

nontarget muscles and other structures. Likewise, surgical ablation of the glabellar complex or the motor nerves controlling the glabellar complex will inevitably affect nontarget tissues to some extent.

2. Relaxation of muscles for facial expression via BoNTA will always cause some degree of relaxation in adjacent muscles due to diffusion of BoNTA from the injection site to nontarget tissues (e.g., injecting the glabellar complex will also effect the frontalis muscle and/or various components of the orbicularis oculi to a lesser extent).

3. Attenuation of a muscle's action by surgical or pharmacologic means inevitably induces some degree of compensable recruitment of nearby muscles to contract. For example, relaxation of the glabellar complex is sometimes associated with recruitment of the nasalis and levator labii alaeque nasi, causing the formation of "bunny lines" on the proximal bridge of the nose.

Therefore, when making observations and designing experiments to affect the perception or expression of emotional states through mechanical, surgical, or neurochemical modulation, it is important to consider the broad spectrum of primary and secondary effects such interventions may incur; these, at least in theory, may affect facial feedback and the underlying neural systems.

Botulinum Toxin in Major Depressive Disorder

Despite the broad range of behavioral, surgical, electrical, and pharmacological treatments, major depressive disorder (MDD) is a debilitating condition with no universally effective intervention. In fact, up to one-third of patients on pharmacologic therapy fail to achieve remission despite multiple antidepressant trials [11]. Therefore, clinicians and researchers continue to seek new and effective treatment options for this condition.

BoNTA has recently been investigated by three similarly designed, randomized, double-blind, placebo-controlled trials and their pooled analysis to determine if BoNTA injection into the glabella has a role in the treatment of MDD [12–16]. In total, 134 subjects, who were diagnosed with stable, mild-to-severe MDD by study psychiatrists or clinical psychologists and had no recent changes to psychiatric medication(s) for the past 28 or 60 days (depending upon the study), were randomized into either placebo or BoNTA treatment groups. All BoNTA cohorts received 29 U injected into the procerus (7 U), medial corrugators (6 U), and lateral corrugators (5 U) if female and 39 U (2 U more per site) if male; Finzi *et al.* administered 40 U total per male subject [14]. An equivalent volume of 0.9% NaCl was injected into the same MFE of those enrolled in the placebo treatment arm. Response to therapy was assessed at baseline and 6 weeks after BoNTA injection using the Beck Depression Index (BDI) and Clinical Severity Score of Glabellar Frown Lines (CSS-GFL) for all studies. Additional depression scoring systems and total study duration (6, 16, and 24 weeks) varied by trial. Other notable differences between these trials included whether moderate-severe baseline frown lines upon maximum effort and active antidepressant medication were required for enrollment. The 24-week trial also included a double-crossover at 12 weeks with similar outcomes to those from the first 12 weeks. All trials attempted to maintain psychologic evaluator blinding with two of the studies covering the glabella and forehead with a cap during psychiatric assessments, and the third not informing psychiatric evaluators on the effects of the study drug. To assess whether potential unblinding may have influenced the outcomes between the two treatment arms (placebo or active treatment), subjects and psychiatric evaluators guessed which treatment arm the subject was assigned at the conclusion of two of these studies. No association was found between correctly identifying the treatment arm and improvement/worsening of depression scores.

In each study and overall, a statistically significant reduction in depression scores was noted at 6 weeks. Approximately one-third of patients in each study achieved remission (BDI $\leq$ 9, Montgomery–Asberg Depression Rating Scale $\leq$ 10, and 17-item version of the Hamilton Depression Rating Scale $\leq$ 7). Their pooled response and remission rates correlated with outcomes of citalopram from the STAR*D trial, which was one of the largest antidepressant trials [15]. No statistically significant differences were noted between response and remission rates of citalopram versus BoNTA. Improved BDI scores were not associated with visual changes in glabellar frown lines by pooled analysis. Additionally, baseline frown lines poorly predicted baseline depression severity or subject response to BoNTA treatment. Interestingly, the long-term, 24-week trial also noted continued improvement in depression scores even after dissipation of BoNTA's paralytic effects. Improved BDI scores were even reported in an individual that disliked the cosmetic effect from BoNTA injection and those without baseline frown lines. As most subjects were female, extrapolations without firm conclusions can be ascertained for male subjects. Given the results of these three studies and their pooled analysis, BoNTA appears to induce a remission or reduction in depression severity by factors beyond aesthetic, patient–provider interaction, or placebo effects.

Following these trials, a Phase 2 proof-of-concept clinical trial assessing Allergan's onabotulinum toxin A in adult females with major depressive disorder was launched. The trial concluded in 2017 revealing a trend towards treatment benefit, but failing to reach its primary endpoint of a statistically significant improvement in depression scores at 6 weeks ($p = 0.053$) compared to placebo. However, statistically significant outcomes were achieved at week 3 ($p = 0.005$) and week 9 ($p = 0.049$). The company plans to proceed with Phase 3 trial development [17].

Proposed Neuropsychiatric Mechanisms of Botulinum Toxin

Hyperactivity of the left amygdala has been linked to anxiety, depression, post-traumatic stress disorder and a heightened fear response. Normalization of this hyperactivity appears to be one of the potential effects of BoNTA injected into the glabella. Functional magnetic resonance imaging (fMRI), which provides an indirect assessment of neuronal activity by identifying changes in cerebral blood, has demonstrated reduced activity in the left amygdala following glabellar injection when imitating angry, but not sad facial expressions, compared to untreated controls [18]. A similar reduction in activity of the left amygdala has been shown following initiation of antidepressant medications. Interestingly, improvements in depression scores have been demonstrated following BoNTA injection of the glabella (MFE of negative emotion – frown), while worsening of depression scores occurred following injection of the crow's feet (MFE of positive emotion – smiling) [19]. However, the exact mechanism(s) by which BoNTA imparts this and other neuropsychiatric effects remains of great debate.

The prevailing proposed mechanisms for this effect include (a) proprioceptive feedback from muscles of facial expression, (b) societal positive/negative feedback via mirror neuron activity and (c) aesthetic preferences, (d) BoNTA migration to the emotional epicenters of the brain, and (e) improved feelings about oneself due to aesthetic and placebo effects, or the interaction of a friendly, sympathetic, nonthreatening, and nonjudgmental professional administering BoNTA. As previously noted, the findings from the randomized, double-blind, placebo-controlled trials reduce the likelihood that (c, e) visual/aesthetic-based (societal or personal), placebo, or patient–provider interaction confounders are the primary mechanism behind BoNTA's neuropsychiatric effects. Therefore, this section will focus on the evidence regarding proprioceptive feedback (facial feedback hypothesis), social feedback (emotional contagion and facial mimicry from mirror neurons), and BoNTA's potential migration to the brain.

Facial Feedback, Emotional Contagion, and Facial Mimicry Hypotheses

The discussion of the facial feedback, emotional contagion and facial mimicry hypotheses are relevant in the discussion of BoNTA as if (a) the "facial feedback" hypothesis, which suggests facial displays of emotion feeds back to physiologically influence/determine one's emotional experience, (b) "emotional contagion," which involves the emotional responses to *someone else's* emotional display, and (c) "facial mimicry," which involves imitation of another's facial response (and in turn, *could* lead back to emotion contagion if the facial feedback hypothesis is correct) do systematically occur, then botulinum toxin injections might lead to changes respectively in: (a) the patient's own emotional experience and physiological reaction; (b) the emotional experiences of others with whom the patient interacts, and (c) the emotional displays of another with whom the patient interacts. In short, botulinum toxin injections might have the potential to affect a large set of processes in the patient undergoing the procedure as well as in those with whom the patient interacts.

Facial Feedback Hypothesis

In simple terms, the facial feedback hypothesis proposes that expressive behavior can alter one's emotional state and how he/she interprets the expressions, actions, and intentions of others [20, 21]. This idea echoes throughout history with examples documented in the ancient narrative of the *Iliad* and even Elizabethan texts like Shakespeare's *Henry V* where soldiers are instructed to construct formidable expressions in preparation of their upcoming exertion in battle [20]. However, this idea reverberates beyond

fictional texts into the scientific literature through the writings of Charles Darwin [22] and Gelhorn's laboratory findings [23] of a decreased responsiveness in sympathetic nervous system and hypothalamus following curare-induced relaxation of animal striated muscles.

Numerous studies have sought to determine whether the manipulation of a subject's facial displays affect his/her emotional experiences. The best of these have carefully tried to manipulate facial displays in a manner that minimizes the participants' awareness that they even are producing an emotional display. Results from these trials generally support the facial feedback hypothesis. For example, Strack, Martin, and Stepper found that having subjects hold a pen between their teeth (simulating a smile) caused them to find cartoons funnier [24] (Figure 26.4), and Larsen, Kasimatis, and Frey noted subjects

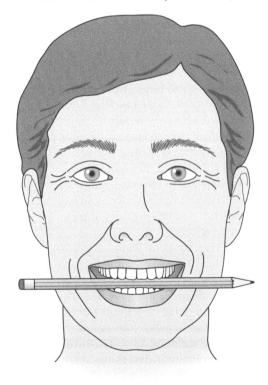

Figure 26.4 Subjects asked to hold a pen between their teeth to simulate a grin found a cartoon to be funnier than did subjects who were not asked to perform this maneuver. *Source:* Alam 2008 [25]. Reproduced with permission of Elsevier.

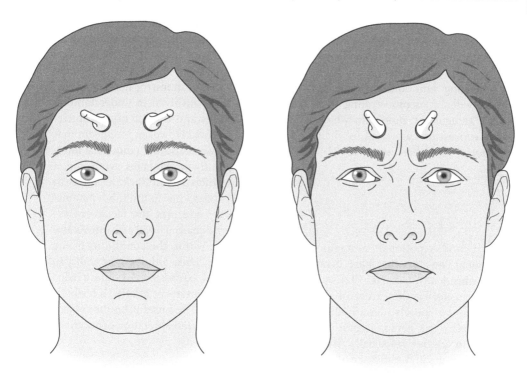

Figure 26.5 Subjects who had two golf tees attached to either side of their foreheads and were asked to try to move these together to simulate a frown concurrently rated unpleasant photographs more negatively than subjects who viewed the same photographs but did not simultaneously attempt the movement. *Source:* Alam 2008 [25]. Reproduced with permission of Elsevier.

rated unpleasant photographs more negatively when attempting to move two tees taped to either side of their forehead together (simulating a frown) [26] (Figure 26.5).

Expanding upon this body of work, Ekman and Levenson imbued the study of facial feedback with laboratory rigor in the 1970s and 1980s [27–29]; these efforts culminated in the widely discussed article published in *Science* that examined physiological responses to facial movements [30]. In this study, six target emotions – surprise, disgust, sadness, anger, fear, and happiness – were evaluated using a "directed facial action task." In each case, a coach provided subjects precise instructions regarding which muscles to contract to replicate the facial expression of a target emotion instead of providing a global command to make a representative emotional expression (e.g., in lieu of posing anger, subjects were asked to: "pull your eyebrows down and together, raise your upper

eyelid and tighten your lower eyelid, narrow your lips, and press them together.") These artificial emotions elicited similar autonomic responses, measured by electrodermal and cardiovascular responses, as the actual emotions re-experienced from the subject's past. Not only did negative expressions differ from positive expressions on autonomic parameters, regardless of the method used to create these expressions, but expressions of particular emotions differed from another by autonomic parameters. These findings provided some of the initial evidence in support of the hypothesis that facial expressions are not merely a manifestation of antecedent internal emotional states, but rather can induce the internal and biological experience of emotions.

There has been some criticism of studies that utilize facial expression coding systems when investigating the facial feedback hypothesis. One problematic claim is that such studies contain cues that lead participants to behave in certain ways. A similar worry is that instructions regarding facial expressions are silly or embarrassing, thus potentially changing emotional responses. Further, the evidence demonstrating the validity of the "categorical" model, in which specific facial expressions are used to elicit specific emotions, is less than complete [31].

Facial Mimicry and Emotional Contagion

Facial mimicry and emotional contagion are two additional concepts that have been demonstrated empirically. Lanzetta [32] was instrumental in exploring the extent of the latter, which can be loosely described as the process whereby one person's emotions are transmitted to another, especially when the transmission occurs in the absence of significant conscious awareness. "Contagion" of this type has applicability for group cohesion (e.g., smiles can instigate acceptance, approval, and bonding) and group survival (e.g., fearful facial displays and vocalizations can alert other group members to danger) [33] as normal subjects display enhanced facial reactions to angry, but not neutral faces, when fear is induced prior to viewing the facial expressions [18].

Facial mimicry, on the other hand, entails the rapid elicitation of spontaneous synchronous facial expressions by others in response to similar facial expressions in the index individual. Such mimicry has been documented in human infants as early as the first few days of life[34]. In adults, more complex emotions are subject to transmission in this manner. These are implicated in emotional contagion, social perception, and the embodied affect [35].

Both facial mimicry and emotional contagion intimately rely upon the activation of mirror neurons as demonstrated on fMRI [36], positron-emission tomography (PET) [37]), and single-pulse transcranial magnetic stimulation (TMS)[38] when viewing various facial expressions. Mirror neurons, which were originally discovered in the premotor cortex of monkeys, discharge when an individual performs a given motor act *and* when they observe others perform that same motor act. The human mirror neuron system is believed to be involved in understanding another's actions and the intentions underlying those actions. However, it appears that mimicry is only one tool for emotional intelligence as a study on Moebius syndrome, a condition in which patients lack the ability to make facial expressions, found these patients could correctly interpret the facial expressions of others equally as well as controls and normative data within the conditions of the experiment [39]. Thus, although the ability to mirror the facial expressions of others helps one express and interpret another's feelings, this skill appears to be a useful, but nonessential component for interpretation of another's emotions.

BoNTA Migration to the Brain

In addition to the indirect effects of neuropsychiatric modulation via the facial feedback hypothesis, facial mimicry, and emotional contagion, BoNTA hypothetically could produce direct effects on cortical neurons through central anterograde or retrograde migration. Although BoNTA has been demonstrated to lack the ability of retrograde migration and transcytosis of tetanus toxin [40], Antonucci *et al.* potentially identified cleaved SNAP-25 proteins in rat brains after injecting their whisker muscles with BoNTA [41]. The conclusions of this study remain controversial as the antibody chosen for western blotting or immunohistochemistry remains incompletely characterized for differentiating cleaved and uncleaved SNAP-25. Additionally, injecting supratherapeutic quantities (150-fold greater than clinically used for the entire glabella) limit clinical extrapolation. A separate investigation, which utilized radioiodinated neurotoxin, failed collaborate these findings [42]. Human correlates have not been studied. Thus, until more evidence arises supporting BoNTA's migratory ability to the central nervous system, the anterograde/retrograde migration of BoNTA does not appear to be the likely underlying mechanism for BoNTA's neuropsychiatric effects.

Future Potential Uses of Neuromodulators in Neuropsychiatry Beyond Depression

As with many other aspects of human biology and neuropsychology, there is a broad spectrum of activity in the mirror neuron system for the human population. While "normal" people can be found at various points within this spectrum, a number of disease states (notably autistic spectrum disorders [43, 44], Asperger's syndrome [45], psychopathic personality disorder [46] and schizophrenia [47]) are characterized by very low levels of mirror neuron activity and have low or inappropriate rapid facial reactions and facial feedback in response to emotional stimuli.

High-functioning individuals with autistic spectrum disorders may be relatively unimpaired in the cognitive assessment of basic emotions, in part because they recruit different neural networks and rely on different strategies to process facial emotions; however, they still show differences in the automatic processing of facial expressions [48]. Tardiff *et al.* observed in an experimental setting that slowing down the presentation of facial expressions improved the ability of autistic children to recognize those emotions [49]. It would be interesting to determine if modulating the degree and rate of facial expressions (e.g., in the parents of autistic children) by treatment with BoNTA would improve the ability of autistic children to recognize and correctly interpret those expressions. Conversely, one would have to consider whether some of these parents have low levels of mirror neuron activity or facial feedback activity themselves [50, 51]. Thus, it would also be of interest to determine whether modulating facial expression by BoNTA in parents

of autistic children would limit the ability of such individuals to maintain empathy [52].

At the other end of the mirror neuron and facial feedback spectrum, individuals, who display excessive empathy and/or expression mimicry, may make those around them become uncomfortable [53]. These individuals with "high self-monitoring" [54] could feel more natural, and be able to internally mirror the feelings of others *more* accurately when facial feedback and associated mirror neuron activity is modulated by treatment of certain muscles of facial expression with BoNTA. Some experimental evidence indicates that reducing facial mimicry may allow an individual to more accurately assess the truth or falsehood of the statements of a conversational partner [55]; recent studies have revealed that excessive emotion impairs cognitive processing and reasoning [56]. Therefore, modulation by treatment with BoNTA may help an affected individual feel more "in control" and better understand others after this tendency has been attenuated. Similarly, those seeking BoNTA due to elevated stress, anxiety or grief may find attenuating negative facial expressions associated with these situations helpful in coping with their situation; in fact, one of the authors has collected over 20 cases where individuals sought BoNTA treatment specifically because they felt treatment improved their coping with such emotions in previous experiences. Perhaps, this self-selected population of individuals are at the high end of the mirror neuron and facial feedback activity spectrum, and being so, derive particular benefit from moderating these systems with BoNTA.

Conclusion

Although BoNTA treatment initially may appear to be an insensitive and shallow approach to the management of neuropsychiatric conditions, scientific investigations indicate a potential role for BoNTA in the treatment of depression and possibly other conditions. Due to the wide variety of non-mutually exclusive mechanisms by which botulinum toxin's paralytic effects on facial displays may induce a change in one's mood, caution should be exerted when interpreting or stating these promising findings.

In addition, when reviewing the available evidence and considering future avenues for research, it is important to remember that experimental observations may or may not have clinical or commercial significance. In general, patients are not interested in getting a "statistically significant degree of improvement," but rather seek a reliable, obvious improvement which they can associate with the treatment. Therefore, when translating clinical observations and scientific experiments related to the effects of treatment on muscles of facial expression with BoNTA into treatment protocols, it will be important to develop proper selection and exclusion criteria for proposed treatments, so those most likely to benefit from treatment can be identified and those unlikely to benefit can be excluded. In so doing, the selective injection of BoNTA into muscles of facial expression may provide long-term therapeutic benefits to those with major depressive disorder and potentially other neuropsychiatric conditions.

References

1 Ekman P. Facial expression and emotion. Am Psychol 1003;48:376–379.

2 Eckman P in A Conversation With: Paul Ekman; The 43 Facial Muscles That Reveal Even the Most Fleeting Emotions. New York Times (Aug 5, 2003). http://www.nytimes.com/2003/08/05/health/conversation-with-paul-ekman-43-facial-muscles-that-reveal-even-most-fleeting.html. Accessed February 27, 2017.

3 Schwartz GE, Fair PL, Slat P, et al. Facial muscle patterning to affective imagery in depressed and non-depressed subjects. Science 1976;192:489–491.

4 Schwartz GE, Fair PL, Salt P, et al. Facial expression and imagery in depression: An electromyographic study. Psychosom Med 1976;38:337–347.

5 Smith CA, McHugo GJ, Lanzetta JT. The facial muscle patterning of posed and imagery-induced expressions of emotion by expressive and nonexpressive posers. Motivation Emotion 1986;10:133–157.

6 Izard, CE. Facial expressions and the regulation of emotions. J Person Soc Psych 1990;58:487–498.

7 Ekman P. Frisen WV, O'Sullivan M. Smiles when lying. J Pers Soc Psych 1988;54:414–420.

8 Ekman P, Roper G, Hager JC. Deliberate facial movement. Child Develop 1980;51:886–891.

9 Oberman LM, Winkielman P, Ramachandran VS. Face to face: blocking facial mimicry can selectively impair recognition of emotional expressions. Soc Neurosci 2007;2:167–78.

10 Mori K, Mori H. Another test of the passive facial feedback hypothesis: when your face smiles, you feel happy. Percept Mot Skills 2009;109:76–78.

11 Warden D, Rush AJ, Trivedi MH, et al. The STAR*D Project results: a comprehensive review of findings. Curr Psychiatry Rep 2007;9:449–459.

12 Wollmer MA, de Boer C, Kalak N, et al. Facing depression with botulinum toxin: A randomized controlled trial. J Psych Res 2012 May;46(5):574–581.

13 Magid M, Reichenberg JS, Poth PE, et al. Treatment of major depressive disorder using botulinum toxin A: A 24-week randomized, double-blind, placebo-controlled study. J Clin Psychiatry 2014 Aug;75(8):837–844.

14 Finzi E, Rosenthal NE. Treatment of depression with onabotulinumtoxinA: A randomized double-blind, placebo controlled trial. J Psychr Res 2014 May;52:1–6.

15 Magid M, Keeling BH, Reichenberg JS. Neurotoxins: Expanding uses of neuromodulators in medicine – major

depressive disorder. Plast Reconstr Surg 2015 Nov;136(5S):111S–119S.

16 Mitwalli H, Dolan C, Bacigalupi R. Botulinum toxin for depression: Does patient appearance matter? J Am Acad Dermatol 2016 Jan:74(1):171–173.

17 Calzadilla, K, Marmur, M. Allergan Reports Topline Phase II Data Supporting Advancement of BOTOX® (onabotulinumtoxinA) for the Treatment of Major Depressive Disorder (MDD). *PR Newswire*. 2017 Apr. Retrieved from http://www.prnewswire.com/news-releases/allergan-reports-topline-phase-ii-data-supporting-advancement-of-botox-onabotulinumtoxina-for-the-treatment-of-major-depressive-disorder-mdd-300435486.html.

18 Hennenlotter A, Dresel C, Castrop F, *et al.* The link between facial feedback and neural activity within central circuitries of emotion – new insights from botulinum toxin-induced denervation of frown muscles. Cereb Cortex 2009;19:537–542.

19 Lewis MB. The positive and negative psychological potential of botulinum-toxin (Botox) injections. Abstract presented at: British Psychological Society Harrogate, North Yorkshire, England, United Kingdom; Apr 9, 2013. Available from http://www.bps.org.uk/bpslegacy/conf_abstracts?&ResultsType=Abstracts&ResultSet_ID=9317&FormDisplayMode=view&frmShowSelected=true&localAction=details. Accessed February 5, 2017.

20 Izard, CE. Facial expressions and the regulation of emotions. J Person Soc Psych 1990;58:487–498.

21 McIntosh DN. Facial feedback hypotheses: Evidence, implications, and directions. Motivation Emotion 1996;20:121–147.

22 Darwin, C.R. *The Expression of Emotions in Man and Animals*. Oxford, England: Oxford University Press, 1998:366.

23 Gellhorn E. The physiological basis of neuromuscular relaxation. Arch Intern Med 1958;102;392–399.

24 Strack R, Martin LL, Stepper S. Inhibiting and facilitating conditions of facial expressions: A non-obstrusive text of the

facial feedback hypothesis. J Pers Social Psych 1988;54:768–777.

25 Alam M, Barrett KC, Hodapp RM, Arndt KA. Botulinum toxin and the facial feedback hypothesis: can looking better make you feel happier? J Am Acad Dermatol 2008;58(6):1061–1072.

26 Larsen RJ, Kasimatis M, Frey K. Facilitating the furrowed brow: An unobstrusive test of the facial feedback hypothesis applied to unpleasant affect. Cognition Emotion 1992;6:321–338.

27 Ekman P. Facial expressions of emotion: An old controversy and new findings. Phil Trans R Soc Lond B 1992;335:63–69.

28 Gladwell M. The Naked Face. The New Yorker (August 5, 2002), pp. 38–49.

29 Gladwell M. *Blink* (Chapter Six, Sections 2 and 3). New York: Little, Brown & Co., 2005:197–214.

30 Ekman P, Levenson RW, Friesen WV. Autonomic nervous system activity distinguishes among emotions. Science 1983;221:1208–1210.

31 Winton WM. The role of facial response in self-reports of emotion: A critique of Laird. J Pers Soc Psych 1986;50:808–812.

32 McHugo GJ, Lanzetta JT, Sullivan DJ, *et al.* Emotional reactions to a political leader's expressive displays. J Pers Soc Psych 1985;49:1513–1529.

33 Hatfield E, Cacioppo JT, Rapson RL. *Emotional Contagion*. Cambridge: Cambridge University Press, 1994.

34 Meltzoff AN, Moore MK. Newborn infants imitate facial gestures. Child Develop 1983;54:702–709.

35 Stel M, Vonk R. Mimicry in social interaction: benefits for mimickers, mimickees, and their interaction. Br J Psychol 2010;101:311–323.

36 Haughton VM, Turski PA, Meyerand B, *et al.* The clinical applications of functional MR imaging. Neuroimaging Clin N Am 1999;9:285–293.

37 Paulesu E, Connelly A, Frith CD, *et al.* Functional MR imaging correlations with positron emission tomography. Initial experience using a cognitive activation paradigm on verbal working memory.

Neuroimaging Clin N Am 1995;5: 207–225.

38 Enticott PG, Johnston PJ, Herring SE, *et al.* Mirror neuron activation is associated with facial emotion processing. Neuropsychologia 2008;46:2851–2854.

39 Rives Bogart K, Matsumoto D. Facial mimicry is not necessary to recognize emotion: Facial expression recognition by people with Moebius syndrome. Soc Neurosci 2010;5:241–251.

40 Dienhardt K, Schiavo G. Endocytosis and retrograde axonal traffic in motor neurons. Biochem Soc Symp 2005;139–150.

41 Antonucci F, Rossi C, Gianfranceschi L, *et al.* Long-distance retrograde effects of botulinum neurotoxin A. J Neurosci 2008;28:3689–3696.

42 Tang-Liu DD, Aoki KR, Dolly JO, *et al.* Intramuscular injection of 125I-botulinum neurotoxin-complex versus 125I-botulinumfree neurotoxin: time course of tissue distribution. Toxicon 2003;42:461–469.

43 Stel M, van den Heuvel C, Smeets RC. Facial feedback mechanisms in autistic spectrum disorders. J Autism Dev Disord 2008;38 1250–1258.

44 Oberman LM, Winkielman P, Ramachandran VS. Slow echo: facial EMG evidence for the delay of spontaneous, but not voluntary, emotional mimicry in children with autism spectrum disorders. Dev Sci 2009;12:510–520.

45 Minio-Paluello I, Baron-Cohen S, Avenanti A, *et al.* Absence of embodied empathy during pain observation in Asperger syndrome. Biol Psychiatry 2009;65: 55–62.

46 Fecteau S, Pascual-Leone A, Thoret H. Psychopathy and the mirror neuron system: preliminary findings from a non-psychiatric sample. Psychiatry Res 2008;160:137–44.

47 Varcin KJ, Bailey PE, Henry JD. Empathic deficits in schizophrenia: the potential role of rapid facial mimicry. J Int Neuropsychol Soc 2010;16:621–629.

48 Wang AT, Dapretto M, Hariri AR, *et al.* Neural correlates of facial affect processing in children and adolescents with autism spectrum disorder. J Am Acad Child Adolesc Psychiatry 2004;43:481–490.

49 Tardif C, Lainé F, Rodriguez M, *et al.* Slowing down presentation of facial movements and vocal sounds enhances facial expression recognition and induces facial-vocal imitation in children with autism. J Autism Dev Disord 2007;37: 1469–1484.

50 Zhao X, Leotta A, Kustanovich V, *et al.* A unified genetic theory for sporadic and inherited autism. Proc Natl Acad Sci USA 2007;104:12831–1286.

51 Wheelwright S, Auyeung B, Allison C, *et al.* Defining the broader, medium and narrow autism phenotype among parents using the Autism Spectrum Quotient (AQ). Molecular Autism 2010;1:10. http://www .molecularautism.com/content/1/1/10. Accessed February 27, 2017.

52 Oberman LM, Winkielman P, Ramachandran VS. Face to face: blocking facial mimicry can selectively impair recognition of emotional expressions. Soc Neurosci 2007;2:167–178.

53 Kühn S, Müller BC, van der Leij A, *et al.* Neural correlates of emotional synchrony. Soc Cogn Affect Neurosci 2011;6(3): 368–374.

54 Cheng CM, Chartrand TL. Self-monitoring without awareness: using mimicry as a nonconscious affiliation strategy. J Pers Soc Psychol 2003;85:1170–1179.

55 Stel M, van Dijk E, Olivier E. You want to know the truth? Then don't mimic! Psychol Sci 2009;20: 693–699.

56 Zinchenko A, Kanske P, Obermeier C, *et al.* Emotion and goal-directed behavior: ERP evidence on cognitive and emotional conflict. Soc Cogn Affect Neurosci 2015;10(11):1577–1587.

27

OnabotulinumtoxinA (Botox®) in Dermatology

Jason J. Emer, MD,[1] Eileen Axibal, MD,[2] Ellen S. Marmur, MD (FAAD),[3] and Heidi Waldorf, MD[3]

[1]*Cosmetic Dermatology and Body Contouring, Private Practice, Beverly Hills, CA*
[2]*Department of Dermatology, University of Colorado, Aurora, USA*
[3]*Mount Sinai School of Medicine, Department of Dermatology, New York, USA*

Introduction

Since the approval of botulinum toxin for medical use in the United States nearly three decades ago, the use of neurotoxin has become a standard of care for the treatment of facial dynamic wrinkles. Of the various formulations of botulinum toxin type A that are available or in development, onabotulinumtoxinA (Botox/Botox Cosmetic; Allergan, Inc., Irvine, CA) is the most commonly used and widely studied. It was approved by the Food and Drug Administration (FDA) in 1989 for strabismus and blepharospasm and started being used for off-label aesthetic purposes in 1992 [1]. The FDA approved onabotulinumtoxinA (BoNTA-ONA) for the treatment of glabellar "frown" lines in 2002 [2] and lateral canthal "crow's feet" lines in 2013 [3]. In 2004, BoNTA-ONA was FDA approved for the treatment of severe axillary hyperhidrosis inadequately managed by topical agents in adult patients [4]. The toxin also continues to be widely used off-label to treat other skin lines and for facial contouring, as well as for palmoplantar and facial hyperhidrosis [5–8]. It is available worldwide and has many non-dermatologic indications including treatment of bladder dysfunction, chronic headache, spasticity, cervical dystonia, belpharospasm, and strabismus [4]. While the use of botulinum toxins continue to expand with new formulations and indications, this chapter will focus specifically on onabotulinumtoxinA and its FDA-approved uses in dermatology.

Efficacy

Years of clinical trials and clinical use have proven excellent efficacy BoNTA-ONA. In 2002 and 2003, two articles published by Carruthers *et al.* reported on a total of 537 patients who enrolled in two separate phase 3 randomized, double-blinded, multi-center, placebo-controlled studies of identical design to evaluate the efficacy and safety of BoNTA-ONA for temporary improvement in moderate to severe glabellar lines [9, 10]. Of those enrolled, 405 patients received BoNTA-ONA and 132 patients received placebo. The total dosage of BoNTA-ONA was 20 U, divided equally into five injection points. Reduction in glabellar line severity was superior in the treatment group compared to the placebo group at all study time points, both by investigator and patient assessment. More recently, three sequential phase 3 studies published in 2014 and 2015 further demonstrated the efficacy and safety of onabotulinumtoxinA for its newest cosmetic indication, crow's feet lines [11–13].

Two pivotal studies were conducted using BoNTA-ONA for the treatment of primary

Botulinum Toxins: Cosmetic and Clinical Applications, First Edition. Edited by Joel L. Cohen and David M. Ozog.
© 2017 John Wiley & Sons Ltd. Published 2017 by John Wiley & Sons Ltd.
Companion Website: www.wiley.com/go/cohen/botulinum

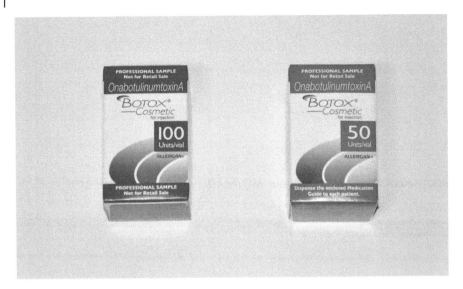

Figure 27.1 Vial types by units. Each vial of BoNTA-ONA contains either 50 U or 100 U. Potency is determined by the amount of saline used for reconstitution.

axillary hyperhidrosis. Naumann and Lowe randomized patients who received a single treatment of 50 U per axilla or a placebo in a ratio of 3 : 1 [14]. During the posttreatment period dramatic improvements were noted in the treatment group with respect to emotional status, ability to participate in daily and social activities, productivity at work, and number of clothing changes per day. The desired effects were rapid and long lasting (at least 16 weeks) with few reported adverse events. Similar results were confirmed in a study by Lowe and Glaser who treated patients with two differing BoNTA-ONA dosages (50 U, 75 U, or placebo) [15]. Though off-label, studies have also validated the efficacy of BoNTA-ONA in both palmar [16–19] and plantar [20, 21] hyperhidrosis.

Storage and Preparation

A vial of Botox® Cosmetic (BoNTA-ONA) contains either 50 U *Clostridium botulinum* type A neurotoxin complex, 0.25 mg human albumin, and 0.45 mg sodium chloride; or 100 U *Clostridium botulinum* type A neurotoxin complex, 0.5 mg human albumin, and 0.9 mg sodium chloride in a sterile, vacuum-dried form without a preservative [22] (Figure 27.1). The initial recommendation to freeze unopened vials (−5°C or colder) has been amended to allow storage in a refrigerator (2–8°C) for 24 or 36 months for the 50 U and 100 U vials, respectively. The product insert recommends dilution with 0.9% sterile preservative-free saline; however, the use of preserved isotonic saline reduces patient discomfort without sacrificing efficacy and has become standard of care [23] (Figure 27.2). The manufacturers also recommend storage of the reconstituted BoNTA-ONA in the refrigerator, toxin administration within 4–24 hours, and not freezing after reconstitution; however, studies have shown that BoNTA-ONA retains its efficacy for at least 4–6 weeks following reconstitution if refrigerated at 4°C [24, 25] and that there is no difference in efficacy of injected Botox after 2-weeks of refrigeration (4°C) or freezing (−20°C) of a reconstituted vial compared with freshly reconstituted Botox [26]. Despite initial concerns about toxin stability, no reduction in efficacy has been found when the vial contents are shaken and foamed during reconstitution [27]. Reconstituted

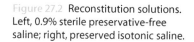

Figure 27.2 Reconstitution solutions. Left, 0.9% sterile preservative-free saline; right, preserved isotonic saline.

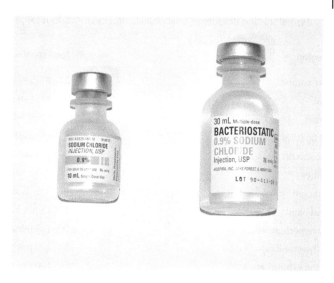

product should be clear, colorless, and free of particulate matter. A publication in 2012 by Liu *et al.* suggested that a single vial of botulinum toxin type A can be safely administered to multiple patients, assuming standard safe injection techniques are followed [28]. This proposition was based a survey of physician members of the American Society of Dermatologic Surgery, which found that most physicians routinely store botulinum toxin for a period of >1 week and use each vial for more than one patient, and not a single case of infection was observed.

Treatment

The onset of BoNTA-ONA has been shown to be rapid within 1–2 days [29]. In two clinical trials, the degree of response by both investigator and patient assessment was similar at day 7 and day 30, with peak effect seen on day 30 [9, 10]. Results from two large studies demonstrated that duration of BoNTA-ONA effect in minimizing glabellar and lateral canthal lines was frequently ≥4 months [30, 31]. The clinical effect is determined by both the number of units of toxin injected as well as the concentration [32–34]. Most practitioners use between 1 and 3 ml of saline to reconstitute for aesthetic

use; A 5 U/0.1 ml preparation is prepared by 2 ml of preservative-free saline into the 100 U vial [35, 36]. Consensus recommendations and package insert validate 100 U/2.5 ml = 4 U/0.1 ml as the most versatile concentration [37]. In a dose-dilution study in which a total dose of 30 U BoNTA-ONA was reconstituted in 1, 3, 5, or 10 ml saline, no differences in safety or efficacy were seen between groups in treating glabellar rhytides [33]. Dosage can be increased to correlate with the size of the treated muscle. Results of a 2009 study by Kane *et al.* demonstrated the efficacy of dosing Dysport based on gender and muscle-mass [38]; while not directly studied, these results could reasonably be applied to Botox. In general, higher concentrations mean low injection volumes, less pain and edema, and more precise placement of product [32]. Delivery of the same number of units in a lower concentration requires a higher volume and therefore has the potential for increased pain and a larger field of effect. This can be utilized to an advantage or may lead to unpredictable side effects nearby or far from injection placement. Dosing units vary by treatment location, as outlined in Table 27.1. The other variable in treatment is needle/syringe type. Some physicians prefer to use a 32-guage needle (A; TSK SteriJect, TSK Laboratory, Tochigi-Ken, Japan) rather

Table 27.1 Typical starting dosages of onabotulinumtoxinA for various target regions.

Target region	Total starting dosage in units[a]
Glabellar compex	20–40 (5–7 sites)
Forehead	10–30 (4–8 sites)
Crow's feet	8–20 per side (1–4 sites)
Vertical lip lines	4–6 (4 sites)
Mouth corners	2–8 per side (1 site)
Bunny lines	2–6 (1–3 sites)
Dimpled chin	2–10 (1–2 sites)
Platysmal bands	10–15 per band (2–10 sites)
Axillary hyperhidrosis	50–100 per axilla (1–2 cm/site; multiple sites)
Palmar hyperhidrosis	50–100 per palm (1–2 cm/site; multiple sites)
Plantar hyperhidrosis	50–100 per sole (1–2 cm/site; multiple sites)

[a] Units are unique to this product.

than the more common 30/31-gauge needles (B; BD Precision Glide, Becton Dickinson & Co, Franklin Lakes, NJ) to help reduce side effects such as pain during injection. Also, an array of syringe types is available for injection and can be chosen based on personal preference (Figure 27.3).

Glabella

The first FDA approved cosmetic indication for botulinum toxin was for treatment of glabellar frown lines using a total dose of 20 s. The glabellar complex includes the procerus, corrugator supercilii, depressor

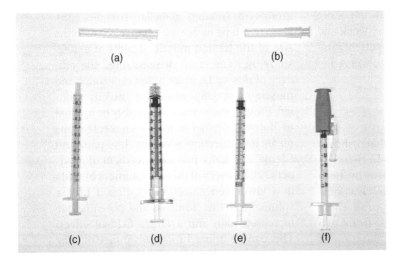

Figure 27.3 Syringes and needles. Some physicians prefer to use a 32-guage needle (a) TSK SteriJect, TSK Laboratory, Tochigi-Ken, Japan, rather than the more common 30-gauge needle (b) BD Precision Glide, Becton Dickinson & Co, Franklin Lakes, NJ, to help reduce side effects such as pain during injection. Also, an array of syringe types is available for injection and can be chosen based on personal preference. (c) Injekt-F Tuberkulin Low Waste Syringe, B. Braun Medical, Bethlehem, PA;. (d) BD Leur-Lok Tip Syring, Becton Dickinson & Co, Franklin Lakes, NJ; (e) BD Tuberculin Slip Tip Syringe, Becton Dickinson & Co, Franklin Lakes, NJ; (f) BD SafetyGlide Insulin Syringe, Becton Dickinson & Co, Franklin Lakes, NJ.

supercilii, and interdigitation of the medial fibers of the orbicularis oculi and frontalis muscles. The procerus is the primary muscle responsible for the horizontal lines of the glabella and the others contribute to the formation of the vertical lines. Numerous injection techniques have been described with early injection incorporating electromyographic guidance to locate the muscle accurately [34, 39]. Most clinical trials have dictated starting doses of 20–25 U of BoNTA-ONA split equally into five injection sites for treatment of the glabellar complex. Additional or fewer injection points may be indicated in certain circumstances such as in men for maintenance of a horizontal brow (two additional) or when products have the ability to diffuse more easily (two fewer) [40–42]. Gender is particularly important and should be taken into consideration as the female brow is typically more arched and the male brow is classically more horizontal (Figure 27.4 and Figure 27.5). Women may require a lower starting dosage than men; in general, men have more muscle mass and thicker, sebaceous skin which may require starting dosages approximately twice that which is used for women [43–45]. Practitioners should evaluate the patient's facial expression at rest and during movement prior to any dosing to assess any asymmetries of positioning, ptosis, and muscular mass.

Orbicularis Oculi

The more recent FDA approved cosmetic indication for BoNTA-ONA (2013) is treatment of the lateral canthal lines, or crow's feet, using a total dose of 24 s (12(on each side, with 4 o at each of three injection sites). Lateral canthal lines are caused by contraction of the orbicularis oculi muscles. These are sphincter-like muscles encircle the eyes and aid in eye closure; they are broad, thin, and superficial, and wrinkles in this region develop from a combination of muscle activity (eye closing and facial expressions) and photoaging. Typically, sites are injected superficially along the lateral orbital rim with 2–5 U of BoNTA-ONA each. To minimize toxin diffusion and paralysis of neighboring muscles (zygomaticus minor, zygomaticus major, and levator labii superioris muscle), typical aliquots are distributed approximately 1 cm apart and lateral to the outer canthus. The usual number of injections is two to five per side and precise location of these points depend on pretreatment analysis, which takes into account the activity of the muscle and orbital line patterns observed.

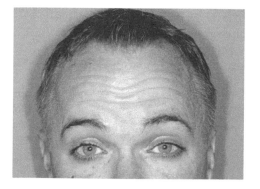

Figure 27.5 Male forehead anatomy. Male forehead rhytides are typically large and broad as compared to females, given an increased distance between the eyebrows and the frontal hair line. Notice the skin is more glabrous, due to increase sebaceous activity. Also, here is a good example of the frontalis muscle as two discrete muscle bellies with insertions more prominent over the eyebrows and with sparing of part of mid-upper forehead. Further, the male eyebrows are more horizontal and less arched as compared to females.

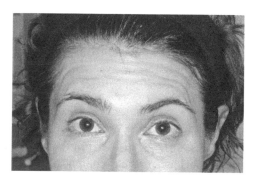

Figure 27.4 Female forehead anatomy. Typical rhytides of the frontalis muscle are evident during forehead elevation with an arched appearance of the eyebrows. Notice the frontalis is one large muscle with broad insertions, rather than two discreet muscles with specific insertions.

Duration of effect in this area is usually less than the upper face and is dose-dependent with higher dosages yielding longer-lasting results. For patients who desire more open eyes (increased scleral show), lower eye lateral rounding, or improvement of infraorbital rhytides, a small aliquot of toxin can be injected into the inferior orbicularis oculi below the midpupillary line [46, 47].

Hyperhidrosis

BoNTA-ONA currently remains the only neurotoxin that is specifically approved by the FDA for the treatment of primary axillary hyperhidrosis, using 50 in each axilla. The Minor test, an iodine starch test, can be done immediately prior to treatment to allow for delineation of affected areas [48] (Figure 27.6). If utilizing the Minor test, is recommended that patients discontinue all antihyperhidrotic therapeutic agents – including antiperspirants – 5 days prior to improve the test's accuracy [49]. Approximately 50 U of BoNTA-ONA are needed for the treatment of one axillae [50], with 20 injections distributed evenly, spaced 1–2 cm apart, in the hyperhidrotic area. In patients with more surface area of involvement, however, additional units are often given so that the total dose per axilla may actually be 60–100 units. Marking the area of involvement with a surgical

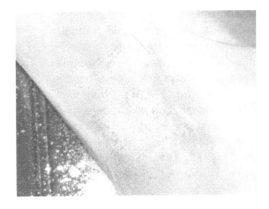

Figure 27.7 Iodine starch test. Iodine starch test is used as an aid for identifying localized areas of sweating in order to concentrate toxin injection for increased clinical efficacy and patient satisfaction.

pen in a grid pattern can help ensure proper distribution of the product. Injections should stay superficial and should be injected next to, not directly on, skin markings to decrease the risk of skin tattooing. Increasing the accuracy of injection placement improves clinical efficacy and patient satisfaction [51]. Although not FDA approved, use of BoNTA-ONA is also common in palmar and plantar hyperhidrosis and is covered in depth in Chapter 23 of this textbook (Figure 27.7).

Safety and Complications

Similar to other BoNTA products, BoNTA-ONA is generally well tolerated. In 2005, Cote *et al.* reviewed all therapeutic and cosmetic, serious and nonserious, adverse events from BoNTA-ONA administration that were reported to the FDA from December 1989 to May 2003 (serious) and December 2001 to November 2002 (nonserious) [52]. Of 36 serious adverse events, 30 were included in the FDA-approved label as possible complications and the remaining six were considered unrelated to the treatment. No deaths were reported among cosmetic users. The most commonly reported non-serious side effects were lack of effect, injection site reaction, and ptosis. A meta-analysis of the number

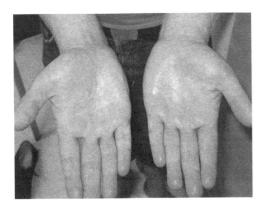

Figure 27.6 Palmar hyperhidrosis. Clammy hands with palmar glistening in a patient with severe hyperhidrosis.

and frequency of adverse events from BoNTA-ONA in 36 studies involving 2309 subjects revealed no severe adverse events [53]. Complications such as pain, bruising, and swelling are mainly dependent on the location (knowledge of target anatomy and avoidance of visible veins) and technique (speed, needle gauge, pressure, and/or ice) of injection, as the periocular, perioral, and lid margins consist or thin, friable skin which is highly vascular with many superficial vessels prone to injury. Most of the available evidence suggests that hematoma and ecchymoses at injection sites occur in less than 1% of injections [54]. Common adverse effects of neurotoxin therapy in cosmetic indications are listed in Table 27.2.

Headache and blepharoptosis have shown to be the most significant treatment-related adverse effects related to glabellar treatment, with headache more likely to be due to injection procedure than the drug itself given that headache occurs with equal frequency in those treated with BoNTA-ONA and placebo [9, 10]. Overall, headaches from BoNTA-ONA injection are mild and require no specific therapy, although a small subset of patients have been reported to develop more severe, debilitating headaches – likely due to micro-trauma from the needle being inserted too deep into the forehead and thus "tapping" periosteum – which are fortunately benign and spontaneously remit within days to weeks with or without treatment (analgesic) [55]. Unintended paralysis of neighboring muscles, or ptosis, is the most significant complication that can occur with cosmetic neurotoxin treatment. Local spread of toxin occurs by diffusion even up to 3 cm in diameter from the injection point [56]. The package insert of BoNTA-ONA reports blepharoptosis occurring in 3% of 405 subjects, whereas an early trial that included injectors with less experience reported blepharoptosis in 5.4% of patients [9, 22]. To limit the incidence of unwanted adjacent muscle paralysis, it is helpful to grasp the specific glabellar muscles prior to each injection to localize delivery and apply digital pressure during injection.

Table 27.2 Common adverse effects of neurotoxin therapy in cosmetic indications.

Upper face
Common:
Bruising/Ecchymosis
Swelling
Ptosis (eyebrow, eyelid)
Asymmetry
Rare:
Interference with eye lid function/physiology
Lower lid retraction / scleral show
Effect on upper lip movement
Atrophy
Globe perforation
Lower face
Common:
Bruising/Ecchymosis
Swelling
Asymmetry
Rare:
Increase or loss of dental show on smiling
Effect on oral muscle strength
Inability to raise or lower lips / irregular lip movement
Difficulty swallowing
Neck weakness
Dry mouth
Drooling
Palmoplantar
Muscular weakness interfering with fine motor function

It is also important to place corrugator injections at least 1 cm above the bony orbital rim, place orbicularis oculi muscle injections at least 1–2 cm from the lateral orbital rim, and place frontalis injections at least 1–2 cm above the upper line of the eyebrow. Of note, at the time of writing of this chapter the use of botulinum toxin in the frontalis muscle is considered off-label yet is commonly performed. In certain situations, it is helpful to consider lower dilutions that give higher localized concentrations and lower injection volumes to help reduce spread or unwanted diffusion. Increased clinician experience can minimize rates of ptosis.

Adverse events associated with treatment of axillary hyperhidrosis with BoNTA-ONA are uncommon. Minimal pain and mild subjective compensatory hyperhidrosis in non-axillary regions in 5% of patients have been described [14]. In the off-label treatment of palmoplantar hyperhidrosis, the most significant complication is the possibility of temporary hand weakness because of diffusion of toxin to the intrinsic hand muscles. This may occur in as many as two-thirds of patients reflecting as minor weakening of finger grip strength that can last for 3–5 weeks [57, 58]. Superficial placement in the high dermis may help reduce muscle effects and increase patient comfort.

To minimize patient discomfort during injections for hyperhidrosis, pretreatment and posttreatment application of ice or ethyl chloride spray, topical anesthetic under occlusion, nerve blocks, and/or frequent changing of the needle tip (as the needle tip may dull after multiple punctures) can be used [59–61]. Vibratory massage devices are also commonly employed to relieve injection pain; the ability of a non-noxious stimulus to suppress discomfort is thought to work through the gate control theory of pain, in which the benign stimulus closes the "gates" to the painful input and prevents the adverse sensation from traveling to the central nervous system [62].

Patient Satisfaction

Numerous studies have demonstrated sustainably high patient-satisfaction rates with

cosmetic BoNTA-ONA treatments [63,64]. A 2015 report by Trinidade de Almeida *et al.* found that long-term, continuous treatment with onabotulinumtoxinA for a mean of 9.1 years was associated with very high patient satisfaction [65]. Several clinical trials in treating upper facial lines have demonstrated significant improvements from baseline and versus placebo in patient self-assessment scores in which the patients rate the degree to which their facial lines bother them, make them look older than they would like, prevent them from having a smooth facial appearance, and/or make them look tried, stressed, or angry when that is not how they feel [66]. High satisfaction rates with BoNTA-ONA treatment results have helped to build interest and create new indications in the noninvasive aesthetic market.

Conclusion

The trend in the use of neurotoxin products for facial aesthetics is towards utilizing the lowest dosage possible for "natural" yet smooth, youthful appearances. For best results, practitioners must have detailed knowledge of the facial anatomy, neurotoxin product characteristics, and must be able to individualize assessments for success. Clinical trials and real-time experience will delineate major differences between the available neurotoxins and their most practical uses in facial aesthetics, as well as other uses such as hyperhidrosis. As the most extensively studied and longest used neurotoxin worldwide, onabotulinumtoxinA can provide safe, effective, and reproducible results – and we expect to see additional FDA approvals for other cosmetic regions (including the forehead) in the future.

References

1 Carruthers JD, Carruthers JA. Treatment of glabellar frown lines with C. botulinum-A exotoxin. J Dermatol Surg Oncol 1992; 18(1):17–21.

2 FDA. BOTOX Cosmetic Approval Letter. 2002.

3 FDA. FDA approves Botox Cosmetic to improve the appearance of crow's feet lines.

September 2013; http://www.fda.gov/
NewsEvents/Newsroom/
PressAnnouncements/ucm367662.htm.
Accessed February 27, 2017.

4 Botox [Prescribing information]. BOTOX
(onabotulinumtoxinA) for injection, for
intramuscular use, intradetrusor, or
intradermal use. Irving, CA: Allergan; 2016.

5 Carruthers J, Carruthers A. The evolution
of botulinum neurotoxin type A for
cosmetic applications. J Cosmet Laser Ther
2007;9(3):186–192.

6 Said S, Meshkinpour A, Carruthers A,
Carruthers J. Botulinum toxin A: its
expanding role in dermatology and
esthetics. Am J Clin Dermatol 2003;4(9):
609–616.

7 Glaser DA, Hebert AA, Pariser DM, Solish
N. Facial hyperhidrosis: best practice
recommendations and special
considerations. Cutis 2007;79(5 Suppl):
29–32.

8 Gregoriou S, Rigopoulos D, Makris M,
et al. Effects of botulinum toxin-a therapy
for palmar hyperhidrosis in plantar sweat
production. Dermatol Surg 2010;36(4):
496–498.

9 Carruthers JA, Lowe NJ, Menter MA, et al.
A multicenter, double-blind, randomized,
placebo-controlled study of the efficacy and
safety of botulinum toxin type A in the
treatment of glabellar lines. J Am Acad
Dermatol 2002;46(6):840–849.

10 Carruthers JD, Lowe NJ, Menter MA,
Gibson J, Eadie N, Group BGLIS.
Double-blind, placebo-controlled study of
the safety and efficacy of botulinum toxin
type A for patients with glabellar lines. Plast
Reconstr Surg 2003;112(4):1089–1098.

11 Carruthers A, Bruce S, de Coninck A, et al.
Efficacy and safety of onabotulinumtoxinA
for the treatment of crows feet lines: a
multicenter, randomized, controlled trial.
Dermatol Surg 2014;40(11):1181–1190.

12 Moers-Carpi M, Carruthers J, Fagien S,
et al. Efficacy and safety of
onabotulinumtoxinA for treating crow's
feet lines alone or in combination with
glabellar lines: a multicenter, randomized,

controlled trial. Dermatol Surg 2015;41(1):
102–112.

13 Carruthers J, Rivkin A, Donofrio L, et al. A
multicenter, randomized, double-blind,
placebo-controlled study to evaluate the
efficacy and safety of repeated
onabotulinumtoxinA treatments in
subjects with crow's feet lines and glabellar
lines. Dermatol Surg 2015;41(6):
702–711.

14 Naumann M, Lowe NJ. Botulinum toxin
type A in treatment of bilateral primary
axillary hyperhidrosis: randomised, parallel
group, double blind, placebo controlled
trial. BMJ 2001;323(7313):596–599.

15 Lowe NJ, Glaser DA, Eadie N, et al.
Botulinum toxin type A in the treatment of
primary axillary hyperhidrosis: a 52-week
multicenter double-blind, randomized,
placebo-controlled study of efficacy and
safety. J Am Acad Dermatol 2007;56(4):
604–611.

16 Pérez-Bernal AM, Avalos-Peralta P,
Moreno-Ramírez D, Camacho F.
Treatment of palmar hyperhidrosis with
botulinum toxin type A: 44 months of
experience. J Cosmet Dermatol 2005;4(3):
163–166.

17 Lowe NJ, Yamauchi PS, Lask GP, et al.
Efficacy and safety of botulinum toxin type
a in the treatment of palmar hyperhidrosis:
a double-blind, randomized,
placebo-controlled study. Dermatol Surg
2002;28(9):822–827.

18 Simonetta Moreau M, Cauhepe C, Magues
JP, Senard JM. A double-blind,
randomized, comparative study of Dysport
vs. Botox in primary palmar hyperhidrosis.
Br J Dermatol 2003;149(5):1041–1045.

19 Solomon BA, Hayman R. Botulinum toxin
type A therapy for palmar and digital
hyperhidrosis. J Am Acad Dermatol
2000;42(6):1026–1029.

20 Vadoud-Seyedi J. Treatment of plantar
hyperhidrosis with botulinum toxin type A.
Int J Dermatol 2004;43(12):969–971.

21 Vlahovic TC, Dunn SP, Blau JC, Gauthier
C. Injectable botulinum toxin as a
treatment for plantar hyperhidrosis: a case

study. J Am Podiatr Med Assoc 2008;98(2): 156–159.

22 Botox [Prescribibg information]. BOTOX® Cosmetic (onabotulinumtoxinA) for injection, for intramuscular use. Irving, CA: Allergan; 2016.

23 Alam M, Dover JS, Arndt KA. Pain associated with injection of botulinum A exotoxin reconstituted using isotonic sodium chloride with and without preservative: a double-blind, randomized controlled trial. Arch Dermatol 2002; 138(4):510–514.

24 Hexsel DM, De Almeida AT, Rutowitsch M, et al. Multicenter, double-blind study of the efficacy of injections with botulinum toxin type A reconstituted up to six consecutive weeks before application. Dermatol Surg 2003;29(5):523–529; discussion 529.

25 Garcia A, Fulton JE. Cosmetic denervation of the muscles of facial expression with botulinum toxin. A dose-response study. Dermatol Surg 1996;22(1):39–43.

26 Yang GC, Chiu RJ, Gillman GS. Questioning the need to use Botox within 4 hours of reconstitution: a study of fresh vs 2-week-old Botox. Arch Facial Plast Surg 2008;10(4):273–279.

27 Trindade De Almeida AR, Kadunc BV, Di Chiacchio N, Neto DR. Foam during reconstitution does not affect the potency of botulinum toxin type A. Dermatol Surg 2003;29(5):530–531; discussion 532.

28 Liu A, Carruthers A, Cohen JL, et al. Recommendations and current practices for the reconstitution and storage of botulinum toxin type A. J Am Acad Dermatol 2012;67(3):373–378.

29 Beer KR, Boyd C, Patel RK, Bowen B, James SP, Brin MF. Rapid onset of response and patient-reported outcomes after onabotulinumtoxinA treatment of moderate-to-severe glabellar lines. J Drugs Dermatol 2011;10(1):39–44.

30 Baumann L, Dayan S, Connolly S, et al. Duration of clinical efficacy of onabotulinumtoxinA in crow's feet lines: results from two multicenter, randomized,

controlled trials. Dermatol Surg 2016;42(5): 598–607.

31 Glogau R, Kane M, Beddingfield F, et al. OnabotulinumtoxinA: a meta-analysis of duration of effect in the treatment of glabellar lines. Dermatol Surg 2012; 38(11):1794–1803.

32 Borodic GE, Ferrante R, Pearce LB, Smith K. Histologic assessment of dose-related diffusion and muscle fiber response after therapeutic botulinum A toxin injections. Mov Disord 1994;9(1):31–39.

33 Shaari CM, George E, Wu BL, et al. Quantifying the spread of botulinum toxin through muscle fascia. Laryngoscope 1991;101(9):960–964.

34 Shaari CM, Sanders I. Quantifying how location and dose of botulinum toxin injections affect muscle paralysis. Muscle Nerve 1993;16(9):964–969.

35 Klein AW. Dilution and storage of botulinum toxin. Dermatol Surg 1998; 24(11):1179–1180.

36 Klein AW, Kreyden OP. Storage and dilution of botulinum toxin. Curr Probl Dermatol 2002;30:126–130.

37 Carruthers J, Fagien S, Matarasso SL, Group BC. Consensus recommendations on the use of botulinum toxin type a in facial aesthetics. Plast Reconstr Surg 2004;114(6 Suppl):1S–22S.

38 Kane MA, Brandt F, Rohrich RJ, et al. Evaluation of variable-dose treatment with a new U.S. Botulinum Toxin Type A (Dysport) for correction of moderate to severe glabellar lines: results from a phase III, randomized, double-blind, placebo-controlled study. Plast Reconstr Surg 2009;124(5):1619–1629.

39 Lowe NJ, Maxwell A, Harper H. Botulinum A exotoxin for glabellar folds: a double-blind, placebo-controlled study with an electromyographic injection technique. J Am Acad Dermatol 1996; 35(4):569–572.

40 Sadick NS. The cosmetic use of botulinum toxin type B in the upper face. Clin Dermatol 2004;22(1):29–33.

41 Rzany B, Ascher B, Fratila A, *et al.* Efficacy and safety of 3- and 5-injection patterns (30 and 50 U) of botulinum toxin A (Dysport) for the treatment of wrinkles in the glabella and the central forehead region. Arch Dermatol 2006;142(3):320–326.

42 Carruthers A. Botulinum toxin type A: history and current cosmetic use in the upper face. Dis Mon 2002;48(5):299–322.

43 Monheit G, Carruthers A, Brandt F, Rand R. A randomized, double-blind, placebo-controlled study of botulinum toxin type A for the treatment of glabellar lines: determination of optimal dose. Dermatol Surg 2007;33(1 Spec No.): S51–S59.

44 Carruthers A, Carruthers J, Said S. Dose-ranging study of botulinum toxin type A in the treatment of glabellar rhytids in females. Dermatol Surg 2005;31(4): 414–422; discussion 422.

45 Flynn TC. Botox in men. Dermatol Ther 2007;20(6):407–413.

46 Flynn TC, Carruthers JA. Botulinum-A toxin treatment of the lower eyelid improves infraorbital rhytides and widens the eye. Dermatol Surg 2001;27(8): 703–708.

47 Flynn TC, Carruthers JA, Clark RE. Botulinum A toxin (BOTOX) in the lower eyelid: dose-finding study. Dermatol Surg 2003;29(9):943–950; discussion 950–941.

48 Swinehart JM. Treatment of axillary hyperhidrosis: combination of the starch-iodine test with the tumescent liposuction technique. Dermatol Surg 2000;26(4):392–396.

49 Grunfeld A, Murray CA, Solish N. Botulinum toxin for hyperhidrosis: a review. Am J Clin Dermatol 2009;10(2): 87–102.

50 Heckmann M, Ceballos-Baumann AO, Plewig G, Group HS. Botulinum toxin A for axillary hyperhidrosis (excessive sweating). N Engl J Med 2001;344(7):488–493.

51 Hexsel D, Rodrigues TC, Soirefmann M, Zechmeister-Prado D. Recommendations for performing and evaluating the results of the minor test according to a sweating intensity visual scale. Dermatol Surg 2010;36(1):120–122.

52 Coté TR, Mohan AK, Polder JA, *et al.* Botulinum toxin type A injections: adverse events reported to the US Food and Drug Administration in therapeutic and cosmetic cases. J Am Acad Dermatol 2005;53(3):407–415.

53 Naumann M, Jankovic J. Safety of botulinum toxin type A: a systematic review and meta-analysis. Curr Med Res Opin 2004;20(7):981–990.

54 Wollina U, Konrad H. Managing adverse events associated with botulinum toxin type A: a focus on cosmetic procedures. Am J Clin Dermatol 2005;6(3):141–150.

55 Alam M, Arndt KA, Dover JS. Severe, intractable headache after injection with botulinum A exotoxin: report of 5 cases. J Am Acad Dermatol 2002;46(1):62–65.

56 Huang W, Foster JA, Rogachefsky AS. Pharmacology of botulinum toxin. J Am Acad Dermatol 2000;43(2 Pt 1):249–259.

57 Klein AW. Complications with the use of botulinum toxin. Dermatol Clin 2004; 22(2):197–205, vii.

58 Klein AW. Contraindications and complications with the use of botulinum toxin. Clin Dermatol 2004;22(1):66–75.

59 Richards RN. Ethyl chloride spray for sensory relief for botulinum toxin injections of the hands and feet. J Cutan Med Surg 2009;13(5):253–256.

60 Smith KC, Comite SL, Storwick GS. Ice minimizes discomfort associated with injection of botulinum toxin type A for the treatment of palmar and plantar hyperhidrosis. Dermatol Surg 2007;33(1 Spec No.):S88–S91.

61 Campanati A, Lagalla G, Penna L, *et al.* Local neural block at the wrist for treatment of palmar hyperhidrosis with botulinum toxin: technical improvements. J Am Acad Dermatol 2004;51(3):345–348.

62 Kuwahara H, Ogawa R. Using a vibration device to ease pain during facial needling and injection. Eplasty 2016;16:e9.

63 Rivers JK, Bertucci V, McGillivray W, *et al.* Subject satisfaction with onabotulinumtoxinA treatment of glabellar and lateral canthal lines using a new patient-reported outcome measure. Dermatol Surg 2015;41(8):950–959.

64 Chang BL, Wilson AJ, Taglienti AJ, *et al.* Patient perceived benefit in facial aesthetic procedures: FACE-Q as a tool to study botulinum toxin injection outcomes. Aesthet Surg J 2016;36(7):810–820.

65 Trindade de Almeida A, Carruthers J, Cox SE, *et al.* Patient satisfaction and safety with aesthetic onabotulinumtoxinA after at least 5 years: a retrospective cross-sectional analysis of 4,402 glabellar treatments. Dermatol Surg 2015;41(Suppl 1): S19–S28.

66 Carruthers A, Carruthers J. Patient-reported outcomes with botulinum neurotoxin type A. J Cosmet Laser Ther 2007;9(Suppl 1):32–37.

Index

Botulinum Toxins: Cosmetic and Clinical Applications, First Edition. Edited by Joel L. Cohen and David M. Ozog.
© 2017 John Wiley & Sons Ltd. Published 2017 by John Wiley & Sons Ltd.
Companion Website: www.wiley.com/go/cohen/botulinum

Printed in the USA/Agawam, MA

July 16, 2021

777800.023